Conversionary Sites

Conversionary Sites

*Transforming Medical Aid
and Global Christianity from
Madagascar to Minnesota*

BRITT HALVORSON

THE UNIVERSITY OF CHICAGO PRESS   CHICAGO AND LONDON

The University of Chicago Press, Chicago 60637
The University of Chicago Press, Ltd., London
Published 2018
Printed in the United States of America

27 26 25 24 23 22 21 20 19 18   1 2 3 4 5

ISBN-13: 978-0-226-55712-0 (cloth)
ISBN-13: 978-0-226-55726-7 (paper)
ISBN-13: 978-0-226-55743-4 (e-book)
DOI: https://doi.org/10.7208/chicago/9780226557434.001.0001

Library of Congress Cataloging-in-Publication Data

Names: Halvorson, Britt, author.
Title: Conversionary sites : transforming medical aid and global Christianity from
    Madagascar to Minnesota / Britt Halvorson.
Description: Chicago : The University of Chicago Press, 2018. | Includes bibliographical
    references and index.
Identifiers: LCCN 2017056177 | ISBN 9780226557120 (cloth : alk. paper) |
    ISBN 9780226557267 (pbk. : alk. paper) | ISBN 9780226557434 (e-book)
Subjects: LCSH: Medical assistance, American—Madagascar. | Faith-based hu-
    man services—Madagascar. | Faith-based human services—Minnesota. | Missions,
    Medical—Madagascar. | Missions, Medical—Social aspects. | Evangelical Lutheran
    Church in America—Missions—Madagascar.
Classification: LCC RA390.M6 H35 2018 | DDC 266—dc23
LC record available at https://lccn.loc.gov/2017056177

Contents

Conversionary Sites in Global Christianities

In Tolagnaro–Ft. Dauphin, the main regional center of southeast Madagascar, a packed dirt path from the main road leads to a three-room clinic with faded lettering on its side. The clinic is Lutheran, but its waiting room is filled with both Catholic and Lutheran patients, as well as those who mainly follow the ways of the ancestors (*fomban-drazana*). The clinic's staff, a single Lutheran doctor and nurse, greet patients in a small *salle de consultation* where a portrait of Jesus hangs over the threshold, a gurney doubles as an examination bed, and a stethoscope and blood pressure cuff sit on an adjacent metal cart. These furnishings, common yet sparse in these particular medical examination rooms, bear subtle traces of other places, noticeable to observant eyes. Malagasy Lutherans in the capital Antananarivo wrote a price in Malagasy *ariary* on the stethoscope and, before that, trucked it from the eastern port city Toamasina. Prior to a long transatlantic journey, it was in the hands of US aid workers, who prayed over and packaged it and, in the process, assigned it a new economic value. In an industrial zone of Minneapolis, crosscut by machine shops and infrequently used railroad tracks, two hundred aid workers collect and sort medical discards from US hospitals, imagining, emailing, and occasionally hosting the Lutheran physicians in Madagascar to whom the discards are sent. Across town, a charismatic Malagasy evangelist–medical doctor instructs US practitioners how to heal problems holistically with the Holy Spirit, translating techniques from a popular revival in Madagascar.

Significant, far-reaching questions come into focus when one examines the religious quality of medical humanitarian initiatives that span world regions. What cultural understandings and practices of medicine and healing underpin such aid programs, and how do those broader fields of therapeutic activity shape the distinctive meanings of humanitarian work? How do medical relief activities transform what counts as participation in a global religious community? This book argues that transnational circulations of medical relief are not simply unidirectional commodity chains, countering popular accounts of the culturally thin, policy-oriented landscape of relief aid. Rather, they take part in more complex, transformative and historically shaped cultural practices of medicine and healing within communities. This is especially the case among global religious communities, for whom medical relief partakes in long-established therapeutic practices of caregiving and healing, as well powerful moral imaginaries surrounding biomedicine's ability to save lives. Religiously-based medical aid shares many qualities with secular medical humanitarianism, as I will explore, but it is also a significantly different enterprise, grounded in and transformed by religious movements.

I suggest in this book that geographically dispersed aid activities, often marginalized as "para-church" work, are actually central cultural spaces in which North American and African Christians define and experience the politics and meanings of contemporary global Christianity. Christian aid programs like the Minnesota–Madagascar aid relationship that I examine are vital to understanding global networks that now link former Christian missionaries and their communities in the United States with members of Christian churches in parts of sub-Saharan Africa. American and Malagasy Lutherans participate today in a series of far-flung aid exchanges and healing services. Yet their ties with one another build on a long-standing US missionary involvement in Madagascar. Though colonial missions are often characterized as an artifact of a distant past, many communities in the United States and sub-Saharan Africa are actively shaping and renegotiating the meanings of these cultural and institutional ties today through a variety of exchanges, including the circulation of medical aid. *Conversionary Sites* explores how Christian aid relationships share complex ties with what came before them, namely colonial-era foreign mission work, and studies how Christians attempt to distinguish humanitarianism as a qualitatively different activity. It contributes a deeper understanding of the role of religion in globalizing medicine and forging durable networks for medical humanitarian action.

Although medical relief arrangements revive ties today between distinct places, such as the Midwest US and southern Madagascar, religion's role in globalizing medicine is not at all new (Feierman 1985; Hunt 1999). Christian missions often introduced colonial medicine in sub-Saharan Africa, as was the case in Madagascar, forging close ties between biomedicine (*fanafody vazaha* in Malagasy) and whiteness or foreignness (Vaughan 1991; Comaroff 1993). Medicine's associations with modernity and viable career pathways for African specialists eventually grew, however, and solidified its role in the evangelistic mission of church institutions. Economic crisis in African states like Madagascar in the late 1970s and early 1980s renewed humanitarian interest in global medicine's resource inequalities. Aware of the sharp discrepancies between what medical anthropologist Julie Livingston (2012, 66) calls the "highly capitalized" spaces of US biomedicine and the realities of "improvising medicine" in many African clinics, some clinicians established programs to send African clinics the "waste" of US biomedicine, or unused medical discards created by planned obsolescence, biomedical innovation, and insurance regulations. The Minnesota–Madagascar aid program is an example of this kind of medical relief. I closely examine this humanitarian model by situating relief arrangements in the cultural and historical conditions through which they have emerged.

These initiatives now form part of secular aid agencies and university global health partnerships, such as those at Duke and Yale (Rosenblatt and Silverman 1992; Mangan 2007; Allen 2017). They diverge in substantial ways, however, from the kind of medical humanitarianism commonly described in the existing literature, especially responses to short-term medical crises and "clinical tourism" or brief medical rotations in foreign clinics (Redfield 2005, 2006, 2013; Fassin 2007, 2008; Wendland 2012b). Medical relief arrangements often involve long-distance circulations of medical commodities with no easily discernible end point, because of the established and enduring inequalities of global medical commerce. They thus differ significantly from in situ interventions that treat the bare requirements of biological life in refugee camps (Agamben 1998) or that proffer emergent care in medical crises (Redfield 2013), as well as from longer-term programs to improve healthcare access by building public health infrastructure (Farmer 2004), or that elicit narratives of serious medical diagnoses from asylum seekers as a "humanitarian exception" for citizenship in France (Ticktin 2011). Relief circulations based on medical resource inequalities, which transpire over years and often feature little face-to-face contact between those sending and those receiving aid, place greater emphasis on social bonds produced through the geographically disparate spaces and material exchanges of the aid endeavor. This minimal form of medical aid is appealing to Christian actors because of the noninterference and cultural distance ostensibly made possible by the relief aid model, in contrast with the face-to-face encounters and cultural imperialism of colonial evangelism.

Building on these insights, I develop an approach in this book to Christian aid spaces as "conversionary sites," or underanalyzed cultural spaces that operate as busy moral crossroads between past and present, as well as between geographically dispersed religious communities and global commodity chains (Guyer 2004; Tsing 2005; Johnson 2007). The term *conversionary sites* calls attention to the value conversions at the heart of the medical relief endeavor, transformations that not only concern the revaluing of medical discards but also entail the reworking of moral, religious, and historical values. For religious practitioners, biomedical relief is a project that seeks to establish equitable ties of partnership between Christians in different world regions but is continually unsettled by the inequalities of the humanitarian endeavor and global medical commerce. Across medical clinics, nongovernmental organization (NGO) offices, aid warehouses, and healing services, religious actors attempt to rework medical discards, moral selves, and even remnants of colonial pasts. Yet they continually face the limits of their ability to fully remake social relations between Malagasy and Americans, particularly through medical materials that were previously *devalued* as waste forms.[1] The book therefore maintains that contemporary biomedical aid from the United States to Madagascar is a multifaceted, cultural, and historical transaction. Indeed, I suggest that this aid program is an ongoing, incomplete *conversion* of the moral foundation and practices and ways of knowing tied to the colonial legacy.

Circulating Things, Not People: Christian Medical Aid and the Colonial Legacy

US Lutherans have had a long-standing foreign engagement with Madagascar through precolonial evangelical missions that began on the island in 1888. For Americans, these religious ties to Madagascar extend even further back in time and space to Norway, for many Norwegian Americans who migrated to the Midwest US in the mid-nineteenth century had connections to the Norwegian Lutheran Church's earlier evangelical missions to Madagascar, which date to 1866 (Skeie 1999; Nyhagen Predelli 2003). It is striking that, by taking part in mission work in Madagascar, many Norwegian Americans worked side-by-side with Norwegians and thus found being in Madagascar a source of diasporic and ethnic national connection to Norway (Halvorson 2008). Through the twentieth century, the Norwegians continued to evangelize and establish church institutions in the southern highlands of Madagascar and, when the Malagasy Lutheran Church was formally founded in 1950, it structurally conjoined churches, seminaries, hospitals, and schools that had originally been part of evangelical ventures linked to the Norwegians and Americans. Today, the Norwegians, like the Americans, are involved in dispensing considerable aid funding in Madagascar through the Norwegian Mission Society, the Norwegian Agency for Development Cooperation (NORAD), and other programs (Hovland 2007).

As I discuss further in chapter 1, as a result of Malagasy efforts to nationalize the Malagasy Lutheran Church, the postcolonial period since 1960 has seen a total reduction in the foreign missionary staff of the Evangelical Lutheran Church in America (ELCA) in Madagascar, with only one paid American on the island in 2005, in comparison with 61 in 1960.[2] The Malagasy Lutheran Church today includes a biomedical health department (Sampan'asa Loterana Momba Ny Fahasalamana, or SALFA) that maintains nine regional hospitals and thirty-nine dispensaries across the island. Like many other postcolonial African states, Madagascar faced economic collapse and indebtedness in the late 1970s. Because of IMF and World Bank structural adjustment and the devaluation of the Malagasy currency (*ariary*), Malagasy Lutheran clinics, like other medical centers, could not afford to purchase medical supplies and thus were unable to provide a basic standard of care. Former missionaries, their families, and Malagasy Lutheran doctors formed two independent Lutheran NGOs at this time in the early to mid-1980s in Minneapolis–St. Paul that collect discarded medical supplies from US hospitals, sort them, and send them to a central distribution center in the Malagasy capital, Antananarivo. Faith-based NGOs thus entered the country during a state economic "crisis," a central facet of humanitarianism analyzed by Fassin (2007, 2008), but have remained involved since

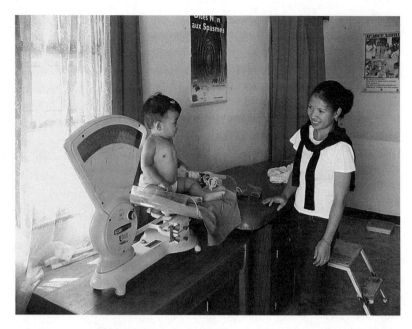

FIGURE O.I. Mother and baby with a US-donated scale, Ambohibao Lutheran Hospital.

the early 1980s as key links to a broader supply chain for Malagasy Lutheran clinics.

Through multisited fieldwork in 2004–6, 2008, and 2014, I have worked as a volunteer laborer in both Minneapolis agencies and examined how SALFA employees process and perceive the aid in Antananarivo, Madagascar, besides participating in worship services and family gatherings with Lutherans in both locations. Today, SALFA employs twenty-one Malagasy Lutheran workers in its Andohalo offices, including aid administrators, public health workers, and clerks, and manages a vast portfolio of foreign aid relationships. Although the US organizations were among its first aid partners, during my fieldwork in Antananarivo in 2014, SALFA had as many as thirty-three separate aid relationships. These partner organizations vary and include large NGOs such as Médecins du Monde, church agencies like Lutheran World Federation, and multilaterals such as the United Nations Food Program. SALFA's current operation far exceeds the US aid partnership and resembles other African medical programs that, as a result of enduring economic inequality and neoliberal reforms, must rely on foreign partnerships to sustain hospitals and clinics. Rather than represent the entirety of SALFA's multistranded aid operation, my aim is to offer a window into the complexity of religiously-based aid by focusing on how the aid alliance between SALFA and Minnesotan Lutherans has developed, and changed, during the decade of my fieldwork.

Both Minnesotan agencies originated through the same initiative among US Lutheran missionary doctors. During my research, however, the two organizations—which I call Malagasy Partnership (established in 1980) and International Health Mission (established in 1987)—continued to diverge in their ideological orientation, the scope of their work, and the size of their personnel. As a much smaller organization focused only on Madagascar, Malagasy Partnership sent to SALFA at the time of my fieldwork four annual transatlantic shipments of medical relief. This relief cargo was shipped to the port city of Tamatave, Madagascar, where it was processed by customs officials and then transported by truck to the SALFA headquarters and warehouse facility in Antananarivo. A Norwegian American man in his fifties whom I call Gene, a former medical missionary in Madagascar and information technology supervisor at a large Minneapolis hospital, ran the organization entirely through volunteer labor, personally taking on all electronic communications with local contacts, biomedical suppliers, and Malagasy Lutheran practitioners.

Gene and his wife, a nurse, had trained Malagasy Lutheran medical laboratory technicians for two years in 1977–78 in the southern villages of Manambaro and Ejeda. This experience, he says, enabled him to fulfill a lifelong "spiritual calling to Madagascar." Gene's uncle had been a missionary in Madagascar from 1960 to 1972, and Gene grew up in a rural farming town in Minnesota, often hearing stories about Madagascar. After his short-term mission work in Madagascar had ended and he and his wife had returned to the United States, Gene agreed to secure parts for an X-ray machine and send them to another long-term medical missionary doctor, whom I call Dr. Fosse, who had been instrumental in establishing SALFA in 1979. Because they continued to receive requests for medical equipment, Gene and his wife filled barrels and crates to send to Madagascar as a service project of their American Lutheran Church (after 1988, the ELCA) congregation's "home bible study cell." They eventually amassed enough donations to rent a small warehouse building for Malagasy Partnership in suburban Minneapolis. During my fieldwork, the agency relied on the close, loyal ties between three core Euro-American families, whose middle-aged parents and adult children had volunteered regularly for more than two decades, as well as the avid participation of two Malagasy émigré families, who attended special sea container packing sessions.

International Health Mission (IHM), by comparison, was established as an independent Lutheran organization in Minneapolis in 1987, which receives only a small amount of funding from the ELCA. Its founders patterned it after the Medical Benevolence Foundation, which formed in 1963 to furnish Presbyterian Church clinics around the world with US biomedical surplus.[3] Like Malagasy Partnership, the agency initially stored medical materials in volunteers' home basements, garages, and storage units and a borrowed space at a local Christian college. After eight years without a permanent facility, IHM purchased its original warehouse building in 1995 in an industrial zone of a northwestern Minneapolis suburb. In 2005 the agency bought a neighboring warehouse and doubled the original size of the facility by breaking down the adjoining wall. IHM shipped fourteen containers of medical relief to Lutheran hospitals in Tanzania, Cameroon, Papua New Guinea, Liberia, and Nicaragua in 2005, and the dramatic expansion of the IHM headquarters signaled its plan to send as many as twenty-eight annual containers to those and other locations, including Lutheran facilities in Bangladesh and southern India.

Though IHM sent sea containers to Madagascar in its early years, at the time of my research it financed a portion of Malagasy Partnership's overseas shipping, pharmacotherapy for patients in small communal treatment centers called *toby* (Malagasy; lit., camp), medical training programs, and medical and dental equipment. IHM employed four full-time staff and managed a US$1.9 million budget in 2006, but it relied predominantly on a 150-person local volunteer workforce drawn from an 18,000-member national mailing list. As many as twenty-five people, primarily Euro-American retirees of self-identified Scandinavian or German descent, staffed each volunteer shift, doing everything from packaging transatlantic sea container shipments of medical materials to installing the electrical wiring in the agency's headquarters.[4] I worked as a volunteer aid laborer in both warehouses for eighteen months and draw extensively from these experiences throughout this book. The IHM leaders and board members, many of whom (during my fieldwork in 2005–6) were former Madagascar missionaries or were children of Madagascar missionaries, knew Gene personally. If they were not volunteers, many Madagascar missionaries with whom I spoke donated money to both these organizations, making them sister agencies with shared religious constituencies. On the other hand, it became clear to me that the agencies had notable differences in their goals and organizational structures, and I point to the implications and effects of these differences throughout the book.

All my US informants identified with being Lutheran but participated in various Lutheran sects with widely diverging theological and social views. At least half were ELCA members, a theologically and socially liberal Protestant denomination known for participating in professional assistance work across the globe under the auspices of Lutheran World Relief. Other informants, including a number of former Madagascar missionaries who became born again after returning to the United States, belonged to the charismatic Lutheran Renewal movement or the conservative Association of Free Lutheran Congregations. As I illustrate further in chapter 2, the combination resulted in a variety of opposing liberal and conservative views among those involved with the two NGOs and also spurred new charismatic alliances between Lutherans in Madagascar and the United States. Yet, in my experience, the medical aid organizations were able to loosely unite conservative and liberal Lutherans because they nurtured the idea that medical aid is both an activity of social justice and an opportunity for witness and left open to individual interpretation which held more prominence.

In addition, the varieties of Lutheranism publicly affirmed in the aid agencies did not adhere closely to one doctrinal view of Lutheran practice but, as I will show, were a more eclectic hybrid that owes a substantial debt to evangelical language and ways of apprehending the personal relationship with God and Jesus in everyday life. The Minnesotan agencies participate in the widely documented late-twentieth-century cultural shift in US Protestantism between mainline denominations, such as Methodism and Lutheranism, and nondenominational and evangelical structures of affiliation and belonging (Wuthnow 1989; Miller 1997; Harding 2000). My informants on the whole exhibited a hybrid identity that drew from evangelicalism but to various degrees still embraced being Lutheran, whether as an institutional affiliation or an ethno-cultural identity linked historically in the US Midwest to Swedish, Norwegian, and Danish descent (Nelson 1980; Gjerde 1985; Granquist 2007). In subsequent chapters, I often refer to *Christians* rather than *Lutherans* to signal the identity categories preferred by some of my US informants; I use the term *Lutheran* when informants do so and when addressing the denominational ties and their histories that link Lutherans in Madagascar and the United States through the current aid program.

Collectively, both US agencies espouse a biblical commitment to "accompany" Malagasy Lutherans from afar by sending medical relief to SALFA but not humanitarian workers or long-term Christian missionaries. The founding of the two NGOs went hand-in-hand with changing approaches to global engagement among US Lutherans (discussed further in chapter 1). With decolonization in Madagascar and waning support for foreign mission work from mainline Protestants in the United States, members of the American Lutheran Church/ELCA began to overtly reject long-term mission work between 1970 and 1990 as a morally corrupt "colonial" practice, imbalanced by Euro-American claims to religious and cultural authority. Institutionally, liberal Lutherans turned to humanitarian relief, short-term missions, nationally run evangelism, and micro-development schemes as more ethical examples of the singular term *global mission*. Today, US Lutherans involved in the aid program predominantly view their own immobility as the most ethical position, in that Americans living in Madagascar for a long period would be viewed as interfering with Malagasy church affairs. Malagasy Lutherans, however, do travel to Minnesota and, in chapters 2 and 5, I explore the role of Malagasy doctors in constructing the meaningfulness of religiously-based aid on US soil. In contrast with colonial mission work, both Malagasy and Americans attempt to create an aid practice ethically informed by, in the words of Tanzanian Lutheran theologian Richard Lubawa, "partnership not paternalism" among national churches (2007, 6). In subsequent chapters, I examine how this ethical ideal is practiced while also investigating the emerging forms of power and authority in Christian aid alliances.

Christian Aid Spaces as Conversionary Sites

My approach to Christian medical relief seeks to understand it from within its own networks and cultural practices (Riles 2000) while appreciating how aid, in the words of anthropologist João Biehl (2010, 154), requires bringing into view "the immanent fields—leaking out on all sides—that people invent to live in and by." That is, aid activities take place in a broader constellation of culturally shaped, dynamically shifting practices of personhood, moral reasoning, religious affiliation, gender, race, and national identity and citizenship. What I aim to show through this approach is that Christian aid arrangements draw meaningfulness from broader landscapes of religious and cultural activity in distinct places, while also being influenced by the traveling forms of governance that characterize aid, such as accountability requirements. The sum of these parts is a view of Christian aid arrangements as multistranded social formations characterized by their position amid localized religious movements and distinguished as much by disjunctures of understanding as by imaginaries of Christian unity and connection.

Yet I have also sought to better understand how medical relief not only draws from the religious movements with which it is affiliated but also transforms those religious communities and individual religious actors in the process. How do Lutheran actors negotiate distinct regimes of value—advanced capitalist and religious moral economies—that shape medical relief work? How do they refashion their Christian identity— and the subjectivities of those with whom they labor—in keeping with prevalent medical humanitarian categories, such as aid giver, patient, doctor, and aid recipient? Lutherans must sort through and accommodate the distinct ideological premises of these value regimes, as well as their moral and political incompatibilities, which uneasily come together within humanitarian spaces. I argue that religious humanitarians enact a range of "conversionary processes," broadly defined, to smooth over the problems and uncertainties that arise in faith-based aid arrangements. Conversions across distinct forms of economic and spiritual value, whether through prayer or by moving materials between formal and informal economies, enable actors in diverse institutional and cultural positions to translate the broad geographic scale and circulations of aid work to their particular aims.

In anthropology, the term *conversion* has often played double duty to illuminate religious and economic processes of transformation, and I draw upon both these meanings in this book. Anthropologists of Christianity have analyzed religious conversion as a sociohistorical and culturally variable process, rather than only an internal psychological one, which involves adopting moral dispositions, religious language, performances of selfhood, and everyday habits of religious community (Comaroff 1985; Harding 2000; Robbins 2004). Among economic anthropologists, the term *conversion* has signaled a transformation in value between economic forms culturally deemed commensurable, often within bounded "spheres of exchange" that place moral barriers to exchange across those categories, as among Tiv society in central Nigeria (Bohannan 1955). Subsequent writers like Jane Guyer (2004, 30) have questioned the idea that these exchange spheres are so tightly restricted and, instead, conceptualized value conversions as open-ended junctures where Tiv worked "stepwise toward the constitution of stores of value that had greater longevity and security." Guyer defines conversions as those cultural practices that "add, subtract, or otherwise transform the attributes of exchanged goods in ways that define the social direction of future transactional possibilities" (30). I adopt some of Guyer's imagery of value conversions as "junctures" and "crossroads" to theorize the conversionary work performed in Lutheran aid spaces. As in Guyer's description, Lutheran aid workers seek to translate and transform value across asymmetric regimes—those of medical commerce, Christian spiritual economies, and humanitarian accountability—and endeavor to parlay those moves into more enduring forms of Christian affiliation and material support.

Yet I contend that these transactions are characterized equally by the limits and disquieting excesses of Lutherans' attempts to work across such disparate value regimes. Because Lutheran aid exists at the crossroads of global medical commerce and global religious communities, I am equally interested in charting the "social alchemy" as aid workers strive to make diverse value forms, such as medical castoffs and gifts from God, commensurable with each other, an unfinished, partial, and ongoing process that can produce moral anxiety (Bourdieu 1977, 195, cited in Guyer 2004, 30). Because Lutheran medical aid centers on the global circulation of medical discards, I analyze how variously placed Lutheran actors attempt to reconcile the capitalist exchange value of the discards with the castoffs' role amid wider, culturally variable projects of religious community, particularly that of building an equitable partnership in response to the colonial legacy. Lutheran medical aid provides an example of what Joel Robbins (2013) calls "value pluralism" as economic, religious, and historical values are uneasily brought together and activated in Christian aid spaces. I conceptualize these value forms as mutually influential, vibrating together as musical chords and sometimes producing cacophony, yet not necessarily equivalent with or capable of being totally subsumed by each other. In my experience, Christian aid is characterized by these moments of recognizing dissonance and, though they have not often been theorized ethnographically, by individual attempts to "make do" at the level of material practice. Indeed, while "making do" can be an imaginative and religiously significant act of improvisation (as I suggest in chapters 2, 3, and 4), it can also be understood as a felt experience of the disunity among these value forms, and, ultimately, of the limits of the conversionary processes I describe in this book.

This approach helps me to connect the fine-grained, everyday work of aid, understood and practiced in various ways by Malagasy Lutheran doctors, US laypeople, SALFA aid administrators, former Madagascar missionaries, and NGO leaders, with the broader sociohistorical projects of religious community in which Lutheran aid is enmeshed. Although the aid relationship does not entail the conversion of my informants to Christianity, most of whom are lifelong committed Christians, it does involve a transformational process in the moral stances, dispositions, expressions of Lutheranism, and styles of interaction compatible with a humanitarian sensibility. Though Lutheran Christian ties were once focused on face-to-face conversions of non-Christians in Madagascar, aid alliances now seek to morally convert American and Malagasy individuals to a Christian humanitarian subjectivity. This subjectivity forms part of a broader effort at equitable partnership, yet aid participants find themselves inescapably entangled in the inequalities and value conversions of advanced capitalism.

Global Christianities as an Ethnographic Subject

As an anthropologist, my approach to global Christianities diverges from studies that focus exclusively on how theological and doctrinal debates in Christian communities shape contemporary forms of global engagement. I am particularly interested in how laypeople, former US missionaries, Malagasy-émigré evangelists, SALFA aid workers, and Malagasy Lutheran medical doctors experience and apprehend their role in such globalizing practices. Indeed, practitioners in Minneapolis–St. Paul and in Antananarivo variously position themselves within a global religious community and use those global connections to foster emerging, fragmented charismatic and liberal branches of Lutheranism, something observed in Protestantism more broadly (see, e.g., Poewe 1994; Miller 1997; Harding 2000; Cannell 2006; Klassen 2011).

Considerably less scholarly attention has been given to the historical connections that continue to shape forms of religious globalization among contemporary North American Protestant and African Christian communities, such as migration to the United States, aid flows, and cultural exchange programs, as well as their corresponding global imaginaries (but see Robert 1997; Bays and Wacker 2003; Wuthnow 2010). Within subsequent chapters, I develop an approach that recognizes global Christian connections as profoundly historical and local cultural practices (Nielssen, Okkenhaug, and Skeie 2011). In making these arguments, I build on a sizable literature in anthropology that conceptualizes Christianities as distinctive local communities of practice, inflected by the historical patterns of textual and theological debate, political and moral discourse, and inclusions and exclusions of broader cultural formations of ethnicity/race, gender, and citizenship (Harding 2000; Robbins 2003b; Cannell 2006; Elisha 2011). Simultaneously, though, my research sheds light on less well understood, enduring regional interrelationships that compose contemporary global Christian connections and warrant further study (Hefferan 2007; Hefferan et al. 2009).

I therefore shift my focus in this book from global Christianity as a given entity to globalizing practices as a foundational part of Christian experience. Global Christianity is often taken to mean either the universalizing aspects of the faith or the global scope of contemporary Christianity, frequently from a Western, historically imperialist perspective (Sanneh 2003; Masuzawa 2005; Robbins and Engelke 2010). But we can also look at how Christians place themselves in a broader religious community extending beyond the interacted and visible one of the present. Using this lens, we can consider how practitioners make finding themselves as part of a global ecumene into one of the core aspects of what it is to be Christian in the contemporary world. This makes global Christian subjectivity into a broader identity claim with cultural and historical dimensions. It also suggests that different Christians culturally understand their positioning in what we can term the global ecumene in distinct ways, or as Robbins and Engelke (2010, 626) put it "both in relation to and against the global frame." These understandings are shaped by the social, historical, and theological concerns that make the category of the global rise to relief in religious practice as a shifting, complex combination of the foreign, nonlocal, outside, absent, and even distant. Looking into these social practices that create senses of the world beyond the immediate context, concretize it, and provide access to certain entitlements or resource flows offers us a window into how relationships are forged between the home churches of past European and US colonial-era missions and independent national churches in parts of the global South.

Religiously inspired aid requires investigating religious experience in out-of-the-way spaces that seem on the surface less overtly "religious," in that they often are considered marginal to centers of clerical and theological authority. As scholars of Christianity have noted, Protestant communities often espouse "language ideologies" that privilege individual spoken and textual engagement with the Word of God. These language ideologies theoretically place diminished significance on material and sensuous forms of worship, which may risk idolatry and threaten modern notions of agency (Keane 2007; Bialecki and Hoenes del Pinal 2011). Yet others have argued that, even as Christian communities may give primacy to the written and spoken word, the Word is a multifaceted concept that can in fact be expressed and known through a range of cultural forms, often in dynamic combination with language, including water, food, material exchanges, music, dress, dance, and ecstatic bodily states (Feeley-Harnik 1994; Keane 1996; Csordas 2002; Coleman 2004; Luhrmann 2004). An important question that emerges from these scholarly conversations is from whose perspective, and from what sites of religious activity, these diverse linguistic and material forms of worship differently come to matter in Christian communities. As Colleen McDannell (1995) puts it, though Protestant Christianity has been overrepresented in the study of Christianity, linguistic practices linked to forms of clerical and theological authority within communities often have been historically taken as the true Protestantism. This has sometimes resulted in skewed views of Protestant Christianities that conflate authoritative proscriptions with everyday practice and neglect the role of power and authority in overshadowing other forms of worship with which linguistic approaches to the Word have always coexisted.

The sites of Christian aid that I describe in this book create spaces for religious experience but rarely feature Bible studies or services common to volunteers' or aid workers' home congregations. Although linguistic forms of worship like prayer remain highly important, aid laborers often looked in my experience to the heterogeneous medical aid that they handled for signs of God's direction. Some studies of Christianity have identified the cultural work of establishing God's presence as a central problem among believers (Engelke 2007). As committed Christians, my informants in Madagascar and the United States seemed less concerned about whether God was present—it often seemed the divine was, if anything, abundantly busy in their lives—and more focused on the hard work of discerning God's will or guidance for their work. Through my fieldwork, I came to understand that, for US lay humanitarians, the unusual materials of medical aid, which ranged from hospital beds to handmade bandages, were in fact material signifiers of everyday religion. Moreover, Malagasy evangelists used bodily imagery as a representational device that offered glimpses of medical aid's long-distance circuits and often unseen recipients. I therefore advocate an approach to Christian aid that analyzes its semiotic or communicative dimensions and, in keeping with my informants' experiences, draws attention to interactions among the material, embodied, and linguistic aspects of aid work (Parmentier 1997; Keane 2003). As I will show, aid labor is an ongoing practice of religious interpretation, from which individual aid workers often draw diverse and sometimes conflicting meanings.

Building on the idea that Christian aid fosters forms of transnational affiliation, we can also ask how these aid alliances differ from secular aid programs, a question I return to throughout the book. Scholars have noted that medical humanitarian structures, from state-based humanitarian programs to transnational medical aid organizations, encourage novel forms of cultural affiliation and belonging. In the wake of the Chernobyl disaster, Adriana Petryna (2004) has argued that Ukrainians embraced "biological citizenship" in order to claim individual entitlements to state compensation for Chernobyl's health effects. In his study of HIV-AIDS programs in Côte d'Ivoire, Vinh-Kim Nguyen (2010, 186) terms the connection fostered between HIV-positive individuals and the transnational AIDS treatment community a form of "therapeutic citizenship" that "confers on individuals specific rights (to health, in this case)." Unlike the individual citizenship claims that Petryna and Nguyen describe, the Minnesota-Madagascar aid program emphasizes a shared moral and religious community in which individual entitlements are still significant but ideologically minimized. In addition, in the Lutheran aid partnership, it is Malagasy Lutheran physicians as medical experts, rather than Malagasy laypeople or patients, who participate in the transformative opportunities for self-fashioning and transnational community provided by the program.

Nonetheless, like the aid recipients in Nguyen's work, Malagasy Lutheran physician-aid brokers adeptly navigate the aid program's narrative practices, often turning their connections into forms of economic and political capital. Moreover, global religious communities nurture imaginaries of belonging and affiliation, which are arguably similar to citizenship. As I will show, some Malagasy Lutheran doctors, for example, work to distinguish themselves from non-Christian clinic patients in rural areas of Madagascar and instead align themselves as Christian citizens with evangelical Christians living in Madagascar and abroad. Thus, although citizenship implies a claim to individual rights not fully borne out here, the Minnesota-Madagascar aid program does engender imaginaries of connectedness and transnational Christian health care that bind people together without extensive physical contact. The Lutheran aid partnership also provides cultural materials for identification and access to economic and political resources, as Nguyen and Petryna both illustrate. Yet in contrast to the citizenship claims outlined by Nguyen and Petryna, these Lutheran Christian forms of belonging, I suggest, are not completely novel but influenced by US and Malagasy cultural histories of foreign interaction.

In short, I analyze aid work in this book as a material and bureaucratic practice of religion, offering distinct creative opportunities for refashioning global religious networks. Yet, by bringing theories of religious practice and religious movements into conversation with preexisting scholarship on humanitarianism, I aim to show how religious actors are adopting contemporary forms of bureaucratic humanitarianism while professionalizing older religious models of charitable assistance. Although scholars have noted the religious genealogies of charity, philanthropy, and notions of universal humanity (Barnett and Weiss 2008; Barnett 2011), contemporary bureaucratic humanitarianism often has been studied as a secular sphere of action (but see Benthall and Bellion-Jourdan 2003; Bornstein 2005, 2012; Barnett and Stein 2012). Religious NGOs, however, are actively seizing the putatively secular language, funding, and bureaucratic protocols of humanitarianism as a way to direct their outreach activities and justify their work to other social actors in a broader political and cultural arena (Benthall 2010). At the same time, the religious actors involved in the Minnesota-Madagascar aid alliance root their work in Christian exchange ideologies, divine and moral sources of authority, and ideals of moral personhood. Giving attention to both these processes helps illuminate faith-based humanitarian initiatives as social processes grounded in and transformed by religious communities, while shaped in ongoing dialogue with the broader aid world.

An Ethnography of Multisitedness:
Methodology and Positionality

This book draws upon more than twenty-four months of primary ethnographic research in the Midwest US and shorter research periods in
Madagascar among Lutheran clinicians, volunteer laborers, healer-
evangelists, and former missionaries. The research initially focused on
the colonial legacy of US foreign mission work in Madagascar. In true
ethnographic fashion, however, my understanding of the subject quickly
began to shift: Medical relief agencies, established to supply Malagasy
Lutheran clinics with medical technologies, were beginning to provide
a renewed source of connection between Malagasy Lutherans and US
Lutherans (compare Wuthnow 2009, Klassen 2011). What I found presented a number of thorny methodological and theoretical questions:
What was it that I was, in fact, studying? And how could I apply ethnographic research techniques to Christian social formations that mainly
rely on building connections between geographically dispersed sites,
rather than on face-to-face encounters? I started to consider the "sites"
of my research as not only geographic or spatial ones, linking Madagascar and Minnesota and interweaving churches, aid offices, and family
gatherings in Antananarivo and in Minneapolis–St. Paul, but also temporal in character for my research participants, enabling them to selectively link past and present. Accordingly, I have worked to conceptualize
transnational Christian aid as multisited and multiperspectival global
networks always deeply contextualized and created in particular spaces
and times.

The research that forms the foundation for this book has stretched
across a decade (2003–14) and placed me in various roles as a participant observer. In order to investigate the labor process and representational practices surrounding medical aid, I worked as a volunteer aid laborer in both Minneapolis warehouses for eighteen months in 2004–6,
sorting, counting, and packaging medical supplies for clinics in Madagascar and other former sites of US Lutheran missionary activity, such
as Lutheran hospitals in northern Cameroon and northern Tanzania.
Cumulatively, I examined the "humanitarian representational practices"
(Malkki 1996, 389) through which the two NGOs discursively characterized their work and enabled collective participation in the provision of

medical care. At the same time, through the flow of goods and conversation in the two warehouses, I studied how these representations became the subject of debate among volunteers and how the very materiality of the medical supplies prompted concerns about the ethics and politics of aid. Further, I examined how people of various positions and cultural identities (e.g., US Lutheran missionaries and volunteers, Malagasy Lutheran medical practitioners, and SALFA employees) perceived medical aid transactions in light of the history of US Lutheran evangelism in southern Madagascar. By examining the medical supplies as material-semiotic forms, I investigated from a variety of perspectives how their material properties and interpretation contributed to the embodied practice of religion and the redefinition of Lutheran worldly engagement.

My fieldwork involved mirroring my US-based informants' own mobility across the Twin Cities and their participation in various religious organizations, some of which overlapped in membership and some of which did not. For example, I took part in a "cross-cultural house church" run by a Malagasy Lutheran doctor and émigré-evangelist, whom I call Gabriel, for the entirety of my Minneapolis fieldwork, from October 2004 through September 2006, except while I was pursuing research in Madagascar in November–December 2005. I interviewed members of the house church, who also regularly attended healing services that Gabriel ran at a local conservative Lutheran congregation that I call Good Shepherd (described in chapter 2), and spoke casually with them on numerous occasions in the handful of St. Paul homes where they met. Gabriel and his family were therefore known among several interconnected Lutheran organizations, churches, and communities in greater Minneapolis–St. Paul whose members did not all traverse the same sites of religious engagement: house church members, former missionaries to Madagascar and their families, volunteers at the two Lutheran medical aid organizations, and members of Good Shepherd Lutheran. In addition, while in Madagascar for research in late 2005, I met with Gabriel's youngest daughter in the capital, Antananarivo, and also spent time at the Ambohibao Lutheran Hospital just outside the capital city, where members of the hospital's chemical dependency unit immediately questioned me about Gabriel and spoke highly of his earlier work with them. In 2014, on a return trip to Madagascar, I spent time with Solofo, Gabriel's youngest son, who had just moved back to Antananarivo from the Minneapolis–St. Paul area. This pattern of involvement in informants' family gatherings and worship services was characteristic of my research practices, and I draw upon this dense web of experiences throughout the book.

My research followed the transnational movement of medical supplies from Minnesota warehouses through Malagasy Lutheran clinics. I spent time in the headquarters of the Malagasy Lutheran health department (SALFA) in Antananarivo in 2005 and 2014 in order to examine how SALFA disburses medical supplies and monetary aid from both US organizations to clinics throughout the island. I interviewed five SALFA employees who serve as liaisons to the US Lutheran aid agencies, and I observed two SALFA medical centers, a dispensary in Tolagnaro in southeast Madagascar and a large regional hospital in Ambohibao outside Antananarivo. Through these experiences, I was able to acquire some understanding of SALFA centers with various clinical capabilities, staffing and specializations, patient populations, and differential access to medical resources.

As with my US research, I spent time with Malagasy informants outside their workspaces and joined them and their families for meals, walks through Antananarivo neighborhoods, shopping trips, and worship services. I studied the Malagasy language as my research progressed and used a combination of English, Malagasy, and French when interacting with informants in Antananarivo, as almost all of them are fully trilingual. When I mention Malagasy Lutherans in this book, I am referring to this small group of SALFA aid workers, doctors, Malagasy Lutheran pastors, and Malagasy émigrés and visitors to the United States with whom I spent time, most of whom are ethnically Merina or Betsileo— two Malagasy ethno-regional groups linked to highland Madagascar and known historically for high rates of Protestant affiliation (Bloch 1986, 39; Larson 1997; Keller 2005, 37–40). Similarly, when I mention US Lutherans, I am referring to the approximately forty ELCA missionaries to Madagascar and their family members whom I knew and interviewed, mainly Norwegian Americans; five NGO leaders and board members in the two Minneapolis organizations whom I interviewed; and approximately fifty US Lutheran laypeople with whom I spent time in the Minneapolis NGOs and other religious organizations.[5] To protect their privacy, I use pseudonyms for all the named individuals in the book, as well as specific churches and the US organizations.

As is clear from my previous description, studying transnational Christian aid required me to be mobile within a Christian aid relationship that, in fact, problematized the privilege and historical inequality of Americans' global mobility. Acutely aware of these issues, I worked when traveling to Madagascar for research to help further my informants' projects. On my trip to Madagascar in 2005, for example, I brought a suitcase of donated surgical sutures requested by Malagasy Lutheran physicians in southern Madagascar, which were needed for procedures in the Manambaro Lutheran Hospital. I also brought a small collection of individual packages sent by Malagasy émigrés in Minneapolis for adult children still living in Madagascar. I returned to the United States with fund-raising pamphlets from the Malagasy Lutheran director of the Manantantely Bible School, who wished to develop US Lutheran sponsors for scholarships to offset tuition costs. I also gave a presentation to participants in the US NGOs in Minneapolis–St. Paul about SALFA's use of medical aid to facilitate communication between the two sites. Besides offering me insight into the very religious networks that compose the subject of my research (compare Riles 2000), these instances created opportunities for me to provide collaborative support for the people participating in my research, furthering their own diverse aims for Lutheran education and medical care.

The research that is the basis of this book is shaped by the dynamic, shifting, and highly variable relationships between my informants and me, which pulled various "strands of identification" into focus while others receded from view (Narayan 1997, 26). In my interactions with US missionaries and their families, I was most often introduced first through the name of my paternal grandfather, who was a US Lutheran missionary to southeast Madagascar from 1932 to 1961, and second as a student of anthropology. American and Malagasy informants frequently questioned me about my father's family history, since I had a recognizable last name. Through my repeated verbal placement amid networks of deceased kin relations who were missionaries, I was depicted by US informants as someone who had been ambiguously "away" (from Minneapolis–St. Paul, missions, Madagascar, and the church) yet had some understanding of Madagascar through family ties. This historical connection built trust with my informants but posed additional ethical dilemmas for me. Though my father's family was deeply involved in Lutheran evangelism in Madagascar for three generations (from 1866 to 1961), my father made a break as an adult with the Christian church and his family's history of involvement in Madagascar. I was not raised as a Christian nor was I personally familiar with the Twin Cities until I began the preliminary research for my dissertation in 2003. My own religious identity has since shifted as well and, through conversion and a shared life with a Jewish partner, I am now a semiobservant liberal Jewish woman.

Reflecting upon his research at the Church of Our Lady of Guadalupe in South Chicago, Robert Orsi (2005) has written eloquently about the ambiguities, anxieties, and existential dilemmas of doing research in a religious tradition with which one is, in some way, familiar. As Orsi (2005, 162) puts it, "There is a muddle of unacknowledged transferences—the fieldworker in one's own discipline is kind of recognizable to practitioners and kind of not, and vice versa, and so each fills in the space of who they think the other is or wants them to be or fears they are, or all of this at once." My fieldwork involved moving between and ambiguously occupying a variety of positions all at once and some more than others, depending on the situation: granddaughter, daughter, student, non-Christian, missionary descendant with a familiar last name, anthropologist. The shifting terrain of these interactions was not a matter of my inadequately accommodating myself to the people with whom I did research (for this would lack honesty and efface difference), but rather it was jointly produced through a "muddle of unacknowledged transferences," as Orsi points out. A crucial problem to me throughout my research and writing has been not to make my research into an exercise in boundary-making (of self and other, Christian and non-Christian, past family involvement and present interaction), but to try to keep these multiple and unresolved aspects of my experiences in view.

My mention of family history and other personal details is not meant to erect such a boundary, but rather to indicate how the ethnographic knowledge in this study is situated, partial, and produced through the relationships between myself and my informants. In particular, my status as a nonbeliever sometimes became a focal point of my interactions with informants, superseding my family history. After I turned off the tape recorder during an interview at a retired Norwegian American missionary couple's house in suburban Minneapolis, one woman retreated into a back room of the house, only to return a few minutes later with a tract that she slid across the dining room table to me. The title in bold black print, "Would You Like to Know God *Personally*?," quickly registered that my status as a nonbeliever had, for this couple, become a significant component of our exchange. But most informants gently asked me questions, opened their lives to me, and, as I came to understand these informants' perspectives on the matter, let God do the rest. In comparison with anthropological tales of the challenges of establishing fieldwork connections, I found my entry to the world of Christian aid in Minneapolis–St. Paul and Antananarivo relatively smooth, and I grew to appreciate that these Christian networks were in fact designed to welcome strangers. I had a more difficult time with leave-taking and the quiet gestures of disappointment signaled by some informants who, I think, had hoped to see me undergo my own conversion process.

In Madagascar, because of my identity as a US *vazaha* (foreigner or white person in Malagasy) with a missionary family history, I emphasized often in conversation that I was an independent researcher. I initially hoped to make clear that I was not connected in any official capacity with the US NGOs, lest my Malagasy informants think I was there to observe their work and report back to the Minneapolis organizations. Although I built rapport with my Malagasy informants, it is quite likely that I was nonetheless, as a white American, associated in some ways with the US history of involvement in Madagascar and with the US NGOs. Signaling their awareness that my aims were different from those of US aid leaders, however, some of my SALFA informants voiced their appreciation of my efforts to seek multiple Malagasy and American views of the aid relationship. For example, Clement, the SALFA financial officer and a self-described lover of books, told me he was glad that I would be writing a book—that books were appropriately substantial—and expressed enthusiasm at being part of the project.

Within this book, I have worked to uphold the trust and generosity shown to me by my American and Malagasy informants, while recognizing the inequalities in global positions and access to resources that characterize the aid relationship. As an anthropologist, I have taken a critically empathetic approach to the aid program, analyzing its disparate practices as cultural activities and pointing out areas where I see imbalances or blind spots of power and authority. These critiques should not be read as condemnations of the aid endeavor nor as signaling an anthropologist's privileged perspective. I find many aspects of the aid program courageous and admirable, as are all forms of activism in the world that seek to rectify social inequality. I believe nevertheless that an anthropological analysis can offer insight into the on-the-ground challenges of Christians' efforts to recognize and remedy inequality in the global communion. It is my hope that this book will contribute to this self-reflexive project within Christian communities and well beyond.

Outline of the Book

The book is organized around six conversionary processes and their limitations, which characterize the medical aid relationship between Christians in Madagascar and Minnesota. The book positions itself in these
social sites in order to show how religious practitioners harness medical
aid and its imaginaries in a variety of transformative moral and political
projects. Each chapter introduces a different facet of humanitarianism
commonly addressed in the literature and then contextualizes it in the
religious logics of Christian aid. These topics are humanitarianism's histories, the political economy of aid, care-giving practices, accountability measures, and the formation of aid broker subjectivities. Simultaneously, this enables the reader to appreciate the different dimensions of
religious experience transformed by the aid relationship: historical con-
sciousness, moral personhood, forms of moral accountability, notions of
care, and negotiations of difference.

Chapter 1 shows how Lutheran actors reorient relations of past and
present as they become humanitarians. Specifically, it examines how,
through the aid relationship, religious actors in Minnesota and Madagascar rework their sense of a shared colonial past, redeeming certain
histories of colonial interaction while actively forgetting or breaking
from other pasts. These ruptures crucially underpin the political ideology that humanitarian work is a more egalitarian and neutral activity,
respectful of Malagasy sovereignty, than the colonial missions that came
before. My research points to how moral worlds are selectively transformed when certain Christian frameworks of global engagement crum-
ble, in this case colonial missions, and seemingly new ones, that of being a religious humanitarian, take shape through their "ruins" (Stoller
2008).

Chapter 2 examines the "biospiritual imaginaries" that underpin Lutherans' increasing attention to healing and medicine as globally connecting religious activities. Bringing together research in Malagasy
Lutheran–led healing services and medical aid organizations in
Minneapolis–St. Paul, I analyze the "bodies multiple" (Mol 2002) of
Lutheran medical work and explore the global imaginaries and forms
of community they foster, as well as their perhaps unexpected ideological fissures and contradictions for Minnesotan Lutheran aid workers.

Taking the reader inside the Minneapolis NGOs, I show how middle-class US aid workers make the organizations into therapeutic spaces for addressing insecurities caused by job losses, financial problems, and health crises, grounding a humanitarian ethic of care in these lived realities.

Chapters 3 and 4 closely study the value conversions and inequalities of global medical commerce that underpin the aid program. In chapter 3, I consider the unique structural position occupied by the Minneapolis NGOs, which both capitalize on and inflect the tensions of waste economies in US biomedicine. The NGOs convert hospital "waste," which often consists of unused medical supplies made obsolete or undesirable by manufacturer use-by dates, into economic value for the US biomedical establishment when they accept those discards as charitable donations. I discuss a key problem faced by US NGO laborers in this conversionary process: they must resolve in their everyday work the moral paradox created by "doing good" through sending medical waste overseas.

Chapter 4 picks up this commodity chain in Antananarivo and examines how SALFA employees differently perceive the valuation of the discards, as well as their US partnership. Drawing from my ethnographic research in SALFA headquarters in Antananarivo, the chapter describes how SALFA administrators nurture and seek forms of spiritual and material benefit from a range of religious and professional networks in which SALFA itself is situated. I suggest that it is important to view Malagasy acceptance of heterogeneous medical discards from the United States as an actively chosen act of value generation. This transaction hinges not so much on value in medical supplies themselves but rather the future potential of Malagasy ties with a variety of foreign donors, including the two US NGOs.

Chapters 5 and 6 investigate how the aid relationship has compelled new subjectivities and forms of governance. Chapter 5 focuses on the emergence and experiences of an elite cohort of Merina and Betsileo Malagasy Lutheran doctors who act as cultural translators or "middle figures" to the two US NGOs (Hunt 1999). The chapter suggests Merina and Betsileo Malagasy male doctors appear as expected aid partners because of their own efforts to render themselves visible through leveraging strategic resources and connections with both NGOs, as well as long-standing forms of ethno-regional and gender privilege within Madagascar. I examine three cultural activities through which Merina and Betsileo physicians rework and perform the category expectations of this emerging aid subjectivity, which exhibits selected qualities of the medical doctor, humanitarian, and foreign missionary.

Chapter 6 charts how aid accountability in Christian aid partnerships selectively combines neoliberal and biblical reasoning on what it means to be morally accountable, creating an emerging religiously informed medical audit culture. Moving in the chapter from the Midwest US to Madagascar, I build a multisited portrait of accountability work as a mobile or traveling form of humanitarian governance (Pandolfi 2010), understood and enacted in culturally distinct ways. Audit procedures lay bare a vexing set of questions for both Malagasy and Americans: What does it ultimately mean to be accountable, and how is accountability assessed? Do accountability requirements between fellow believers contradict basic contemporary principles of global religious communion, evoking shadow histories of colonial evangelism and its inequalities?

The conclusion asks how Malagasy and Americans reckon the time duration or end of medical relief. Many Malagasy and Americans express concerns about the long-term foreign presence and "dependency" of the medical relief model, a subject about which scholars of humanitarianism have written extensively. What is aid's end, and what futures can be imagined through its termination? Intertwining these imagined futures with the present moment of aid, the conclusion considers how aid circulations are diverse projects of world-making for religious actors.

CHAPTER ONE

Remembering and Forgetting through Medical Aid Work

The storyteller is the figure in which the righteous man encounters himself.
—Walter Benjamin (1968, 109)

Madagascar has long held a prominent place in the geopolitical imagination and imperial projects of US Lutherans in the Midwest. (See figure 1.) Today these century-long ties between Lutherans in the US Midwest and in southern Madagascar have been revived through a medical aid program that sends shipments of U.S.-procured medical supplies to church-run clinics in Madagascar. The aid program thus builds on the history of US Lutheran ties to Madagascar but also seeks to establish a new kind of professional aid relationship that respects Malagasy sovereignty and national authority. Yet how do people involved with contemporary Christian aid arrangements that emerged from colonial foreign mission work, such as the Minnesota-Madagascar aid program, regard their own history? This chapter closely examines how Lutherans in Minneapolis–St. Paul and in the Malagasy capital Antananarivo apprehend the colonial mission past. It reveals that the past is a crucial, often overlooked, resource in the cultural process of becoming Christian humanitarians and in crafting the moral foundation of religiously-based aid.

In this chapter, I pursue a central question: How do certain connections and values of history come to matter in the present for Lutheran humanitarians, while other linkages are erased or muted? I understand the past as a relational value, intimately bound to a sense of the present and continually being made and remade in relation to "present" endeavors, rather than as a container or context for current aid work. I take inspiration here from critical postcolonial studies and, specifically, Ann Stoler's (2008) assertion that imperialist projects are never entirely new but take shape from the "ruins" of what came before. This approach to Christian aid alliances reveals the dynamism, variability, and political qualities of history making and its ongoing, vital role in shaping the dominant sensibilities of aid work. For former US Lutheran missionaries and their U.S.-based supporters, becoming humanitarians has meant reworking histories of mission involvement in Madagascar in particular ways that segment time and morally cleanse the late-colonial period, but not the early colonial past. In the process, former missionaries attenuate their ties to the early colonial past that, in fact, played a strong role in laying the groundwork for current medical humanitarian projects through the introduction of biomedicine in Madagascar. By contrast, Malagasy Lutherans working at SALFA's Antananarivo offices do not cleanse their contemporary aid work of colonial influences. Rather, they identify instances of colonial continuities in the foreign support they seek and the organizational structures they navigate to operate Lutheran medical institutions in Madagascar.

The Lutheran aid program emerged under specific political and economic conditions in Madagascar, as I described in the Introduction. As long-term US missionaries were leaving Madagascar in the late 1970s, the Malagasy economy collapsed after a period of state-endorsed socialism under President Didier Ratsiraka. In the midst of this "economic crisis" and subsequent austerity measures imposed by World Bank structural adjustment, Malagasy Lutheran doctors and former US medical missionaries established in 1979 the Malagasy Lutheran health care department or SALFA to coordinate medical and technical support for individual Lutheran clinics across the island. Many of these Lutheran hospitals had found it increasingly hard to obtain basic medical materials because of widespread commodity shortages, weak currency, and diminished international trade under Ratsiraka's administration. Former medical missionaries organized two NGOs in Minneapolis in the early-to-mid-1980s—IHM and Malagasy Partnership—to send medical relief to SALFA in Antananarivo. Since then, this humanitarian arrangement has continued. With increasing economic hardship during the intervening thirty years in Madagascar, the aid alliance has become part of the long-term functioning of SALFA, which today provides support to forty-eight clinics across the island. Many former US missionar-

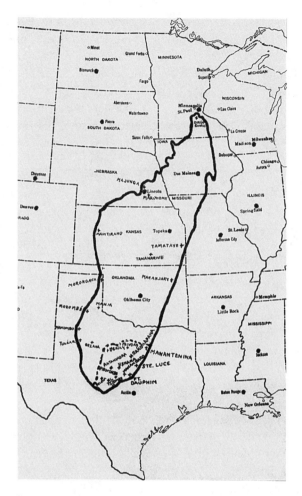

FIGURE 1.1. The book *Zanahary in South Madagascar* (1932, 31) by American Lutheran missionary Andrew Burgess features this map, superimposing Madagascar on the middle section of the United States.

ies and their families now voluntarily work for or financially support the two Minneapolis-based NGOs.

The social and political transformations I have described are not limited to Lutheran Christian ties between Madagascar and the United States but form part of a much broader phenomenon that occurred across African states in the 1980s and 1990s. Scholars have documented the rise of a neoliberal order at this time that shifted political power

away from centralized states to NGOs and religiously-based organizations (Bornstein 2005; Ferguson 2006). By neoliberal order, scholars refer partly to World Bank and International Monetary Fund
structural adjustment plans in postindependence states like Madagascar that favored market liberalization and required austerity in government spending on public services like health care in exchange for
high-interest loans (Peterson 2014). Such structural reforms created a
greater role for NGOs and other transnational alliances in the provision of social services like health care. Though neoliberalism is an umbrella term with widely varying meanings that can sometimes obscure
as much as they reveal (Ganti 2014), I use the term in this chapter to
draw attention to how preexisting religious organizations in Madagascar responded to state-based market reforms and, in subsequent chapters, explore the ambivalent cultural relationship of Lutheran aid participants with individualist discourses of accountability "conducive to
neoliberalism" (Rudnyckyj 2009, 130). Building on the idea that neoliberalism encompasses shifting techniques and relationships of governing, rather than only market reform in a limited or state-based structural sense, some writers have characterized these loose, horizontally
organized, transnational configurations as new political alliances in African nations that, after the 1990s, have increasingly displaced prior, colonialist orientations to citizenship and sovereignty (Nguyen 2010; Piot
2010, 8).

The Minnesota-Madagascar aid alliance offers some interesting qualifications to this thesis. Although Lutherans' aid interventions took the
shape of NGO alliances that were fostered under the rising neoliberal
order of the 1980s and 1990s, their partnership emerged directly from
the structures and encounters of colonial evangelism. In addition, in various ways, colonial pasts still come to matter for both Americans and
Malagasy from within these "newer" NGO-based alliances. This evidence suggests the existence of hybrid configurations in African states
that are neither rooted only in colonial structures of political rule nor
emerging merely from neoliberal transformations in governance but
complexly cut of the cloth of both. Also, as Wacquant (2012) has argued,
neoliberalism is not characterized by the total evisceration of the state
but the reconstitution of it through a variety of market reforms that support the interests of a political elite. This reengineering process can be
visible in market liberalization programs in Madagascar since the 1980s
that have, in turn, sustained the Minnesota-Madagascar aid program;

these state-based market reforms are, as Wacquant (2012, 73) writes, a "space of . . . struggles over the very . . . priorities of public authority," a subject with a contentious and multistranded postindependence history in Madagascar. Together, the Lutheran aid initiative calls for ethnographic techniques attuned to how people perceive such programs as continuous and discontinuous with what came before them.

Anthropologists have argued that a proliferation of late-twentieth-century cultural experiences of discontinuity and rupture, ranging from migration to the rise of an international aid regime, can be traced to market liberalization and its widespread effects (Comaroff and Comaroff 2000; Ong 2006). I build in this chapter on these far-reaching conversations on late-twentieth-century cultural experiences of displacement amid shifting forms of affiliation and increasingly powerful transnational structures of governance. I am particularly interested, however, in how, even in cultural practices that emphasize disjunctures with what came before them, such as the Lutheran aid alliance, discontinuity is, in some ways, an ideological position that is never perfectly realized and requires ongoing practice. That is, the claim of newness and difference itself forms part of the political power of these transnational alliances. Therefore, I explore how the relationship between cultural continuity and discontinuity is perceived by individual actors themselves—in this case, between the current aid alliance and the colonial history of Lutheran involvement in Madagascar—and examine what kind of cultural work this selective recognition of affinity and disjuncture with the past enables in the medical aid program, and for whom.

In what follows, I organize the chapter as a multilayered dialogue between individuals' contemporary reflections and the colonial history of US-Malagasy interactions. In this process, I aim to show how contemporary reflections serve or critique particular narratives of the past and feature specific forgettings. My approach endeavors to shed light on how "humanitarian sensibilities" take root in global religious communities (Haskell 1985). They are social formations that shape and require a variety of cultural values and practices for their existence, including in this case specific narratives of the past. In turn, my use of the term *humanitarian* is meant to signal how, through these practices, Lutherans take part in the culturally pervasive process of making their actions, narrated views, and selfhood compatible with the moral order of the broader aid world. Not all of my Lutheran informants adopt the term *humanitarian* as an identifier for themselves, since some view it as too secular a label to adequately characterize their biblically inspired aid work. Nevertheless, I suggest here and in subsequent chapters that, through their medical relief organizations, they exhibit a humanitarian sensibility and draw heavily from the bureaucratic protocols, technocratic measures, ethical standards, discourse, forms of subjectivity, and funding sources of the broader aid world.

Among these activities, recognizing how Christian aid workers place their own work in time is a crucial part of understanding the cultural and moral logic of Christian aid arrangements. At strategic moments in the chapter, I draw in "forgotten" histories of colonial involvement using archival documents to provide critical alternatives to current US notions of the colonial past. Forgetting here is a culturally patterned, rather than necessarily individual, process that supports the formation of a humanitarian identity in the present time; forgetting thus plays a culturally productive role and is not simply an omission (Connerton 2008, 63). Bringing together these dissonant views mirrors the way that various versions of the past continually erupt, rather unpredictably, in contemporary aid efforts, as I will show throughout this book. To begin, I briefly situate the Minnesota-Madagascar aid program in the early colonial biomedical encounter in southern Madagascar. Given the immense scope of this subject, my aim is to provide a selective portrait of American and Malagasy medical interactions in southern Madagascar to show the colonial and cultural conditions through which Lutheran medicine was introduced, often in sharp contrast to the practices of Malagasy medicine (*fanafody-gasy*). This medical infrastructure, as it has been enculturated, refused, and reworked in diverse ways across Malagasy communities, constitutes part of the foundation of SALFA's current operation and the aid program.

Revisiting the Role of Colonial Missions in the Globalization of Medicine

Today, the Minnesota-Madagascar aid relationship builds on a century of interaction between Malagasy and Americans in southern Madagascar. Since 1888, US Lutherans have sent about 385 missionaries from Minnesota and the Upper Midwest to southern Madagascar.[1] Norwegian American Lutherans were already well aware of Madagascar when they migrated to the Midwest United States, primarily from 1860 to 1900

(Gjerde and Qualey 2002, 2). Along with South Africa, Madagascar had been one of two primary "mission fields" of the Norwegians (Nyhagen Predelli 2003). The Norwegian Missionary Society began evangelism programs in highland Madagascar in 1866, as had other European church societies. Merina Malagasy Queen Ranavalona II opened the country's borders to missionaries and other foreigners in 1861.[2] Ranavalona II went on to make Protestantism a state religion in 1869, a move that strategically aligned the Merina state with the British Protestants of the London Missionary Society and other international societies in reaction to increasing French attempts to annex Madagascar (Nyhagen Predelli 2003, 21).

Following the Norwegians, Norwegian American Lutheran churches dispatched missionaries in 1888 to the region in Madagascar south of the Tropic of Capricorn, or south of Anantsono–St. Augustine in the west and Manantenina in the east, in the land primarily of Mahafaly, Tandroy, and Tanosy people. In the ensuing decades of French colonial occupation (1896–1960), Lutherans built outposts, churches, dispensaries, and schools in the southwest and southeast; when combined with institutions built under the auspices of the Norwegian Lutheran mission in the southern highlands, these became part of the institutional foundation in 1950 for the national Malagasy Lutheran Church or FLM (*Fiangonana Loterana Malagasy*). Today, the FLM counts nearly three million members and forms one of the island's four largest Protestant churches in a national population estimated to be about 50 percent Christian (Feeley-Harnik 1997, 87; Keller 2005, 40).[3]

Medicine was a substantial component of early mission work in Madagascar, but Americans faced specific French colonial restrictions on how it could be pursued. After French colonial occupation of Madagascar in 1896, US medical doctors and other foreigners were prohibited by the French from practicing medicine in Madagascar without training in "tropical medicine" in France, a policy that increased French administrative control of colonial welfare institutions. Only one American Lutheran Free Church missionary doctor, J. O. Dyrnes, completed this requirement in 1899 and established a dispensary in Manasoa in southwest Madagascar.[4]

Yet even amid French colonial prohibitions, Americans followed the institutional rise of medicine in the United States and the broader movement among European and US foreign mission societies in making medicine an "all but universal" component of mission work by World War I

(Walls 1996, 212). In southeast Madagascar, US missions did so primarily through the work of single female missionary nurses, trained at the Lutheran Deaconess Hospital in Minneapolis, who were not subject to the French colonial regulations. From the 1880s well into the 1950s, these nurses dispensed medications from their homes on mission stations, accompanied evangelists to tend to the sick and ailing in outlying villages, and led extensive health and hygiene presentations by "flannelgraph" or during sewing and embroidery lessons.[5] Some carried copies of *The New Standard Formulary* (1920), a pharmacopoeia guide with which they prepared basic medicines (Vigen 1979, 48). Missionary pastors themselves, using the little medical training they received in seminary, usually brought with them to rural villages during evangelism trips a small medical kit, which included aspirin and later antimalarial medications. I heard stories from retired missionary pastors in Minnesota who continued to do so well into the 1980s.

In the late nineteenth century, foreigners entered a therapeutic environment that already included several kinds of Malagasy medical specialists, such as the *ombiasa* (Malagasy, healer-diviner) and *mpsikidy* (Malagasy, herbalist). During the late nineteenth and early twentieth centuries, European and US biomedical practices produced an influential cultural divide between *fanafody vazaha*, or literally foreign, white, and European medicine, and *fanafody-gasy* or Malagasy medicine, the latter being an epistemological object brought into existence by the biomedical colonial encounter (Sharp 1993). What came to be referred to as Malagasy medicine or *fanafody-gasy* is part of a broader complex of ritual practices in Malagasy communities rather than a medical system in the Western sense. These practices center on the ongoing work of achieving a kind of equilibrium in Malagasy relations with the ancestors (Malagasy, *razana*) and in social relationships with other people, rather than only identifying and treating discrete bodily symptoms. Individuals consult *ombiasa*, who attribute illness to a range of factors both inside and outside the individual body, including an offense against the ancestors or the breaking of a social taboo (*fady*) observed by one's kin group or social position. Treatments can include offerings of food for the ancestors, an herbal remedy prepared by a *mpsikidy*, treatment by a bone setter, or wearing on one's body or placing outside the house a protective talisman, known as an *ody*, to guard the ailing from external illness-causing agents (Sharp 1993; Harper 2002).

Among late-nineteenth- and early-twentieth-century US Lutheran missionaries, much ink was spilled on portraits for US audiences that characterized the *ombiasa* and Malagasy medicine (*fanafody-gasy*) as unreliable and nonmodern in contrast to biomedicine. As mediators between the living and the ancestral dead and not only healers in a limited sense, *ombiasa* were perceived as the primary obstacle for introducing the Gospel.[6] US missionaries contended that *ombiasa* fostered fear of the ancestral dead among Malagasy, from which only Christian conversion would liberate them; *ombiasa* were alleged to capitalize on this fear with, in the stark words of missionary cleric P. A. Bjelde, "cruel deceits" (1938, 32).

This pejorative phrase simplified a number of more contradictory and complex positions that missionaries occupied in relation to *ombiasa*. Many early-twentieth-century Malagasy converts and dispensary patients consulted both *ombiasa* and Christian nurses and medical doctors, something noted repeatedly by Norwegian American doctor J. O. Dyrnes in his diaries. In one early-twentieth-century reflection, Dyrnes wrote, "At first the people came to the doctor for his treatment, and then went home and drank their own traditional medicines. To them it seemed that the more medicine they took, the quicker they would be well. Gradually, however, many have learned to take my advice on the matter" (cited in Ose 1979, 26). These lines attest to the slow biopolitical work pursued in small medical outposts like Dyrnes's clinic in Manasoa; for forty years, he and others instilled a hierarchy of medicinal treatments through subtle and not-so-subtle disciplinary measures. For example, as a medical doctor and consecrated pastor, Dyrnes preached a holistic Christian approach to healing. He implied to patients that healing effectiveness required asking for forgiveness for sins and seeking Christian salvation. On occasion, he did not dissuade Malagasy visitors' perception that their sickness may be a "punishment from God as well as a call to repentance," as he recorded in Norwegian of his June 9, 1914, visit with a wayward Christian man named Jonatana.[7]

Colonial mission medicine, however, built on the long-standing symbolic and ritual power of Malagasy medicine in several ways, showing a more complex process of Malagasy appropriation and localization of Christian medicine through familiar cultural categories (Larson 1997, 970). For instance, as biomedicine was introduced, allopathic medications became known as forms of *fanafody* along with other substances, including "the rich pharmacopoeia used by moasy [also *ombiasa*] and other indigenous practitioners" (Sharp 1993, 205). Though US Lutheran missionaries attempted to distinguish Westernized medicines from the many varieties of *ody*, including love medicine (*ody fitia*) and bad medicine (*fanafody ratsy*) or sorcery (see also Graeber 2007b, 76), Malagasy and biomedical healing practices were also linguistically and culturally intertwined, as biomedicine derived some cultural authority through its association with the ritual power accorded to *ody*.

US Lutheran missionaries also tacitly recognized the cultural authority of *ombiasa* and other Malagasy medical specialists by seeking to convert as many as possible in the precolonial and early colonial period (1888–1914), as well as later, and then upholding them as model converts. *Ombiasa* themselves found new channels of identity making and social community through Christian affiliation, often at times of great hardship according to mission records. According to the story of Tongalaza, a Tandroy "sorcerer" or *ombiasa*, after his son's death and his own bout of life-threatening pneumonia, he converted and took the Christian name Petera while throwing his *ody* in the forest, where, in the words of one missionary, "he knew they could not be found by others" (Dahl 1934, 20).[8] Mission photographic records, like written missionary narratives, indicate that public moments such as these—disparaging and literally casting off the implements of *fanafody-gasy*—were common elements in staging and performing the ontological boundaries between mission medicine and Malagasy medicine. Yet, as I have suggested, the early-twentieth-century colonial medical encounter also relied on, coexisted with, and selectively appropriated the practices and symbolism of *fanafody-gasy*, showing a more complex interrelationship.

US medical activities in southern Madagascar in the late nineteenth and early twentieth centuries, including their devaluing of Malagasy medicine, also took place in the context of a French colonial biopolitics and contributed to it. A cornerstone of French policy in Madagascar was an oppressive system of taxation that required forced labor of colonial subjects who could not pay their taxes. Though the French often lacked the means of enforcement (Feeley-Harnik 1991, 128), the system was enshrined in the civil code or *indigénat*; the labor requirements were condemned by the International Labor Organization in 1930 but not changed until 1946 (Randrianja and Ellis 2009, 161). Alongside its labor policy, the early French colonial administration instituted medical schools, dispensaries, and hospitals to increase the birth rate and decrease mortality, particularly among ethnically Merina Malagasy, who were viewed as racially superior in the eugenicist colonial policy (Harper

2002, 136; Andersen 2010). These labor and medical policies have been read together as linked parts of a French colonial biopolitics, which viewed Malagasy colonial subjects primarily as a labor pool (Harper 2002, 137; Andersen 2010, 428). Christian missionaries' nursing care and work to teach hygiene, referred to collectively as "hygienic and medical measures" in one 1898 colonial document (cited in Harper 2002, 138–39), was viewed by the colonial state as part of this interwoven tapestry of legal and political means of administering the Malagasy population.

The pursuit of mission medicine itself was thus not a culturally neutral pursuit but a politicized one in the French colonial context. Indeed, in subtle yet influential ways, Americans' medical work often instructed the domestic and moral order of bodily participation in a colonial system of labor; by modeling a Christian bodily habitus that emphasized self-discipline, accountability, hard work, and healthfulness through hygiene, nutrition, and teetotalism, they interwove the pursuit of biomedicine and Christian identity with the values of capitalist production promulgated by the colonial state. US missionaries were not directly providing a labor force for the colonial regime. Nevertheless, mission schools and churches did teach a work ethic and forms of individual responsibility and bodily habitus compatible with, and necessary for, the expansion of, the colonial economy.[9] This circumstance was encoded in many other late-nineteenth- and early-twentieth-century European and US missionary encounters across the globe and is therefore not unique to the experiences of US Lutheran missionaries in southern Madagascar (see, e.g., Comaroff 1985; Meyer 1996; Keane 2007). Part of the reason is that European and US Protestant missionaries' religious understandings were influenced by and had in some cases shaped the emergence of industrial capitalism in their home societies (Comaroff and Comaroff 1992).

The current aid relationship is arguably the heir of a far-reaching series of early Malagasy-US colonial interactions. Individual US Lutheran missionaries variously perceived medicine as a "concrete expression of Christian charity" (Bjelde 1938, 41), a form of development and progress, an opening for the Gospel, a form of ministering to the soul, and a way to build personal relationships with non-Christian Malagasy villagers. Yet underpinning these medical and health-based activities of foreigners was a colonial orientation toward Malagasy culture as deficient or in need of reform (Vaughan 1991, 56). Though US missionaries were noncolonial foreign actors without territorial control of the island and its population, such representations are equally part of colo-

nialism because they created a foreign depiction of Malagasy culture
that suited Western imperialism (Vaughan 1991). Among US Lutherans,
such representations were central components of culturally introducing biomedicine in Madagascar and establishing a long-standing healing conflict with the *ombiasa* or Malagasy ritual practitioner, an ontological divide that continues to inform the contemporary aid program
(see chapter 5). It is difficult for the aid relationship to fully extricate itself from these earlier practices because of the thoroughgoing way that
colonial-era interactions shaped the understandings of medicine now deployed in the aid program. Colonial mission medicine supported a vast
biopolitical apparatus that created through its practice culturally specific
notions of the subjectivity of the patient (Vaughan 1991, 56), the biomedical body, and biomedical illness categories, upon which institutionalized Lutheran medicine in Madagascar and the US-Madagascar aid program now rests.

Deploying "Colonial Missionaries" and
Creating a Humanitarian Sensibility

During the first three months of my field research, however, I noticed
that the former Madagascar missionaries and aid workers whom I knew
in Minneapolis–St. Paul sometimes distanced themselves from their US
Lutheran predecessors by pejoratively using the terms "colonial missionaries" and "colonial days." On my weekend visit to her house, Margaret,
a retired missionary and ELCA member, who lived in southeast Madagascar from 1959 to 1987, told me the previous missionary generation
had "a little bit of that colonial attitude" and admitted finding "embar-
rassing" their writing on Madagascar. She described her work with Malagasy Lutheran women's aid societies as a two-way process of mutual
learning; she pointedly added that, in contrast to prior US missionaries, her generation understood that "missionaries are not there to change
people's culture because culture is not what makes someone a Christian." On another occasion, a short-term medical missionary, Gene, who
voluntarily operates Malagasy Partnership, was reflecting on the comments made the previous day by another visiting missionary. This visitor
had said in front of both of us that retired US missionaries should make
more return visits to Madagascar to assist Malagasy Lutherans in church
affairs. When I asked Gene what he thought about this suggestion, he

paused and then replied, with what I took as a critique, "Gives me a colonial twinge."

As I came to understand, Madagascar missionaries, their adult children, and the social networks of which they were a part were subtly reforming their cultural and religious role to be more in keeping with that
of a humanitarian or aid giver, using extensive, pointed references to
"colonial missionaries." In turn, their contemporary commitment to assist churches overseas through NGO work and other service projects became the "moment of retrospective significance" from which those missionaries and their coworkers perceived and recast the colonial past
(Trouillot 1995, 26). Many former Madagascar missionaries like Gene
and their adult children helped found or began working with the two
medical aid agencies in the 1980s, shifting their relationship with the
FLM to that of an aid laborer or financial contributor. Prior to that time,
this group of approximately fifty retired, primarily elderly US Lutheran
missionaries filled a range of positions as "foreign workers" in the FLM,
from ordained pastors to nurses and hospital administrators; spent various lengths of time in Madagascar, with some living on the island up to
forty years; and primarily left Madagascar in the 1970s and 1980s.[10]

Though both IHM and Malagasy Partnership boasted a vibrant network of Lutheran lay volunteers, many of whom had no family ties to
Madagascar, these missionaries and children of Madagascar missionaries were disproportionately represented in positions of authority
at both agencies.[11] Indeed, I was initially brought to IHM at the insistence of one of these former missionaries, a widower in her late seventies named Lois. Lois's adult daughter and son-in-law, a medical doctor,
were among the medical missionaries to establish IHM after working at
the Manambaro Lutheran Hospital in southeast Madagascar.[12] In 2005–
6, nearly half of the IHM board members or up to six people were children of Madagascar missionaries and former Madagascar missionaries.[13]
Across a variety of religious and family activities, including church services, home-cooked meals, and aid work, I saw how they were gradually transforming themselves into Lutheran humanitarians and deploying certain discourses of the past as a cultural resource to aid in this
process. These seemingly mundane conversational remarks offer insight
into cultural and political transformations *within* Christian communities
that have paved the way for aid arrangements between world regions,
while offering religious actors like former missionaries new rhetorical
tools of self-making (Battaglia 1995).

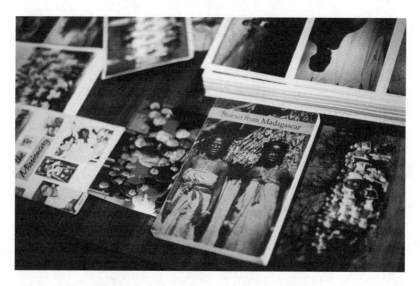

FIGURE I.2. Books on display, Madagascar missionary gathering, Wisconsin.

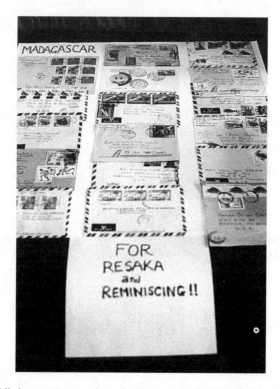

FIGURE I.3. Missionary correspondence for "conversation" and reminiscing, Wisconsin.

I look at the narrative practices of former missionaries and their supporters as a form of moral reasoning, which establishes moral boundaries between the colonial past—often referring to the early colonial interactions I have described—and current Lutheran projects and selves,
including aid endeavors. By naming and placing amoral colonial actions
in the past, literally using a temporal signifier to segment historical time,
speakers attempt to morally cleanse their lifework and the present moment from similar moral dilemmas. Yet, rather than have one clearly defined set of meanings, I noticed that the colonial discourse had a shifting
set of moral referents, often folding back on missionary-supported aid
endeavors and on the missionaries themselves. Rose, a retired missionary nurse and wife of Dr. Fosse who had just been appointed to the IHM
board in 2006 after living in Madagascar for nearly forty years, privately
expressed some concerns to me about the agency's growing aid program
and added emphatically, "We don't want to be called neo-colonials!"
The IHM executive director Curt once gave the example of an unethical medical agency that carelessly sent all "its technology" overseas and,
paraphrasing Matthew 7:15–23, portrayed this kind of relief work as a
"child of colonial days in another clothing."[14] Still others with whom I
spoke individually named those they saw as "colonial" among the sizable community of retired missionaries, these judgments occurring out
of earshot and in the presence of seemingly neutral parties like myself.

At the time, many Madagascar missionaries were reading primatol-
ogist Allison Jolly's 2004 book *Lords and Lemurs*, which profiles the
historical relationship between a French family, the de Haulmes, and
Tandroy Malagasy in southern Madagascar, where these missionaries
lived for many years. Several took issue with Jolly's portrait of US Lutheran missionaries, such as Pastor Torvik, who was described in one
scene as using a forbidding "voice that saved sinners from hellfire"
(Jolly 2004, 149). For these informants, Jolly's portrayal had evoked a
stock "colonial missionary" character—stern, punitive, unyielding, and
culturally and racially insensitive—from which this generation and individual people sought to differentiate themselves. In describing "old
colonial days," the fifty-year-old eldest daughter of a retired clerical missionary who donated money to IHM said some missionaries "imposed
their way of life" on the Malagasy people with whom they came in contact. "I knew missionaries like that," she said, referring to her childhood
in southeast Madagascar in the 1960s and early 1970s, "but my father
wasn't one of them."

American uses of the term *colonial* identify a range of forms of un-equal power and cultural imperialism as key moral problems, including conflating culture and religion, acting ethnocentrically, usurping Mal-agasy cultural and religious authority, and showing disregard for Mala-gasy national sovereignty. The colonial discourse voiced by Madagascar missionaries-turned-aid-workers suggests that late-colonial Madagascar missionaries and their fellow aid workers, in contrast to morally troubled "colonial missionaries," were always already diffusely "humanitarian." From their perspective, they espoused the values of Malagasy sover-eignty, partnership, and mutual exchange now regarded as ethical stan-dards by the home church. Reforming their own subjectivity through the colonial discourse pushes such humanitarian values into the late-colonial past in which they worked and implies that this "time," as well, was al-ready "humanitarian" and not "colonial." Yet by placing problems of un-equal power in the colonial past, this framework downplays the political and economic inequalities introduced through aid programs, as well as aid's continuities with the missionary past. Moreover, this culturally con-structed series of connections between the late-colonial past and the cur-rent aid program prompts questions about the degree to which this "time" laid the groundwork for the aid program and what dimensions of late-colonial Malagasy and American interactions are forgotten or laid aside in this American reworking of the past. To explore these questions, I turn now to an examination of the nationalization of Malagasy Lutheran med-ical institutions and the slightly earlier process of building Lutheran med-ical institutions in southern Madagascar in the 1950s and 1960s.

Late-Colonial Interactions and Nationalism of Malagasy Lutheran Medical Institutions

Significant late-colonial political and cultural shifts can be observed in the relationship between Americans and Malagasy, and these changes continue to influence the current aid relationship. Although mission-aries originally discredited much of the work of Malagasy medical spe-cialists, such as *ombiasa* or ritual healers, it became more common to embrace Malagasy culture as a source of medical and even scientific wis-dom in the second half of the twentieth century, a sharp change from early-twentieth-century missionaries.[15] Gene, the founder of Malagasy

Partnership and a short-term medical missionary technician in Madagascar from 1978 to 1979, told me that his wife was the first missionary to enlist a Malagasy midwife for the birth of their son in 1979, a realization that surprised him at the time. When US aid workers now reject "colonial ways," they have in mind these early-twentieth-century missionary approaches that devalued Malagasy culture. US missionaries now characterize the late-colonial and early postindependence years as times of partnership and collaboration with Malagasy Lutherans. Upon close inspection, however, Americans still initially held disproportionate religious and cultural authority of medical institutions in those years, though Malagasy and Americans had been building a professional class of Malagasy Lutheran medical workers for several decades. It was not until 1979 that the two US-instituted Lutheran hospitals in southern Madagascar had Malagasy medical directors: Dr. Noel Rakotomavo at Manambaro and Dr. Justin Ravelonjanahary in Ejeda.

The nationalization of church-run Lutheran medical institutions—a key element of the SALFA medical network—was thus a slow process that did not completely unfold in the late-colonial or even early post-independence years, but considerably later into the 1970s. Americans like Gene and Dr. Fosse were part of joint Malagasy-US initiatives to create professional pathways for Malagasy Lutheran nurses, doctors, and laboratory technicians, so that the Americans could, as they put it, "work themselves out of a job." For example, in 1978, Gene was brought to Manambaro Hospital in southeast Madagascar to train a class of Malagasy medical laboratory technicians. His mandate from the US church office was to bring the medical laboratory instrumentation at Manambaro to the level of a small hospital in the United States within two years. This was a tall order, he said, because there had been few resources and little training for laboratory work. His students were relying on outdated 1941 laboratory texts left by a predecessor. Gene quickly improvised in light of the commodity shortages of the time and ended up teaching the practical chemistry of laboratory work; to stain microscope slides, for instance, he created a solvent from an organic cleaner he found in a hospital out-building.

Other programs to train Malagasy medical professionals had been in place for considerably longer in the two US-instituted hospitals at Manambaro in the southeast and Ejeda in the southwest. In 1956, a US Lutheran missionary nurse, Viola Lewis, began a nurse training program at

Manambaro with twelve Malagasy men and four women in the first class
(Vigen 1979, 53). The course included study in anatomy, physiology,
nursing ethics, microbiology, and disease etiology, in addition to pract-
icum placement in the hospital. For the next twenty years, graduating
nurses, which varied from two to twenty-six per year, went on to work in
private and government-run clinics, not only in the Lutheran hospitals.
US-led training programs also began in the late 1950s and early 1960s
for laboratory and X-ray technology, which Gene resumed in the late
1970s. By 1971, most of the Manambaro Hospital's top leadership, drawn
from the local Lutheran synod and the hospital's governing board, were
Malagasy, including the medical director, administrator, synod leader,
hospital chaplain, and a representative for the hospital staff, which to-
taled seventy-two employees (Vigen 1979, 66).

Though Americans and Malagasy began training programs in the
late-colonial and early postindependence years for a range of Malagasy
Lutheran medical professionals, Americans still held prominent medical positions at Manambaro and Ejeda until the mid- to late 1970s.[16]
The reasons for this are multifaceted: A number of Malagasy doctors
had left Madagascar to practice elsewhere in the 1970s because of the
widespread commodity shortages that hindered medical care. In addition, some Americans espoused problematic, Eurocentric views of Malagasy as more prone to institutional corruption in the 1950s and 1960s
and thus may have disfavored Malagasy hospital leadership on that basis
(see chapter 6). It appears, however, that money was equally if not more
a factor in why missionaries sometimes remained in their positions.[17]
Missionaries were free medical labor for the hospital, because their salaries were paid by the ELCA. They also brought with them access to US
church grants such as donations for equipment, building repairs, and the
hospital's "poor fund."

Current Malagasy Lutheran employees of SALFA told me that US
missionaries' departure had meant that church-run institutions had, for
the first time, to come up with a full salary for a Malagasy employee,
which stretched institutional budgets or quickly became unsustainable
(see chapter 4).[18] Lutheran hospitals sometimes had to offer smaller salaries than what they hoped and had difficulty attracting qualified Malagasy doctors, many of whom were from the capital city region, to remote,
rural hospitals. In this context, missionaries often became resource man-
agers and seekers of external grants to fill in gaps when US church funding dried up, making their role considerably more bureaucratic (compare

Beidelman 1974, 243–44). When combined with state economic collapse and structural adjustment reforms, this is precisely how the US aid partnership came into being in 1979 between SALFA in Antananarivo and the two Minneapolis-based NGOs begun by former missionaries.

Midcentury Institutionalization of Lutheran Medicine

As I described earlier, US missionaries practiced medicine only on a small scale through dispensaries and nursing care until the 1940s. It was not until the mid- to late colonial and postindependence years that US missionaries and Malagasy church leaders in southern Madagascar built two hospitals in Manambaro (1954) and Ejeda (1960), shifting their approach to a less "personal" and more institutional and "technical" form of mission medicine (Vaughan 1991, 74). The French colonial administration granted permission to build these two sixty-bed hospitals in the late 1940s. Many of the retired US medical missionaries involved in the two Minneapolis medical NGOs view the aid program as an outgrowth of this midcentury process of institutionalizing and nationalizing Lutheran Christian medicine in southern Madagascar, in which they were directly involved. When they refer to the moral hazards of "colonial days," they do not mean this midcentury period of institutionalizing medicine, even though it largely also occurred during French colonial rule. As I show in the following section, the institutionalization of Lutheran medicine also participated in colonial politics, namely a shifting French approach to rural populations in southern Madagascar.

Colonial Surveillance and Late-Colonial Medicine

The French gave US Lutherans permission to build the Manambaro Hospital in November 1947, a significant year in Malagasy history.[19] The most violent Malagasy uprising against French colonial rule began to unfold in spring and summer 1947. An estimated eighty thousand Malagasy lost their lives in the insurrection, and the French jailed many suspected leaders, including some Lutheran pastors based in the southeast, for more than a decade (Cole 2001; Harper 2002, 89). French administrators brought in Senegalese soldiers to quell the rebellion. Scholars observe that, in several regions including parts of the southeast, the aftermath of the 1947 uprising lasted until the mid-1950s because of the severity of the French response (Cole 2001; Harper 2002).

The French appear to have approved the two US hospitals at this time not simply because of a loosening of French administration but rather from a transformation in the style and form of indirect rule. It could be observed that biomedical development in southern Madagascar was a vehicle that increased French colonial surveillance of those very rural populations thought, in some cases, to have planned and taken part in the 1947 rebellion (see Harper 2002, 89).[20] After decades of colonial taxation, forced labor, and land seizure, rural populations were led to believe that, after World War II, French colonial policy toward Madagascar would loosen and change, particularly after Charles de Gaulle promised as much in a 1944 address (Randrianja and Ellis 2009, 173). Soon after, however, French administrative control of the island was reinstated, with an increasing French focus on rural development. Randrianja and Ellis (2009, 169) write, "It was a mix of international and local factors—the Second World War and the post-war international situation, later combined with the alarm call of Madagascar's 1947 insurrection—that eventually persuaded the French metropolitan government to pay more attention to Madagascar's rural sector." Bringing the Lutherans' work in rural communities in southern Madagascar into a closer relationship with the colonial state could be understood to serve French interests in several respects, as Protestant churches had long been a site of Malagasy nationalist organizing (see chapter 5).

Current US discourses of the colonial imply that Americans had increased their solidarity with Malagasy congregants and respect for Malagasy authority and sovereignty over French *colons* in the mid- to late colonial period. This could certainly be borne out on an individual basis. When taking into account the structural position of the US missions, however, the situation in practice appears more complex, with missionaries overtly and institutionally aligning their work more closely with the colonial state while indirectly continuing to critique it and supporting efforts to nationalize the church. Expatriate relations between the French and Americans had settled by the 1940s and 1950s into a begrudgingly cool alliance, perhaps because of the geopolitics leading up to and shaping World War II and its aftermath.[21] The US evangelical missions were structurally compelled under French colonial rule to manage relationships with both Malagasy congregants and French *colons*. The current colonial discourse, however, obscures the complexity of Americans' relations with the French at this time and oversimplifies the multifaceted moral positions that Americans appear to have held in the late colonial period. Moreover, the institutionalization of Lutheran medicine in the 1940s through the 1960s—upon which the current aid program builds— would also not have been possible without the earlier biopolitical work of establishing biomedicine's cultural authority.

In sum, though US medical missionaries and Malagasy Lutherans in-stitutionalized medicine in the late colonial period in southern Mada-gascar and increasingly took a bureaucratic approach to their work, it was also initially part of a context of shifting French approaches to colo-nial administration, particularly its attempted surveillance of rural pop-ulations. Moreover, while nationalizing the church was a late-colonial priority of Malagasy and Americans, several church-run institutions largely remained under US control until the 1960s and 1970s, making the late-colonial and postindependence years also a time of dispropor-tionate US religious and institutional authority. These issues are largely forgotten in the contemporary "colonial" discourse voiced by some US aid workers, which locates political and cultural inequality between Americans and Malagasy in the early colonial period and associates the late colonial period with more positive, supportive, and egalitarian ties between Americans and Malagasy Lutherans. As Paul Connerton (2008, 63) writes, "What is allowed to be forgotten provides living space for present projects." Forgetting here participates in what Connerton refers to as a discarding process during which details and knowledge that do not suit a new identity are cast off through small acts that seem incon-sequential or disconnected but do in fact evince a shared logic, whether or not it is overtly recognized. These forgettings also show the ideologi-cal work performed by the cultural category of the "colonial"; it enables current aid providers to make connections with the late colonial period but reject problematic moral ties to early and mid-twentieth-century colonial work.

Shifting Approaches to Lutheran Global Relations

These discursive moves align former Madagascar missionaries-turned-aid-givers with local forms of Lutheran Christianity seen as compati-ble with aid work. By distancing themselves from the structural racism and cultural imperialism associated with colonial missions, they also re-spond to criticisms of US Lutheran foreign involvement that emerged in their own home church, the American Lutheran Church (after 1988, the

Evangelical Lutheran Church in America or ELCA), which became recognized nationally and by other Christians as a liberal Protestant denomination in the second half of the twentieth century (Erling 2003).
Amid widespread critique of foreign mission work across African states
in the 1970s, including Madagascar, the ALC–ELCA decreased funding for US missionaries in Madagascar and increased support for a range
of activities, including humanitarian work, which began to be referred
to as part of the church's "global mission." This term worked to dissociate mission work from US imperialism and highlighted the underlying idea that every Lutheran church pursued mission work, rather than
only North American and Western European churches (Robert 1997).
A main ELCA statement, for example, observes rather expansively,
"Churches in the North are being called to be accountable for the legacy of the modern missionary movement which lived within, benefited
from, and was influenced by its historical context(s) of colonial expansion, slave trade, the Enlightenment, and legalistic elements of Pietism"
(Division for Global Mission 1999, 14). The same statement goes on
to note, "An important step on the way to mutual ground in relationships in mission is healing the pain and injuries of the imperialist and
colonialist past" (18). Long-term missionaries' gradual expulsion from
the church ritually attempted to cleanse or heal the institution of these
moral problems. With the end of the missionary movement, faith-based
NGOs have become the global actors that missionaries once were in
the ELCA (Bornstein 2005; Wuthnow 2009). It is interesting that, while
long-term missionaries became symbols of this morally suspect "past"
approach to global engagement in the home church, they have also been
at the forefront of instituting these NGO-based religious alliances, as
in the Minnesota-Madagascar aid program, using their extensive foreign
contacts.

New Biblical Models and Accountability for the Colonial Past

Since the 1980s, the ALC–ELCA and other Lutheran churches in the
United States and abroad have embraced a biblical model of global faith
known as accompaniment from Luke 24:13–35. Accompanying instructs
the ethical ideal of separate national churches supporting each other
from afar. The contemporary prominence of the accompanying model
can be understood as a response to the legacy of colonialism, since it

posits national sovereignty and respectful cultural exchange as key spiritual and humanitarian values. Aid arrangements theoretically espouse these values because they are thought to be politically neutral and to not directly interfere in Christians' operation of their church institutions. Though not everyone directly quoted Luke 24, leaders of both Minneapolis NGOs frequently spoke of their work as that of "accompanying," "walking with," and "assisting" church leaders overseas. Accompanying is an example of what the anthropologist Charles Piot (2010, 75) calls a "horizontal, networked form of sociality," which has become increasingly common across contemporary Christian communities. Melissa Caldwell (2017, 75–76), for example, observes that, among faith-based aid workers in Moscow, accompaniment language is widely used to express solidarity with aid recipients and evoke a relationship based on shared humanity.

For the Lutherans I know, the biblical story of Luke 24, upon which the accompanying model is based, instructs specific values of sociality that inform the Minnesota-Madagascar aid alliance. In this passage, Jesus secretly joins the disciple Cleopas and a friend as they walk on the road to Emmaus. Jesus disguises himself as someone else, a stranger, thus remaining in certain respects unseen but still present to his companions. When they arrive at an Emmaus home, Jesus finally reveals himself to his companions when they break bread together but disappears from sight immediately thereafter. The Matthew 28 commission to preach the Gospel "to the nations" is a biblical text that underpinned the foreign mission movement and has been characterized by some as justifying imperialism. In contrast to this, Luke 24:13–35 was often interpreted by liberal Lutherans in my experience as calling into question Americans' global mobility. For agency leaders like Gene, for example, it reinforced the idea that Americans should send humanitarian aid and invisibly accompany fellow Christians from afar but not travel overseas for long-term work. US Lutherans running the aid organizations wished to be visible as moral actors, serving the needs of foreign Lutherans as in the passage's pivotal act of commensality (breaking bread). They also aimed, however, to be unobtrusively present to their partners as Jesus was on the road to Emmaus.

The model of accompanying from Luke 24 has been adopted not only by US Lutherans but by some Malagasy and Tanzanian Lutherans with whom US churches now have aid relationships.[22] In 2005 I attended an address at the ELCA's primary seminary in St. Paul by visiting Tanzanian Lutheran theologian Richard Lubawa, himself a proponent of a Tanzanian-Minnesotan companion service program called *Bega kwa Bega* (Shoulder to Shoulder in Swahili). In his spoken address, as well as the written version from which I cite here, Lubawa used widely touted statistics to illustrate that the "actual nerve centers" of the Christian world are shifting from north to south because of the rapid spread of charismatic and nondenominational forms of Christianity during the past thirty years in parts of Africa, Latin America, and Asia (see Jenkins 2002). He went on to proclaim, "Christian mission must be one of service (not epitomized by structures or attitudes of dominance)." Lubawa drew directly from Luke 24:13–35 to characterize Christian life as a walk or "long journey, just like the disciples of Jesus on their way to Emmaus." He further explained, "This is a journey that involves the reordering of memories so that the past can no longer terrorize the present; a journey that is full of questioning about the meaning of life; a journey that struggles with issues, crises, and pains of our time; a journey which gives us the opportunity to listen and reflect on the challenges of Jesus who walks with us answering our questions and leading us unto the right direction in the future." Lubawa's interpretation of the bodily journey of Luke 24 politicizes "accompanying" and makes the individual Christian path to salvation a walk that exists deeply in the problems and inequalities of the world. Like the ELCA statements cited earlier, Lubawa reasons that current Lutheran Christian aid relationships bear the injuries and "pains" of the past, from which they must break. Yet, rather than a total rupture, Lubawa's language implies that turning to the future also requires a kind of sorting of the past in the present, or a "reordering of memories" as he puts it. As I explore later in the book, accompanying provides an ethical framework for an egalitarian relationship between global churches yet, in the context of the Lutheran medical relief endeavor, paradoxically tends to obscure recognition of the historical and market-based hierarchies through which aid flows.[23] Accompanying nurtures a view of solidarity and partnership that, among US aid providers, often lays aside the historical inequalities upon which the aid program is built. In the next section, I examine how US aid workers reorient past and present through identifying partnership as non-"colonial," further aligning themselves with the perspective of Lubawa and other influential contemporary Lutheran norms of global companionship.

Language as Ethical Practice: Demarcating Partnership as Noncolonial

Although both Minneapolis organizations stressed the equality of their partnership with overseas Lutheran churches, building on the biblical model of accompanying, they did so in different ways. Gene, the founder of Malagasy Partnership introduced earlier, criticized the perspective of fellow believers who referred to overseas clinics as "mission hospitals." He avoided the term *mission* in part because it implied to him that the hospitals were under the authority of the US church. Malagasy nationals ran SALFA institutions, he said, and must be recognized as the authorities of their health care system. Gene worked to form direct relationships with Malagasy Lutherans, without relying upon US Lutheran intermediaries. Malagasy Partnership, he pointed out, was "one link in a chain" of God's construction. It built upon the easy access Americans had to medical surplus and attempted to redistribute some of these goods for the benefit of Christians elsewhere. In addition to his full-time job in information technology at a large Minneapolis hospital, Gene personally conducted all the organization's email communication with SALFA liaisons and medical suppliers in the United States. Malagasy Partnership volunteers were able to form relationships with individual SALFA employees (described in chapter 5) through Gene's personal familiarity with them, with the SALFA clinics, and with the Malagasy language.

IHM likewise constructed its role as that of a "helping" assistant to health care programs of Lutheran churches in other countries. The chair of the IHM board of directors in 2005–6, Janet, a former medical missionary to Madagascar and child of missionaries, expressed her desire to not be a "*vazaha*" (foreigner/stranger/white person in Malagasy) who remained in Madagascar, indirectly signaling a sensitivity to Malagasy perspectives.[24] Rather, she wanted to ensure that Malagasy nationals controlled Lutheran institutions, and she repeatedly described IHM's work as "supportive." In a recorded conversation, I once used the phrase "take over" to refer to Malagasy nationals taking charge of Lutheran health care institutions. My sentence came out, however, sounding ambiguously as though IHM was "taking over" Malagasy health care programs. Janet caught this and quickly corrected in her turn of talk: "not take over," she emphasized gently before I clarified, "but support." In addition, I asked Janet whether she had designed preventive health care programs through IHM, a cause for which she said she felt a responsibil-

ity. In her turn, Janet responded, "I haven't designed preventive health
care programs through IHM, but have been supportive of those efforts
financially through IHM." IHM should be a "faithful partner," she said,
appearing acutely aware of the role of language itself in publicly verifying the moral tenets of partnership. Linguistic distinctions become a
contested space in the formation of a new identity; culturally patterned
forgettings of the sort I have described require, according to Connerton
(2008, 64), both "the emergence of a new type of vocabulary . . . [and] . . .
the disappearance of a now obsolete vocabulary."

When considered together, the two US discourses that I have described—that of colonial missionaries and that of partnership—create a
split between the (less moral) early colonial past and the (more moral)
humanitarian present, building on humanitarianism's widespread cultural appeal and even "moral untouchability" (Fassin 2010). Among
American NGO leaders, being a Christian humanitarian partly happens through demonstrating one's allegiance to these humanitarian values in everyday language and signaling a sensitivity to issues of power
and equality, in contrast with early colonial missionary work.[25] Scholarship on humanitarianism implies, though, that the current aid program
may have inherited a more diffusely influential set of understandings
from these earlier approaches, even laying aside the direct genealogy between the current aid program and colonial mission work. Nineteenth-
century Christian charity, abolitionist campaigns, public health, and
even "welfare provisions" for medicine under colonial rule (Bornstein
and Redfield 2010, 16) played a role in shaping notions of universal humanity, the inhumane, progress, and the ethics of care for distant or unknown strangers, now taken for granted as the basis for much contemporary humanitarian work (Haskell 1985; Laquer 1989; Barnett and Weiss
2008; Feldman and Ticktin 2010). Lutheran aid workers tend to overlook
these genealogical threads and instead align substantial components of
their current work with the post–World War II secular humanitarian
model; a primary reason is that early colonial medicine did not respect
state sovereignty and national authority and, as I have suggested, bears
a substantial moral burden from which Lutherans now wish to distance
themselves.

These twentieth-century cultural transformations and genealogies of
humanitarian care result in several contradictory orientations for Lutheran aid workers. Post–World War II aid organizations increasingly
identified secularism as a precondition for professionalism, separating

aid work from its religious and charitable origins and building a bureau-cratic infrastructure, ideally to increase credibility. In what Redfield (2010, 60) calls the "humanitarian orthodoxy" of the International Committee of the Red Cross, aid work rested on a foundation of secular, Enlightenment values, particularly impartiality in aid dissemination, political neutrality, respect for state sovereignty, and the establishment of a theoretical "state of exception" in which humanitarian actors worked separately from state governments and from wartime conflicts. Today, Lutherans observe neutrality and state sovereignty in their aid work, following certain qualities of the post–World War II model of the Red Cross. Simultaneously, though, they retain a commitment to religiously-based aid. Although Lutheran clinics in Madagascar treat patients regardless of their religious affiliation, they do attach evangelical messages to aid dissemination, as Malagasy Lutheran physicians sometimes witness to clinic patients (see chapter 5).

Moreover, though Lutherans hinge their contemporary global alliances on a respect for state sovereignty, scholars have documented how international humanitarian activity, ranging from relief aid dissemination to trauma rehabilitation programs, often weakens the centralized state (Terry 2002; James 2010). Some argue that humanitarian operations introduce a new form of governance or "mobile sovereignty" that has neocolonial dimensions (Ghosh 1994; Pandolfi 2010). Even neutrality itself has been analyzed as a principle that, as a result of the numerous, ongoing decisions aid agencies must make, is never fully achieved on the ground and, in fact, often furthers specific political agendas (Redfield 2010, 53). Among former Madagascar missionaries and fellow aid workers, neutrality or noninterference is an important moral stance because of what is culturally perceived as the imperialism of early- to mid-colonial evangelical missions. Moreover, the comments of Gene, Rose, Curt, and Janet intimate that each current initiative bears the moral risk of turning "colonial" if it embraces practices that threaten Malagasy sovereignty and cultural authority. They imply that it is necessary to police current programs for their hidden colonial quality. This points again to the US colonial discourse as an absent presence in contemporary aid, a moral specter, and suggests its social purpose far exceeds its historical references. I now turn to how Malagasy Lutherans at SALFA headquarters in Antananarivo ascertain the aid program's continuities with the colonial past.

SALFA and the Colonial Legacy

During my ethnographic research in Antananarivo, Malagasy Lutherans described SALFA as part of the nationalism or *malgachisation* of
church and state institutions in Madagascar in the 1970s. Yet, in contrast to US efforts to break with the early colonial past, they also openly
pointed out colonial continuities they perceived in SALFA's operation.
The SALFA financial director is Clement, a dryly witty Merina Malagasy man in his fifties. I talked with Clement about SALFA in his Andohalo office on several occasions. When I asked him in 2014 about how
SALFA has changed since he began work there in 1987, he interestingly
cast SALFA into a much broader political and national history, intertwining the story of SALFA with the history of the postindependence
state. He wanted me to know that SALFA's work was often crippled by
the fact that, in his mind, Malagasy people were focused 70 percent on
their own "personal social crisis," emerging from and intersecting with
recurrent national political crisis in Madagascar. By personal social crisis, he meant Malagasy concerns over *"securité,"* such as finding employment; having adequate money, food, and medicine; and avoiding increasing crime and violence in Antananarivo and elsewhere (which was on
the rise after Madagascar's 2009 coup). He attributed these crises not
merely to globalization, but to the aftereffects of sixty years of French
colonization.

SALFA, he said matter-of-factly, is a continuation of the medical missionary system. The dismantling of the Norwegian and US missionary establishment led to a greater concentration of authority among Malagasy
leaders. According to Clement, between 1979 and 2000, SALFA was
nonetheless a hybrid outgrowth of both the medical missionary system
and national Malagasy leadership. It is only since 2000, he emphasized,
that SALFA has been a fully Malagasy organization. To him, SALFA
has been in transition since 2000, trying to find its footing financially,
administratively, and philosophically. It was not only the ALC–ELCA
that delayed this transition. Clement pointed out that it was repeatedly
stalled by FLM leaders, who were ill prepared to lose US funding, a
topic I return to in chapter 4.[26] In short, Clement implied that SALFA
should not be viewed as a long-established organization, but as one that
is still emerging from a complex colonial and missionary history.

Other SALFA employees painted a complex portrait of SALFA's

autonomy, as well, suggesting current continuities with foreigners' colonial involvement in Madagascar. Mr. Albert Rajoanary, a former SALFA director appearing to be in his mid-late fifties who now runs a large medical aid agency called Salama (Malagasy, well), may have felt more at liberty to be critical of SALFA's foreign connections than current employees. During a 2014 conversation in his Andohalo office, he told me that, in the last few years, IHM in Minneapolis had sent sea containers of medical supplies for the Manambaro and Ejeda Hospitals in southern Madagascar directly to Tolagnaro–Ft. Dauphin in the southeast, a port that can now accept shipping containers. This move sidestepped the SALFA offices in the capital city. In these cases, Mr. Rajoanary was under the impression that the sea containers were the result of arrangements made between clinicians in those southern medical centers and US aid workers, something that weakened SALFA's centralized authority. Albert also felt that, when he was the head of SALFA, IHM sometimes proposed specific project ideas (funding the training of nurses at the Malagasy Lutheran Nursing School, for example), and had separate meetings in Antsirabe with nursing school officials. Some of the direct relationships between Malagasy Lutheran practitioners, such as the nursing school director, and Americans likewise circumvented the SALFA headquarters in Antananarivo. Bringing together these observations, Albert smiled with an amused expression and said that many foreigners involved in Madagascar (e.g., Norwegians, Danish, Americans, French) during the last century—the colonial period? I asked, and he nodded—have specific, separate things that they want to fund now. These were the politics historically, as these actors claimed different areas for evangelism and administrative control. Although separate aid endeavors can be interpreted as a way to retain focus and expertise, Mr. Rajoanary suggested that he perceived Europeans' and Americans' desire to maintain separateness, rather than collaborating on a joint venture, as an example of the ongoing influence of these historically based colonial politics.

Colonial imprints are also felt by SALFA affiliates in other areas of SALFA's operations, such as in the institutional configurations it has inherited from the mission church. The SALFA network arguably has limited authority to evaluate the programs or clinical outcomes of SALFA medical centers or impose regulations on how various medical aid resources are used. Part of its limited authority stems from the decentralized structure of the FLM under which SALFA is situated. The FLM is divided into twenty-four synods; synods are regional decision-making bodies common to Lutheran polity, which historically decentralizes authority through these semiautonomous councils. They were introduced by US Lutheran and Norwegian Lutheran foreign missionaries as part of the organization and decision-making structure of the mission church, which was then folded into the FLM when it was established as an independent body in 1950. Mr. Rajoanary strikingly said that several FLM synods now see the hospitals as a *"pompe financière"* (financial pump), with which to churn much-needed money into the church. Each synod elects the administration of the local hospitals under its jurisdiction, and so hospital administrators may espouse views at odds with the SALFA centralized system. SALFA does not have authority over those administrators, nor the synod leaders in each region. Most of the twelve hundred SALFA employees across the island (e.g., custodians, doctors, nurses, orderlies) are overseen and paid through the hospital administration, the synod leadership, or a combination, as determined by their size.

In contrast to US discourses of the colonial, the Malagasy Lutherans with whom I have spoken orient relations of past and present differently. They make less of a sharp break between the present moment and the colonial missionary past, with some, like Clement, making the colonial past a precursor to but not determinant of the present. Other people, like Mr. Rajoanary, point to unexpected traces or resurfacings of the colonial in the present-day operations of SALFA, which draw forth an ironic feeling of déjà vu. Some of these SALFA affiliates are like Mr. Rajoanary in aligning themselves with the charismatic *fifohazana* (awakening in Malagasy) movement (see chapter 4). Pentecostal and charismatic Christian movements like the *fifohazana* often require their adherents to adopt a born-again Christian identity and to theoretically disallow prior narratives of selfhood, non-Christian religious practices, and even kinship ties, thus fomenting what Joel Robbins (2003a, 226) has called a "temporal politics of discontinuity." Charismatic movements like the *fifohazana* thus create religious forms of affiliation that can supersede other ethnic, national, and kinship identity claims with which they coexist (Poewe 1994; Nielssen and Skeie 2014).

In light of this, it is notable that, at least in this case, SALFA aid workers maintain both a charismatic Christian and a Malagasy identity and retain a critical evaluation of the past (and possibly present) actions of foreign Christian actors. In other words, they do not indicate that their shared Christianness with US Christians, some of whom are charismatics, nullifies their different experiences as Malagasy Christian citizens. (Another Malagasy informant and *fifohazana* revivalist, Josette, did, however, tell me she is Christian first and Malagasy second.) The fact that Malagasy Lutherans who work at SALFA headquarters do not morally cleanse the present of the colonial means that they may retain awareness of such historical continuities as a source of cultural critique of contemporary aid arrangements. In the following final section, I move further into the SALFA operation and briefly trace the political conditions under which SALFA was founded, which reignited Malagasy Lutherans' ties to Americans and other foreigners.

SALFA's Formation and Nationalism in Madagascar

Since the 1970s, Malagasy Lutherans have established national control of church institutions yet, because of the economic collapse in Madagascar in the late 1970s, have turned to foreign actors, including US Lutherans, for support in running those institutions. Today, SALFA provides medical supplies and financial support to forty-eight Lutheran institutions of various sizes, some of which were established under colonial rule. It is primarily Merina Lutherans, however, one of Madagascar's twenty recognized ethno-regional groups, who have emerged as leaders and partners to the US NGOs and, as I describe in chapter 4, who largely compose SALFA's workforce in Antananarivo. This Merina-Anglo Protestant alliance displaces the connections US Lutherans built earlier with Tandroy, Tanosy, and Mahafaly people in southern Madagascar during the prior century and reinforces forms of Merina political and economic domination. Furthermore, although US mission institutions have since been dismantled, the aid relationship introduces new forms of regulative power through accountability measures, which I discuss further in chapter 6.

The political conditions under which SALFA formed are relevant to explore because they show how church entities carved a national position that favored international alliances and, counter to the Malagasy state's nationalization strategy, increased free-market reforms. By the mid-1970s, the government of Didier Ratsiraka had embarked on an economic nationalization plan, bringing shipping and food-export companies, banks, and other enterprises under state control, and endorsed a form of state socialism as other African states were doing at the time, such as Zambia under Kenneth Kaunda (Ferguson 2006, 118). Rapid economic nationalization was opposed by a Merina-dominated entrepreneurial and civil servant middle class that experienced volatility in their status as the value of the Malagasy franc decreased and imported goods became harder to access during the mid- to late 1970s (Gow 1997; Graeber 2007b, 29). Ratsiraka's nationalization strategy nonetheless fell apart for lack of sustainable revenue. By 1979–80, the republic had turned to the International Monetary Fund to stave off a debt crisis and borrow foreign capital for the government's development plan, which included substantial layouts for education, the military, and infrastructure (Gow 1997, 420; Graeber 2007b, 22; Horning 2008, 423).

Because of the need to make payments on these high-interest loans, though, many of these plans never came to fruition. Debt servicing became a large component of the national budget, outstripping the government's ability to provide public services. Indeed, as Gow (1997, 421) reports, while the national debt was US$300 million in 1978, only two years later it had grown to US$1.3 billion. As a result of the devalued currency, the government could not import basic commodities and, as I heard from Malagasy and Americans, foreign goods like cooking oil, gasoline, spare parts, medicines, and medical supplies vanished at the time or became the purview of a thriving black market. (Recall that Gene began Malagasy Partnership by securing parts in the United States in 1979 for an X-ray machine.) These economic conditions increased unemployment, banditry, and theft of cattle and rice, as well as overall economic insecurity for many Malagasy (Graeber 2007b, 13, 17, 176; Randrianja and Ellis 2009, 198; Cole 2010, 42). In 1978, the Council of Christian Churches of Madagascar united to voice a national critique of Ratsiraka's economic policy and, in particular, opposition to the national control of church-run schools (Raison-Jourde 1995; Keller 2005; Randrianja and Ellis 2009).

SALFA originated in this contentious context of church-state relations in Madagascar to connect Lutheran clinics with foreign patrons and external channels of medical resources, effectively establishing some degree of autonomy from the state's economic policies. Raison-Jourde (1995, 297) writes that "it has only been possible for the churches to take on this role thanks to particularly large injections of cash from abroad, especially by the Lutherans and Catholics. The churches have brought in NGOs, something completely unknown in Madagascar before the 1970s." Though SALFA emerged from a multifaceted process of redefining the relationship of church and state under Ratsiraka's administration, it became a clearinghouse for foreign aid under structural adjustment reforms because it resembled on-the-ground, national coordinating NGOs favored by foreign donors and built on long-standing Lutheran ties to Norwegians and Americans. To ensure debt repayment in Madagascar, as elsewhere in the world, the IMF kept renegotiating the terms of loans and, in 1985, imposed additional conditions, such as further austerity in government spending, currency devaluations and liberalization or opening of the market to foreign investors—known globally as the lot of "structural adjustment reforms."[27] SALFA thus originated on the cusp of a long process of market liberalization in postindependence Madagascar but was also deeply influenced by the contentious political relationship of church and state under Ratsiraka.

SALFA also built on a wave of African nationalisms sweeping the continent in the 1970s, known in Madagascar as *malgachisation*. Church institutions like the Christian Council were part of this political process of *malgachisation* that unfolded in the 1970s, sometimes in parallel with and other times in open conflict with the state. In 1971 Malagasy Christians abrogated a 1913 agreement, signed by foreign missionary societies, which had specified where in Madagascar each European and US Christian group could base its evangelical and institutional operations. This resulted in a loosening of the regional "territories" and regional identities that had long characterized individual Protestant churches in particular, such as the FLM's association with Norwegian and US involvement in the southern highlands and the southern part of the island. With the approval of the FLM's governing board, SALFA was founded in 1979 by a group of Malagasy Lutheran physicians and a few US missionary doctors who remained in the country. The man whom I call Dr. Fosse, a longtime Norwegian American physician, was SALFA's first director and used his foreign connections to establish a pipeline of supplies to SALFA clinics. Dr. Fosse was raised in southwest Madagascar by US missionary parents and went on to practice medicine from 1965 to 2004, receiving a commendation from the Malagasy Republic for his service to Malagasy medical care.[28] Malagasy Christians' focus on establishing national organizations in the mid- to late 1970s, in contrast to the regional identities of the mission churches, influenced SALFA's formation as well. It aligned Lutheran medical institutions all across the island that had previously been considered separate because of their historical ties to the Norwegian and US missionaries.

Though foreigners like Dr. Fosse were involved in SALFA's formation, SALFA and entities like the Christian Council have also served as potent symbols of the national prominence and indigenization of Christianity in Madagascar since the 1970s (Gifford 1998). The Malagasy Lutherans whom I know hold the view that SALFA formally brought together the FLM with the *fifohazana*, which dates to 1894 and had not before been recognized as part of the established church. Several of the revival's prophets, including its Betsileo founder and former *mpsikidy* (herbalist) Dada Rainisoalambo, were ritual practitioners or children of those who practiced *fanafody-gasy* (Malagasy medicine). When they converted or aligned themselves with the revival, they strikingly rejected the veneration of the ancestors, a part of Malagasy communities across the island, and instead established a holistic healing practice that placed Christian teachings in conversation with relational Malagasy illness etiologies—or practices that can externalize as much as internalize illness causation. As a cross-denominational movement, the *fifohazana* today includes more than two hundred *toby*, or camps, across the island, where revivalists combine charismatic Christian and biomedical approaches to healing. Some of the *fifohazana*'s healing camps are loosely affiliated with the FLM and receive some medical support from SALFA, including medical supplies and consultations from Malagasy Lutheran physicians. As I explore further in chapter 4, many SALFA employees feel that SALFA today embodies a special political and spiritual role that results from its close ties with the nationally significant *fifohazana* movement and, particularly, its famous twentieth-century Prophetess Nenilava ("tall mother" in Malagasy). The fact that the *fifohazana* has been viewed as a distinctly Malagasy expression of Christianity boosted their sense that SALFA, too, is a nationally significant and Malagasy-controlled Christian institution.

The Malagasy Lutheran health department or SALFA is an institution that today fits the humanitarian sensibility of the US-Madagascar aid relationship that I have described. Though it is not formally an NGO, it is a fully Malagasy-run, nonstate, church-based entity that espouses the principles of Malagasy national autonomy now widely held as humanitarian values by US Lutheran aid workers as well. Rather than being an outgrowth of structural adjustment reforms, Malagasy church institutions like SALFA took shape through the slightly earlier context of an anticolonial *malgachisation* or Malagasy nationalism in the 1970s and an effort to critique and create autonomy from the economic poli-

cies of the government of Didier Ratsiraka. It is interesting that this specific kind of religious nationalism, often led by Merina and Betsileo Malagasy elites, fostered both a distancing from the structures, authority,
and expressions of Lutheranism associated with foreign missionaries
and a building of strategic alliances with those foreign actors to maintain church institutions. This tension arguably lies at the heart of the
aid alliance. It raises a series of moral and ethical questions of authority
and autonomy, which I continue to explore in subsequent chapters: Does
the aid relationship destabilize Malagasy authority through reintroduc-
ing foreigners' participation in the operation of Malagasy church institutions? What elements of the aid partnership recall structures of the missionary past and which do not, and from whose perspective?

Conclusions

Scholars have observed that humanitarian sensibilities are bound to dynamic, changing social conventions that establish what it means to lead
a moral life, what constitutes morally reprehensible behavior, and what
interventions are considered socially appropriate for helping strangers
(Haskell 1985). My research shows how the moral code of contemporary ELCA Lutherans—and, specifically, what activities, dispositions,
and values appropriately manifest this moral personhood—is tied to the
effects of colonialism. Since the 1970s and 1980s, many liberal Protestant churches in the United States and Western Europe have adopted a
model of global Christianity that emphasizes nationally led evangelism,
extols the virtues of cultural exchange between Christians in different
world regions, and champions aid programs because they ostensibly
maintain the sovereignty of each national church. Former missionaries to Madagascar and their families have largely followed suit, embracing this humanitarian ethic and establishing two medical relief NGOs
upon their arrival home in the United States. Malagasy Lutherans likewise nationalized the FLM's medical institutions in the 1970s and 1980s
and now operate an umbrella organization in Antananarivo to coordinate foreign aid.

Yet I would suggest that religiously-based aid is more than a new approach to Christian relations between US Lutherans and Malagasy Lutherans that replaces or breaks from what came before. Lutheran aid
work is a form of historicization in that it entails a politics of rework-

ing the past.[29] As Lutheran Christians in both regions align their work with a humanitarian sensibility, the aid endeavor itself enables the reorientation of past and present. Some Americans narrate a break with the colonial past, a temporal and moral process of moving away from and "forgetting" certain kinds of early colonial interactions in Madagascar. This discourse nurtures the political ideology that humanitarian work is a more egalitarian and neutral activity, respectful of Malagasy sovereignty, than the colonial missions that came before. It features a variety of forgettings that I have sought to draw into the chapter. On the other hand, I have shown that SALFA employees in Antananarivo espouse diverging relations of past and present through which they may retain a critical lens on the colonial history of contemporary aid arrangements. As I will show in subsequent chapters, Lutheran aid work is a moral practice focused on the ongoing, unresolved work of reorienting relations of past and present, which resurfaces in many different forms. This effort to convert the past through the present constitutes part of the moral foundation of this religiously-based aid partnership.

Humanitarianism thus encompasses a fuller range of everyday history-making activities among humanitarian actors than is sometimes recognized. These practices may seem detached from the humanitarian endeavor, but they establish the moral ground through which it grows and thrives. For former missionaries to Madagascar, being moral actors in the current model of global Christianity means actively creating social distance from morally corrupt French *colons* and "colonial missionaries," while showing their facility and fluency with certain humanitarian values (respecting Malagasy sovereignty and authority, assisting Malagasy institutions, and establishing cultural competency). In the process, former missionaries and current aid providers recuperate late-colonial initiatives as compatible with a humanitarian sensibility but not early or midcolonial mission work. The figure of the colonial missionary constitutes part of the political power of this particular form of global Christianity, because it renders visible imperialism and ideologically places it in the past (Stoler 2006, 100). This culturally constructed contrast between colonial missionaries and what came after has the effect of depoliticizing contemporary aid efforts, even as they carry forth their own forms of regulative and political power (see chapter 6).

The role of medicine in this process is especially noteworthy. In her book *Spirits of Protestantism*, anthropologist Pamela Klassen (2011, xxii) observes that the Canadian liberal Protestants with whom she conducted research have come to recognize "medicine as a tool of conquest" in early-twentieth-century foreign mission work. Today they embrace the exploration of non-Western healing modalities as one step toward healing the "pathologies of colonial domination" (xxii). Although some of my informants certainly espouse such views, they have not on the whole come to critique biomedical modernity, nor necessarily Protestants' global role in medicalization, as Klassen's have done. Rather, biospiritual imaginaries have taken on a heightened role as a source and medium of connection between Christians in the United States and Madagascar. US aid workers build upon the moral appeal and universalizing dimensions of medical humanitarianism, conceptualizing it as a compassionate and humane act rather than an overtly politicized one (Redfield 2010, 59). In the next chapter, I expand on these themes and explore how cultural imaginaries of the medical body serve a central religious role in the aid program–fulfilling the tenets of accompanying–yet provoke unexpected ideological tensions among Lutheran aid workers in Minneapolis–St. Paul.

CHAPTER TWO

Becoming Humanitarians

Bodies Multiple in Communities of Aid

The two Minneapolis medical aid organizations, which I call Malagasy Partnership and IHM, constitute important spaces of social
and historical transformation between national churches. Both agencies
facilitate shifting cultural orientations among US Lutheran laypeople
toward the moral subjectivities of humanitarianism by fostering forms
of participation in the Minnesota-Madagascar aid endeavor. Within the
Minnesotan organizations, volunteers often assemble these moral positions and selective views of global Christian relations through the actual
materials of medical aid work, which extensively feature the body as a
"source and object of cultural meaning" (Lester 2005, 46). Thus, US volunteers' own bodily participation in aid activities is, I argue, a significant
"conversionary site" in the Lutheran medical aid alliance. Volunteers'
bodily involvement is a space of contested meanings and values because
of the agencies' position as a crossroads between, among other cultural
forces, market-driven biomedicine and Christian practices of charitable
assistance. Through their aid work and other faith-based medical activities, US laypeople, on whom I focus in this chapter, navigate these and
other ideological disjunctures specific to the medical relief project.

Scholars themselves have debated the complex relationship between
care-giving endeavors, like the Lutheran aid alliance, and the unequal
market conditions that necessitate humanitarian aid. In *Markets of Sorrow, Labors of Faith*, Vincanne Adams (2013) has termed the moral basis for charitable action an "affect economy." Faith-based aid workers'
felt need to help with post-Katrina reconstruction work in New Orleans
is, in Adams's words, "both the residue and the product of failed mar-

ket arrangements" (124–25). Andrea Muehlebach (2012) has similarly argued that, among Italian volunteers in Milan, volunteerism is a moral corollary to the market. Charitable work is often understood by Italian volunteers to be motivated "not by self-interest but by fellow feeling, not by a rational entrepreneurial subject but by a compassionate one" (6). Muehlebach, Adams, and other writers suggest that these affective motivations underpinning charitable and humanitarian work—being caring and compassionate, relational and giving—are partly made by and advance a neoliberal market that is ostensibly defined as their opposite (Bornstein 2005; Ticktin 2011; Caldwell 2017). Put another way, although being compassionate is not only a product of market liberalization, unremunerated volunteer work—and the cultural elaboration of the moral spaces and subjectivities of volunteerism—ambivalently rectifies *and* enables a variety of unequal market activities.

In a comparable fashion, the Lutheran medical aid alliance stems from and attempts to remedy global inequalities in access to medical resources. As I described in the previous chapter (and discuss further in chapter 3), both organizations—Malagasy Partnership and IHM—redistribute US medical surplus to foreign Lutheran clinics, including those in Madagascar, Tanzania, and Cameroon. Through their activities, the Minnesotan agencies often promote overarching messages of biomedical progress and biomedical efficacy—or the notion that greater access to medical technologies will improve institutional functioning and patient health in foreign clinics. Thus, even as the aid program recognizes the inequities of globalized medicine, this organizational mission also reinforces the value of a market-based approach to institutionalized medicine in which medical effectiveness is linked to a built-up medical infrastructure of technologies and equipment deemed current. US volunteers in both organizations often find forms of religious experience in the salvific qualities of biomedicine and in the medical materials that they handle, as I will discuss. Yet through my own eighteen months as a laborer in both Minnesotan agencies, I also gained awareness of how US volunteers' struggles with the cost and effectiveness of medical care within their own families highlighted disjunctures between the biomedical success narratives of Lutheran aid and the therapeutic, caretaking role of Christian communities. Thus, I focus in this chapter on two seemingly opposed yet mutually reinforcing moments in US volunteers' process of becoming Christian humanitarians: Through their own bodily participation in aid work, volunteers invest in the globalized, biomedical imaginaries of the aid relationship. Simultaneously, I show how they paradoxically use those imaginaries and their involvement in the Lutheran aid endeavor to develop more holistic approaches to Christian caretaking within their own communities that destabilize the preeminence of biomedicine.

Lutheran therapeutic alliances have heightened the cultural significance of the body and medical materials as *things that mediate* or link and shape global relations among Christians. Thus, imaginative attention has been cast locally on these materials, as they have become significant components of the religious practice of aid. I suggest the embodied and material activities of Lutheran medicine loosely shape what I call *biospiritual imaginaries*—influential affective and moral depictions of Christian medicine's global reach and technological prowess (DelVecchio Good 2001, 397; Wendland 2012b, 112). For US Lutherans in particular, biospiritual imaginaries, though differently interpreted by variously positioned actors, collectively make medical work a spiritually meaningful activity, linking Christians in distinct world regions. They do so primarily through religiously evocative part-to-whole imagery, whether of medical instruments to the medicalized body or the individual body to the global church body. For US Lutherans, part-to-whole relations tend to aid's manifold disjoints and gaps, from uncertainties over the eventual use of the medical materials to the market processes to which they contribute. To be clear, these disjoints do not disappear but, through religiously evocative part-to-whole imagery, their presence is often recoded as a sign of the complexity and vastness of divine action. Through aid's mediating materials, agency discourses and long-standing practices of Lutheran foreign engagement, US volunteers thus make imaginative connections to a broader, transnational therapeutic community with seen and unseen dimensions.

As I will show, biospiritual imaginaries draw strength from a broader set of Christian therapeutic activities in Minneapolis–St. Paul that instruct the global significance of faith-based medicine. In keeping with the selective, historically organized regional ties of global Christianity that I described in the previous chapter, conservative US Lutherans have begun looking to rapidly growing, transdenominational Malagasy Christian movements such as the *fifohazana* as a source of knowledge on Lutheran approaches to healing and medicine. The *fifohazana* today features a well-established network of two hundred healing camps (Malagasy, *toby*) across Madagascar that combine biomedical and charismatic Christian healing modalities, including drug therapy, prayer healing, and exorcism. A small number of Malagasy *fifohazana* revivalists, trained as lay preachers or shepherds (Malagasy, *mpiandry*), have migrated to the Twin Cities since the 1990s. During my fieldwork, one Malagasy Lutheran pastor-émigré and physician led healing services patterned on the *fifohazana* at a local Minneapolis Lutheran congregation. Supporting the biospiritual imaginaries I have described, medicalized views of the body and the biotechnologies of institutionalized medicine feature prominently in the healing services, but they ultimately affirm a religious hierarchy of Godly authority over the human pursuit of healing and medicine.

By analyzing Malagasy-led healing services in Minnesota in relation to medical aid work, I aim to challenge the cultural notion of aid as a one-way circulation. The Malagasy-led healing services show how African migrations to North America have shaped how US Christians imagine the global context of and motivations for aid giving. They also enable insight into Christian medical aid as a practice grounded in and understood through transnational religious movements, particularly African Independent Churches with prominent healing theologies like the Malagasy *fifohazana*. In what follows, I first situate the medical NGOs in a broader religiously-based landscape in Minneapolis–St. Paul through which medical aid work acquires significance. By analyzing agencies' promotional materials and volunteers' labor with biotechnologies, I demonstrate how US volunteers foster a biospiritual imaginary that underpins medical aid work. As the chapter proceeds, I trace a more far-reaching set of therapeutic practices, including prayer and caretaking, which characterize Christian communities of aid but are commonly excluded from institutionalized biomedicine. I suggest the Minneapolis agencies are themselves overlooked therapeutic communities for US volunteers, who struggle to care for ill relatives, unemployed adult children, and fellow volunteers with serious medical diagnoses or those taking care of other people. To show the bidirectionality of the aid relationship, I conclude the chapter by focusing on healing services led in Minneapolis–St. Paul by Gabriel, a Malagasy *fifohazana* revivalist. Gabriel's healing services engender the view that Christian prayer healing and biomedicine are compatible, globally connecting activities while also familiarizing US laypeople with a holistic Christian approach to the treatment òf affliction.

Mapping the Religious Landscape of Lutheran Medical Relief

IHM and Malagasy Partnership began as part of the same initiative in the early 1980s of supplying medical materials to SALFA. Since that time, the agencies have diverged considerably in the scope of their aid programs. While Malagasy Partnership continued to ship four containers of medical materials to SALFA in Madagascar during my fieldwork in 2005–6, IHM had expanded its operations to send medical supplies and monetary aid to Lutheran hospitals in as many as eight countries, including Cameroon, Tanzania, and Liberia. IHM employed a full-time office staff of four in 2005–6, though volunteer labor was essential to the functioning of the organization. In combination with an eighteen-thousand-member mailing list, the organization relied upon a 150-person volunteer workforce that was predominantly elderly, retired, and economically middle class. Volunteer workers commuted and shared car rides from their homes across the neighborhoods of the Twin Cities to a sprawling northwest Minneapolis suburb, where the one-story, brick IHM warehouse sits amid a host of small manufacturing shops, auto repair businesses, and distribution companies. Approximately twenty volunteers reported for each scheduled weekly shift. Each person was assigned to one of sixteen specialized workstations devoted to electrical repair, linen inspection, laboratory equipment, and medical-supply fine sorting. Most volunteers were third-generation Americans, who self-identified as ethnically Norwegian, Swedish, Icelandic, or Danish.

At IHM in particular, the elderly Lutheran volunteers prized expressions of humility and often discussed the moral hazards and inappropriateness of self-aggrandizing behavior. I first began working at IHM because, while I was attending a reunion in western Wisconsin for my research among former Madagascar missionaries, I met Lois, an enthusiastic retired missionary to Madagascar from 1952 to 1982. Lois gently avoided my invitations to sit down for a conversation and instead enjoined me to accompany her to IHM for her weekly volunteer shift. I initially wondered whether she simply saw me as a pair of able hands to further the IHM cause, doing something more efficacious than talking about work. It became apparent to me, however, that her work communicated volumes in a more socially appropriate manner than would an

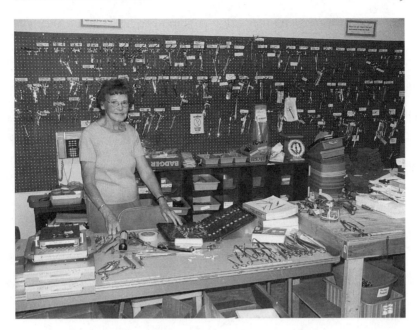

FIGURE 2.1. Iris, a Madagascar missionary from 1951 to 1975 and a trained nurse, specialized in sorting surgical scissors at IHM.

interview. When a layperson once praised Lois in my presence on her "interesting life" and told her she needed to write her life story, Lois, at that time in her late seventies or early eighties, smiled uncomfortably and half-heartedly offered that she would do so when she "couldn't move around anymore."

Malagasy Partnership, by comparison, rented a small warehouse behind a fenced-in auto scrapyard in a northern Minneapolis suburb, which was decorated inside with Malagasy *lamba*, a Madagascar map, a white board with handwritten prayer requests, and photographs of SALFA clinics and physicians. Volunteers at Malagasy Partnership were mainly two generations, or the fathers and children, of three Euro-American middle-class families attending the founder and former Madagascar missionary Gene's ELCA church in a northern Minneapolis suburb. Two Malagasy émigré families, including that of Pastor Gabriel, whom I discuss later in the chapter, volunteered for special container packing sessions, which usually occurred four times per year. Though I never had access to the amounts of specific donations, numerous Mada-

gascar missionaries and their adult children privately told me they donated money to Malagasy Partnership, as well as to IHM. On the whole,
though, regular volunteers were mainly laypeople and, with the exception of Gene, those without a connection to Madagascar or the Madagascar missionary network. Children of the three families regularly brought
their teenage friends, those considered spiritually searching, or friends
from church to the warehouse, whom they wove into the operation.

The two Minneapolis-based medical aid agencies identified as Lutheran but exhibited a variety of sectarian affiliations and fusions of
evangelicalism and Lutheranism. Malagasy Partnership was directly affiliated with the founder Gene's ELCA congregation, and IHM drew
volunteers from across several Lutheran denominations, including the
liberal ELCA, conservative Association of Free Lutheran Congregations, and charismatic Lutheran Renewal. These denominations diverge
markedly on a number of social and theological issues, including the
sanctification of same-sex marriages and inerrancy or critical interpretation of the Bible. Such divides played remarkably little role, however,
within the aid organization. In agency newsletters, wall signs, and spoken addresses at special events, I noticed that IHM leaders in particular
left ambiguous their own allegiance with specific versions of Lutheranism. This can be interpreted as a strategic move to nurture rather than
close off diverse orientations to the body, healing, and medicine among
the agency's large volunteer and donor base, as well as its paid staff and
board. IHM volunteers may also have found common ground among
themselves through being Lutheran, which historically has served as
an ethnocultural identity in the Upper Midwest (Nelson 1980; Gjerde
1985; Granquist 2007). Malagasy Partnership volunteers, who were on
the whole younger, talked more frequently of being Christian and several told me that, echoing a widespread evangelical discourse, spirituality was ultimately "a God thing" (and not a Lutheran thing). Young
volunteers listened to Christian rock on the warehouse radio while they
worked, some became college members of Campus Crusade for Christ,
and still others attended evangelical colleges, such as Wheaton in Illi-
nois. Identifying the various constituencies involved in the two agencies
shows how biospiritual imaginaries, even in Minneapolis–St. Paul, are
multisited social formations. That is, cultural meanings and rationales
for medical aid emerge from, and in turn influence, diverse quarters of
religious practice, personal experiences, employment, neighborhood associations, and volunteers' family relationships.

Bodies Multiple: Dis-membering and
Re-membering the Christian Body Politic

One of my first tasks as a volunteer laborer at IHM in Minneapolis was to organize and package the warehouse's eyeglasses bin. Some of the bin's sixty-two discarded eyeglasses had been carefully stored in their original cases, a variety of cushioned pouches with colorful designs, while others were haphazardly piled in dusty plastic bags. As I wiped each pair with a wet rag, I found myself thinking about the people to which these eyeglasses had once belonged. Twin Cities–area hospices, hospitals, and private individuals had donated the eyeglasses to IHM when a patient passed away or when someone no longer needed a particular prescription. That day, I worked alongside Harriet, an elderly, retired Euro-American Lutheran missionary nurse who had devoted sixteen years to IHM since retiring. Harriet was the medical professional normally staffing the sorting room, and she answered volunteers' questions about medical supplies' purpose, the majority of whom had no medical experience. At the time, I commented on the unusualness of the eyeglasses; besides not being an institutionalized medical supply, as were most of the donations we handled, they clearly carried traces of their prior owners, whether in dust, design, or even fingerprints. Harriet nodded in agreement but added that the eyeglasses were a valued clinical donation. She recalled receiving boxes like the one I was packing while she worked for thirty-six years at a Lutheran hospital in Ngaoundéré, northern Cameroon, and described fitting the glasses to Cameroonian patients using a machine that detected their prescription strength.

As we can see from my work with IHM's eyeglasses, multiple bodies are quietly evoked in the medical aid project, including the medicalized patient body, possible donor bodies, aid laborers' and their loved ones' bodies, imagined aid recipients' bodies, and even the spectral bodies of now-past foreign mission work activities. I came to understand how these "bodies multiple," to take inspiration from Annemarie Mol's (2002) study of bodily multiplicity in Dutch medical practice, created a varied and ontologically distinct tapestry of bodily images that volunteers like myself navigated through their own bodily participation in aid work. These bodies multiple could signal opposing, or at least dissonant, values and relations for the aid endeavor, as I explore further in the next section. To manage meaning, agency discourses and group prayers sometimes linguistically framed the religious meanings that volunteers might take from their aid work, showing the hierarchical relationship between language and other semiotic forms like material things that often obtains in Protestant communities (Keane 2007). Together, these interwoven semiotic materials recast aid labor as a form of bodily piety that, in an incremental and piecemeal fashion, made volunteers into participants in the global church.

Aid Labor as a Form of Bodily Piety

In both Minnesotan organizations, discourses on the body and the hands fostered among volunteers specific "somatic modes of attention" (Csordas 2002, 244). These learned bodily dispositions, common in religious communities, alerted aid workers to unseen connections between the everyday tasks of aid labor and a vast, global scale of divine action (Luhrmann 2004). For example, at Malagasy Partnership, group prayers commonly closed work sessions and dedicated the labor as a service to God. After a long work session one evening, Theo, an engineer and one of the three founders of Malagasy Partnership, thanked God in prayer for allowing him "to be a part of the body" through his work at the agency. Theo's language suggestively glossed the activity we had just undertaken that evening—sorting and packaging hundreds of biotechnological parts, from needles to tracheotomy tubes—as a form of participation in the global church body. At IHM, hand representations often were used to refer to the involvement of unseen actors in the medical aid endeavor while enabling individual laborers to map connections between their own bodies and this vast collective. For example, IHM's motto, "Helping the Hands that Heal," productively suggested that, through their labor, IHM volunteers' hands were folded into a sea of healing hands that encompassed foreign doctors' medical care and potentially also Jesus's earthly healing work. Building on this language and other sources, one IHM worker, a retired medical laboratory technician, pointedly described his aid work to me as a way to "worship with the hands."

Religiously evocative body-based symbolism fused the bodily labor of aid workers with the unseen circuits and clinical spaces of transnational aid. Hand representations, for instance, often signaled to individual volunteers that they could be subjects and objects of divine action in the world, as is common in US Christian imagery (Morgan 1998, 164; Chi-

dester 2005, 52). Fostering possible associations between the medical instruments that volunteers handled and their own bodies, the IHM website
proclaimed, "We are an instrument through which your love and compassion are channeled for both the health and hope of God's children in
the world!" An IHM flyer that instructed how to make "hospice kits" for
advanced AIDS patients suggested individuals' donations to the project
extended their "reach" into the lives of others: "Our prayers and generosity can reach far into the lives of those who have been affected [by HIV-
AIDS]." The hands thus indexed human abilities to overcome divides of
time and space—or imaginatively transcend human bodily limits—when
individuals aligned themselves with God's will. Since the Minnesota
agencies exist at the crossroads of medical commodity chains and geographically separate Christian communities, many aspects of the medical
aid endeavor were physically inaccessible or obscured from view for most
volunteers. By symbolically mapping links between laborers' bodies and
these seemingly inchoate processes, hand representations concretized
and contained the unseen clinical worlds, medical procedures, and market processes to which the aid laborers contributed but that they sometimes had trouble envisioning or imagining. This embodied imagery built
upon widespread cultural references in modern Western philosophy and
history, in which hands often have symbolized far-reaching market processes and divine providence, perhaps most famously in Adam Smith's
"invisible hand" of the market in *The Wealth of Nations* (1776).

Collectively, through the biospiritual imagery I have described, aid
labor was understood in both agencies to be a form of bodily participation in the global church. Through prayer language, conversational remarks, and agency discourses, linguistic framings worked to order the
various bodily images that emerged from aid work and propose possible religious interpretations for them. Thus, even though the materials
of aid labor emphasized the value of biomedicine, they also nurtured the
sense among volunteers that aid work was itself a space of religious play,
where what was visible at any given time could reference a vaster, unseen scale of God's work. Indeed, the unusual materials of medical aid
labor—sutures, bandages, surgical lights, respiratory tubing, and much
more—fueled a biospiritual imaginary among volunteers that, because
of their heterogeneous and fragmentary qualities, emphasized the par-
tialness of vision and an awareness of unseen wholes. Part-to-whole relations of this sort in turn amplified the mediating or linking role of medi-

cal materials. These biotechnologies and the abundant body symbolism that surrounded them fostered creative leaps of interpretation for volunteer laborers between the seen and unseen, medical objects and spiritual processes, and parts and wholes.

The cultural mechanisms and material conditions of affective participation in the Lutheran medical relief program are thus significantly different from other kinds of medical humanitarianism. Other scholarship on medical humanitarianism has found that such interventions extensively feature and elicit the bodily illnesses and bodily suffering of those individuals that are the target of humanitarian aid, often through restrictive images and narratives (James 2010; Nguyen 2010; Ticktin 2011). In her work on asylum seekers aiming to obtain papers in France through the government's humanitarian illness clause, Miriam Ticktin (2011, 90), for example, shows how state doctors and nurses judged asylum seekers' moral legitimacy through a state bureaucratic process that "institutes and protects what is considered an apolitical suffering body." As Ticktin (2011, 13) puts it, biological claims that explicate bodily suffering are central to medical humanitarian "regimes of care" as they engender compassion and make people appear worthy of aid, combining "affective and biological registers." Although the Lutheran medical relief program similarly elicits compassion among its US supporters through Malagasy doctors' circulated clinical narratives and occasional references to patients' bodily suffering, as I will address, the Minnesotan agencies strikingly used volunteers' own bodies to register the religious and humanitarian significance of the aid endeavor. This reverse focus on aid workers' bodies often had the effect of rendering invisible individual foreign clinic patients as recipients of medical relief, as I will discuss. But it produced a powerful affective investment for individual workers, as each act of labor could be understood as a process of self-incorporation into the global communion and a bodily affirmation of Christian commitment.

Moreover, seemingly secular and static medical tools, from catheters to X-ray machines, were continually positioned in the Lutheran aid endeavor as dynamic, mobile, and intersubjective forms that nurtured relationships with God, foreign physicians, and, more rarely, foreign clinic patients (see chapter 3). This recalls what Erica Bornstein (2005, 72) has described among World Vision child sponsor relationships, wherein seemingly "impersonal" monetary remittances between North American child sponsors and Zimbabwean youth are transformed through the organizations' evangelical discourses into "embodied human relationships with alive, unpredictable spontaneous others." Yet in contrast to Bornstein's (2005) work, Lutheran biospiritual imaginaries featured the material culture of institutionalized biomedicine and in doing so complexly implicated aid givers as subjects of care as well. Labor activities in the Minnesotan agencies, which valorized the technological sophistication and specialized knowledge of biomedicine, could also elicit volunteers' stories of their own and their loved ones' experiences as medical patients, as I discuss later in the chapter. Thus, Lutheran aid labor is an intersubjective, embodied process that resembles what Liisa Malkki (2015, 124) has referred to, exploring the significance of knit aid bunnies among elderly Finnish aid givers, as the "enchantment in imagining distance and proximity, anonymity and intimacy." The bodily experiences of Lutheran aid blur yet do not erase the self–other divide common to transnational aid provision.

In sum, the Minnesotan volunteers with whom I worked were taught to see their own bodies as instruments of divine agency and glimpse the Christian body politic through medical aid's fragmentary body parts and biotechnologies. These interpretations seemed to overshadow what I also heard, as someone less well versed in Christian discourse, as the imperialistic undertones of IHM's US-derived portrait of transgressing borders and extending "hands" into foreign spaces. Indeed, the hands have long been both a cultural icon of beneficence (though sometimes also of beneficence's paternalism), as in "lending a hand," and of interference and aggression, as in "forcing someone's hand."[1] Although these imperialist qualities never received comment, some clues to why lie in the embodied understandings I have described. US volunteers often portrayed God as the entity entering foreign spaces in "outreach." Volunteers participated vicariously in these scales of aid through their embodied labor but, concurrently, confirmed God's role as the ultimate border-crosser of the aid program. We could revisit this as not only a religious understanding but also a political claim that runs through Lutheran aid (see chapter 6): it reciprocally fashions Americans as culturally and politically neutral, building on humanitarian aid's claims to neutrality more broadly (Redfield 2010). That is, by heightening God's intervention and involvement in humanitarian relief work, US aid workers indirectly shape themselves as ethical, postcolonial actors who, in contrast to colonial missionary predecessors, do not interfere in Malagasy church affairs (see chapter 1). Yet they often avoided scrutiniz-

ing the power dynamics activated in the unequal American ability to
"reach" into foreign spaces.

Hidden and Spectral Bodies of Christian Global Relations

At IHM, although official discourses made visible to lay volunteers certain bodies and embodied activities, they left less visible foreign clinic
patients as aid recipients in Madagascar, Tanzania, Cameroon, and elsewhere where IHM sent aid. On the IHM warehouse walls, decorating the
various workstations, was a collection of seven framed signs. Each sign
began with the same tagline, FROM THIS PLACE, in large capital letters
atop a green-toned global map; it ended with a statement that described
a different organizational aim or accomplishment. Signs conveyed a variety of messages such as "We spare health care workers frustration by
checking and repairing equipment before it is sent" and "We help spread
the Gospel by equipping clinics in remote areas." These signs maintained the diverse Lutheran orientations to medical aid mentioned earlier. In addition, emphasizing the active US contribution to overseas
medical care, the signs sutured the "here" and "there" of the medical aid
program, but in doing so largely flattened the latter into one undifferenti-
ated category. In this visible framing of the agency's work, clinic patients
had a diminished or minimal role.[2] The relative invisibility of clinic patients strengthened a specific set of connections between US volunteers
and foreign Lutheran doctors, who were conceptualized as the recipients
and dispensers of medical aid (see chapter 5).

The agency's focus on the technical needs of doctors and foreign
medical institutions has gone hand-in-hand with its professionalization.
As I discuss in the next chapter, IHM adopted a variety of ethical protocols, including quality standards, to distinguish itself as a professional
aid agency in contrast to previous Lutheran and other, less recipient-
motivated Christian forms of charitable giving. Although lay volunteers
were often encouraged through these promotional materials to think of
medical doctors as the primary recipients of aid, various views nonetheless persisted among IHM supporters about exactly to whom they were
building a connection: clinic patients or medical doctors. This became
evident in correspondence between agency leaders and supporters living
outside Minneapolis–St. Paul. Many US Lutheran donors and church
groups based elsewhere in the United States contributed from afar to the
agency's popular handwork projects. IHM's four handwork projects in-

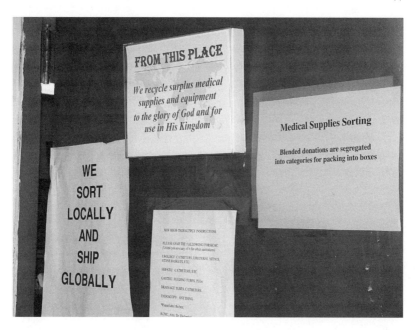

FIGURE 2.2. A "From this place" sign on the IHM sorting room door, prior to the warehouse renovation.

cluded assembling two kinds of medical care kits for mobile health care teams working outside Lutheran hospitals in Tanzania, Madagascar, and Cameroon. Bandage making, however, was arguably the most popular project, judging by the sheer number of crocheted and knit bandages— designed to provide the second layer of protection on a dressed wound— that arrived daily at the warehouse from all across the United States.[3] This project, with its religiously evocative focus on "healing wounds," called forth among IHM supporters the symbolism of bodily suffering; for some, the project fueled a sense of connection with foreign patients yet problematically tended to limit their identity to that of suffering strangers.

One Tuesday afternoon, the IHM volunteer coordinator Dagmar read an email correspondence aloud to six of us seated around the lunchroom table. A year earlier, she had met a young male Lutheran pastor at the Southwest Wisconsin Synod meeting and introduced him to the crocheted bandage project as an IHM representative. The Wisconsin pastor's email to Dagmar was noteworthy for the way that it, perhaps because of the pastor's theological training, articulated a multilayered religious discourse of bodily wounds and linked it to the bandage-making act. The pastor wrote, "The beauty of this project is that it gives you a hands-on connection with suffering people who are living half-way around the world. It also gives me a chance to pray for them while I work at making the bandages . . . [and] helping to bandage a wound; I am thankful that God has opened a way for me to connect with a wounded brother or sister." The pastor's correspondence assembled the multiple bodies often implied in agency promotional materials—the individual believer's laboring body, the medical patient's body, the global body, and the wounded body of Christ—and made them available to the reading and listening audience. Like the IHM volunteer mentioned earlier, the pastor clearly viewed his satellite work for the agency as an act of worship, rather than mere labor.

The pastor's email shows how the bandage-making act could be interpreted by IHM's vast network of US supporters, numbering as many as its eighteen-thousand-person mailing list, through a long-standing Christian discourse of bodily suffering. As a trained seminarian, the pastor sketched an individual patient body already saturated with the cultural and biblical meanings of wounds, suffering, and salvation and characterized this Christlike body as the object of medical aid. His interpretation, which received tacit approval in the IHM warehouse through Dagmar's revoicing of his words, suggested that Christian medical aid is a connective and compassionate activity in the world because it responds to human suffering. Religious historian Amanda Porterfield (2005, 4) calls Christianity a "religion of healing" because of the formative way Christian thinkers across centuries have imputed "meaning to suffering." By linking sufferers symbolically with the wounded Christ, many have suggested that redemption comes from suffering and that suffering itself is an important source of Christian "communion" (Porterfield 2005, 4). Christian humanitarian work then rests to some degree on the moral redemption gained from tending to suffering in the world.

A vast set of writings, however, have cast equal attention on the reductive and troubling imagery of bodily suffering in Christian communities, particularly in late-nineteenth- and early-mid twentieth-century US and European Christian mission work in sub-Saharan Africa. Discourses of woundedness, found in the writings of famous British medical missionary David Livingstone and many others, were particularly influential in morally justifying colonial medical work as a multilayered project of healing the perceived social and individual pathologies in African societies (Vaughan 1991, 57). In the history of Christian medicine in Africa, the wound is thus not a neutral symbol but one that evokes a particular kind of racialized body. Vaughan reports that many early-twentieth-century missionary journals featured stories of individual patients undergoing wound care in East African mission clinics (61). Through this extensive written corpus, certain narrative outlines of the "African patient" emerged and were reinforced among Christian audiences in the United States and Europe. Suffering bodies have long been the imagined object of Euro-American Lutheran evangelism and care, and contemporary bodies of Lutheran medical aid provision do not exist outside this historical and cultural context. Christian communities thus congregate around certain culturally and historically shaped imageries of the body. Even as some individuals like Gene and the IHM board member Janet openly questioned such representations, attempting to culturally unmake or discard them (see chapter 1), IHM could not control the wide range of bodily associations evoked in its work among its large, internally diverse US constituency.

The two medical aid NGOs thus negotiated the presence of these spectral bodies among their own supporters, sometimes indirectly invoking them through their religious discourses while at other times more explicitly challenging such generalized and problematic visions of aid recipients. In my experience, the two Minneapolis NGOs took different approaches to personalizing rather than generalizing the recipients of medical aid. Although Malagasy Partnership volunteers knew Malagasy Lutheran physicians and administrators by name (as I discuss in chapter 5), IHM volunteers were less likely to know foreign Lutheran doctors individually. While Gene kept Malagasy Partnership a small agency, which sent medical materials only to Madagascar, IHM has expanded since 1987 to send medical materials to up to nine world regions. A tension existed between those IHM volunteers, such as foreign missionaries, who more intimately knew the places and people to whom the agency sent aid, whether in Madagascar, Tanzania, or Cameroon, and the US congregants who composed the majority of IHM volunteers and often had no experience in the places where IHM sent medical materials. For some IHM supporters, then, African Christians were both individuals from whom to learn in Minneapolis–St. Paul, as in the case of the Malagasy healing services, and, as in the pastor's email, more distant and anonymous strangers in need, thus reproducing problematic stereotypes of Africa and Africans. Bodily symbolism and bodily discourses bring with them historically and culturally sedimented understandings of Christian global relations. This created an unforeseen problem at IHM in particular, where the body served an especially central role in lending religious significance to the work and aligning (or subdividing) a diverse group of supporters.

I have argued so far that multiple bodies, including partial and fleeting views of recipient bodies, the divine body and the global Christian body, permeated the Minneapolis warehouses, particularly the material activities of individual laborers. Yet the spectral bodies of US foreign mission work were not the only body-based representations that disrupted the dominant narratives of the aid endeavor. Other bodies, less visible and more intimate—the ailing bodies of volunteers' family members—were often the focus of volunteers' relationships with each other in the Minneapolis warehouses. I found that aid work served a therapeutic role for US volunteers themselves, many of whom struggled with their own or their family members' health problems, job losses, inadequate medical insurance, or other kinds of economic insecurity. These intimate interactions fueled parallel, diverging meanings of health and well-being that subtly cast into question the agencies' narratives of biomedical success.

Insecure Bodies in the Minneapolis Aid Organizations

Volunteers' and their loved ones' insecure bodies often became the subject of conversation in the aid warehouses, whether as a result of aging, ill health, job losses, or mounting medical bills. These bodies fell outside the agencies' official discourses on the purpose of its work and took shape in the social community that volunteers created among themselves. Thus, in the aid warehouses, a secondary narrative of care, viewing individuals as holistically immersed in webs of social relationships, took root and informally ran parallel to the agencies' expressed purpose. Here I describe how volunteers' diverse caretaking acts for each other occupied as significant a role for these workers as the agencies' ostensible medical humanitarian goals. Their acts included prayer, public recognition of volunteers' extensive support and emotional caretaking for family members and the therapeutic value of work itself.

Humanitarian Intimacies

After beginning my research in the Minneapolis organizations, I quickly became aware that many volunteers were caretaking extensively for other people, particularly ill spouses, siblings, and adult children, shadow roles they fulfilled in addition to their volunteer shifts. Harriet, the retired missionary nurse mentioned earlier, modestly described herself as a "chauffeur for [her] ninety-one-year-old sister" who had no other living relatives and lived in a local care facility. One elderly man regularly left the warehouse before the noon lunch period shared by volunteers: he once explained that he missed this communal event because his elderly wife could not be left alone at home for more than a few hours. At Malagasy Partnership, Gene expressed being squeezed between caretaking responsibilities for his elderly father and his three children. Confiding in the group one evening, Gene explained that his parents' health continued to worsen. Gene's father had fallen three times and fractured his hip. Gene asked the group for prayer for his parents and conveyed the difficulty he had meeting his family responsibilities. His youngest daughter had just graduated from college and was searching for a job, and his parents required regular visits from him in a small farming community that was a two-hour drive from Minneapolis.

Volunteers supported each other in many ways, listening, supplying food and check-ins for those who were ill, and providing what Klaits (2009, 12) calls "words of consolation." Still other volunteers brought attention to the limits and cost of biomedical care itself as a source of emotional stress. In one volunteer meeting at IHM, Leonard, a retired mail carrier, spoke up to say that he had a prayer request. Leonard's son Daniel had been diagnosed with bone cancer. In pragmatic terms, Leonard recounted that his fifty-three-year-old son had had a "rod placed in his knee and one in his arm from the shoulder to the elbow" to replace weakened bone matter. Leonard's son was participating in a four-thousand-member drug trial that introduced a new medication to fight bone cancer. "They didn't find it quick enough," Leonard said, referring to the cancer. "We'll see if the pill works, but otherwise they'll do chemotherapy. There's six of us going down on Saturday to see him." Can your wife go along? someone asked Leonard, aware of his wife's poor physical condition and her need for regular physical care and supervision. Leonard said that she would, but her presence would require them to stop regularly between Minneapolis and Des Moines, Iowa, where his son lived, extending the trip an additional half-hour. Another person asked whether Leonard's son had children. "He has three by marriage," Leonard responded, pausing. "He's in good spirits. But he had only three years to go until retirement." The weight of Leonard's report, coming from someone who rarely spoke in the context of group meetings, seemed to hang in the air.

Public recognition of individuals' hardships sometimes produced a broader reflection on the volunteers' moral bonds and support for each other. After the few moments of silence that followed Leonard's remarks, the IHM office manager Mark offered, "Well, we're family here, so we need to pray for our own families." In a March 2006 prayer circle at Malagasy Partnership, Theo similarly thanked God "for binding us together here as a family." Though this language is arguably commonplace in Christian communities, kinship terms enabled individuals to socially reflect on and shape what their relationships meant and entailed, thus constructing the aid agencies as moral communities. Aid workers' group prayers established a moral community attuned to the holistic individual, or a person embedded in webs of relationships. They focused on the treatment of a variety of afflictions, not only biomedically defined illnesses but also the emotional burdens of caring for others, and used prayer to comfort individuals and address those ailments. In the context of the NGOs, I could not help but notice that volunteers' experiences exposed gaps between the agencies' emphasis on biomedical solutions and volunteers' encounters with the limits of biomedical care, as well as uneven access to medical care in the United States and elsewhere. Although volunteers did not verbally identify these as ideological disjoints, their own caretaking practices for each other tells a slightly different story—as they interpret Christian care as a more holistic practice of healing a variety of social ills—and allows us to see the aid agencies as therapeutic spaces.

Humanitarian Insecurities and Christian Caregiving

Malagasy Partnership and IHM volunteers can be characterized as middle class, with a range of professional and blue-collar occupations represented within each collective group.[4] Among the three families mainly comprising Malagasy Partnership, the fathers who were regular volunteers each had professional occupations, including that of an engineer and an information technology supervisor. Of the nine regular volunteers at Malagasy Partnership, however, two were unemployed young adults who were living with their employed parents while searching for jobs. At IHM, nearly twenty Euro-American volunteers worked at the warehouse during each shift, with more than 150, mostly occasional, volunteers in total. Most volunteers were retired and ranged in age from sixty-five to ninety. One elderly man was a retired skilled laborer who had worked at the heating equipment company Honeywell. Several women were certified as nurses in the 1950s but had primarily stayed home to raise children and were now widowed. Male volunteers included a retired mortician, a radio technician, a dentist, and a United Postal Service driver. Some but not all were fortunate to have family houses that had accrued value during the previous twenty years in middle-class, suburban Twin Cities neighborhoods. Many lived on small pensions and Social Security checks that they stretched through careful budgeting.

Several informants, however, were deeply embedded in financial and health problems that extended across the generations, involving in some cases their parents and adult children, and they viewed these issues as

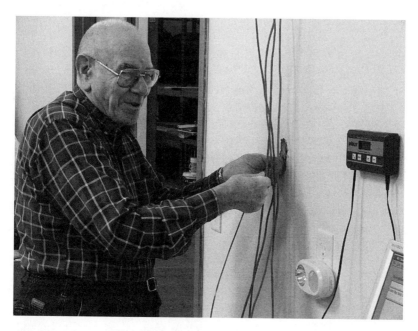

FIGURE 2.3. Bob, a retired skilled laborer for Honeywell, installing the electrical wiring for IHM's warehouse expansion.

collective responsibilities arising from the moral obligations of kinship. Some of their financial difficulties stemmed directly from the neoliberal policies that have been increasingly instituted in the United States, such as layoffs, "flexible" or temporary contract employment, reduced eligibility for health insurance, and prohibitively high-cost health insurance. Even before the 2008 recession, forms of insecurity linked to neoliberal policies were apparent and differently distributed among the volunteers of IHM and Malagasy Partnership. Since 2008, Minneapolis–St. Paul has been lauded by economists as one of the strongest US "post-recession economies" (Vomhof 2010). Yet the area's workforce was subject to years of downsizing practices similar to what has occurred elsewhere in the United States (Besteman and Gusterson 2010, 6). During the last thirty years, ostensibly middle-class US families have had to develop joint strategies to cope with a narrowing field of economic opportunity, and this places added weight on parent-child bonds as sources of financial and emotional support.

As I argue in this book, communities of aid in the United States are thoroughly entangled in economic processes. Though international aid organizations of course focus their efforts outside the United States, they can less visibly operate as places where people plumb problems in their own society, including economic inequality. This is particularly the case for the kind of humanitarianism upon which I focus. Unlike forms of charity, philanthropy, or aid work that rely on wealthy donors or benefactors, the medical aid NGOs in Minneapolis–St. Paul mainly support themselves through small private cash donations. The IHM executive director Curt told me in an August 2005 interview that 80 percent of the agency's money at the time came from individual donations of US$5 and $10. Some large aid organizations, such as World Vision, create opportunities for individual professional careers as administrators, field agents, and program coordinators (Bornstein 2005). IHM paid four employees at the time of my research but, in contrast with other, larger agencies, relied mainly on a sizeable volunteer workforce. Malagasy Partnership was run entirely on volunteer labor. The volunteers in both agencies handle institutional medical discards that have substantial economic value, which I discuss in the next chapter. Although it can definitely be argued that the volunteers accrue social capital from the moral act of "doing good" in the world (Graeber 2007a), they do not benefit financially in any immediate way from this largesse. Meanwhile, the Minneapolis volunteers were themselves sometimes disenfranchised by a US medical and insurance regime that made it difficult for them to pay health insurance premiums or support children with steep medical bills.[5]

Humanitarian action and US lay humanitarians' experiences of social insecurity thus sometimes go hand in hand, rather than being fully opposed activities. Although the possibility of doing unpaid volunteer work precludes debilitating economic precarity, volunteerism does not always equal economic stability. In popular and scholarly writing on international humanitarian aid, these perspectives have until recently been less visible because of a focus on the experiences of aid professionals like field agents and administrators or on aid as a one-way transaction (but see, e.g., Bornstein 2005; Muehlebach 2012; Adams 2013; Caldwell 2017). Looking across both sites of providing and receiving aid illuminates a broader cross-cultural phenomenon, widely documented in the anthropology of Christianity, of Christian communities as therapeutic spaces for dealing with, and attempting to rectify, the problems of neoliberalism, particularly gaps in social services like health care. Although the meanings of caregiving are culturally variable within Christian communities, it is noteworthy here—as in other examples of aid as Christian caregiving among Ugandan Catholic nuns (Scherz 2014) and Baitshepi Church members in Botswana (Klaits 2010)—that relational caretaking builds moral community among US Lutherans. In an environment of disintegrating social support, to care affirms the moral value of the Lutheran aid endeavor as an affective space of compassion and love. Though the NGOs privilege biomedical approaches to bodily care, volunteers' own activities suggest they identify a more holistic body at the center of Christian caretaking, thereby recognizing some of the limits of biomedicine. Lutheran volunteers' care for each other and for their family relations deeply inform the meanings of aid among volunteer laborers in both NGOs, grounding prevalent humanitarian terms in these lived realities.

In my experience, prayers most directly positioned aid as a globalized Christian therapeutic practice tending to a variety of social and individual "ills," including job security, health, and well-being. Acts of prayer enabled the imagination of a Christian body politic that included Malagasy Lutheran doctors and administrators, drawing on the selective, regional US Midwest Lutheran history of imagining the Christian world (see chapter 1). Inside the small office of the Malagasy Partnership building was a white "prayer board" with a list of prayer concerns hand-written in colored marker. Through the prayer board, Malagasy

Partnership volunteers' needs for support with a variety of struggles, from unemployment to ill parents, existed in a shared visual field with prayer requests for Malagasy doctors and administrators, their families, and their patients. In addition, as part of what Gene called a reciprocal "prayer covenant," the Minnesota group prayed for Malagasy physicians and SALFA employees each Thursday night, knowing they would just be awaking in Madagascar to begin a new day of work.

When I asked Gene about the prayer covenant with SALFA employees (such as the SALFA financial officer Clement; Jeannine, a SALFA office worker who handled the arrival of the sea container in Tamatave; and Dr. Remy, a physician in Antsirabe), he observed that he knew Malagasy Lutherans were praying for him, as well. "They know that my dad's been having health problems. They'll sometimes send us a message to ask if we know where Clement is . . . [Laughs] . . . because of the close communication. It's been that close and it just built." Gene's joke commented on a lived experience; that is, combined with the collapse of space-time allowed by email, the prayer covenant fostered for him an intimacy and closeness that could feel "like" physical closeness, as if he was just around the corner from Clement's office. Gene explained that, ultimately, he saw the Malagasy Partnership operation as "supporting [Clement]," who he said is the main reason that SALFA is still operating (for reasons I explore in chapter 4). These exchanges, though fleeting, speak to the growth of transnational alliances that construct Christianity as therapeutic and focused on the body, healing, and medicine (Klassen 2011).

These therapeutic qualities of Christian community have been well documented in the literature on African Christianities (see, e.g., Pfeiffer 2002; Comaroff 2009; Klaits 2010). In the final section of this chapter, I provide a portrait of holistic healing services in Minneapolis, patterned on the Malagasy Christian *fifohazana* and led by a Malagasy pastor and physician whom I call Gabriel. I examine how Gabriel instructs US Lutheran laypeople in new modes of engagement with the body while, as I found among US aid workers, widening the scope of possible afflictions and treatments beyond biomedicine. Healing services thus constitute one site among several in Minneapolis–St. Paul, including the medical aid NGOs, where US Lutherans and their Malagasy coreligionists are reimagining ties between national churches through the lived analytic of the body and a shared focus of faith-based medicine. The biospiritual imaginaries of Lutheran medical initiatives thus feature several cross-cutting influences, including the heterogeneous materials of aid work and the direct influence of African Christian revivalists on North American Christians.

Malagasy Christian Healing Services in Minneapolis–St. Paul

Minneapolis–St. Paul is a US metropolitan area that has, by some measures, experienced 628.4 percent growth in the African-born population between 1990 (3,788) and 2000 (27,592) alone (Logan and Dean 2003, cited in Takyi and Boate 2006, 56). Although these statistical portraits should be viewed cautiously as selective social constructions, this and similar widely cited depictions of the Twin Cities' changing demographics have bolstered US Lutheran evangelical views of the homecoming of the "global church." The faith-based medical activities that I have described advance the view that global Christianity is today what Akinade (2007, 98) calls a "multicentered reality, made up of interconnecting networks and communities." For some, African migrations through the 1990s and 2000s to Minneapolis–St. Paul have made the Twin Cities a global city, or a prime example of this multicultural Christian world in microcosm. That is, decentering Western Christian structures of authority, US Lutherans emphasize the important bidirectionality of the crisscrossing networks composing global Christianity: Americans can learn new approaches to Christian practice from African Christians even as African Christian hospitals rely on US medical aid.

Malagasy Lutheran migrants to Minneapolis–St. Paul have been central actors in shaping these views among US Lutherans. A small population of Merina Malagasy Lutheran revivalists who have come to the Twin Cities for educational opportunity, whether in the area's Christian seminaries or in university graduate programs, have been involved in translating *fifohazana* practices to Minnesotan Lutherans since the late 1990s. Merina refers to a Malagasy ethnic group residing primarily in highland Madagascar, historically known for high rates of Christian, particularly Protestant, religious affiliation (Bloch 1986, 39; Larson 1997; Keller 2005, 37–40). As discussed in chapter 1, although the revivalist I profile is Merina, most US Lutheran missionaries lived and worked in southern Madagascar, where they associated with people identifying with other Malagasy ethnicities, such as Tanosy, Tandroy, and Mahafaly. Rather than maintain those historical connections, faith-based therapeutic initiatives have thus crafted new bonds between Merina Malagasy Lutheran elites and US Lutherans, a topic I return to in chapter 5. I focus in this section on healing services led by one Merina Malagasy émigré who is a pastor in Minneapolis–St. Paul to closely examine how such events translate Malagasy Christian practices of bodily healing to a Euro-American audience.

Although the body holds an important role in faith-based medical activities linking Christians in diverse world regions, bodily forms of worship, such as prayer healing and trancelike ecstatic states, are also one axis in acrimonious theological and sociopolitical disputes between liberal and conservative Lutherans in Minneapolis. The healing services are an example of new alliances between charismatic revivalists like those affiliated with the *fifohazana* movement and charismatic Euro-American Lutherans (see also Okome 2007). Pastor Gabriel's healing services were, in fact, initiated by a former US Lutheran missionary to southwest Madagascar whom I call Walter. Upon returning home in the early 1970s, Walter became born again and established a now-influential charismatic Lutheran movement in Minnesota called Lutheran Renewal. Good Shepherd Lutheran, where Gabriel led services, had at that time just left the ELCA and joined the Association of Free Lutheran Congregations, a conservative Lutheran branch known to be friendly to charismatic practices. During this transition in 2006, Walter, a vocal advocate for the "success" of African charismatic revivals, particularly the *fifohazana*, hired Gabriel, a recent seminary graduate, with the hope that his work would enliven the languishing congregation.

The medical aid NGOs collectively draw volunteers from across these Lutheran denominations, and the religious meanings they understand or attribute to these body-based activities can thus vary widely. Evangelism itself is one among many subjects of debate between conservative and liberal Lutherans; ELCA Lutherans institutionally prioritize social justice work today as a manifestation of the social gospel whereas conservative Lutherans tend to continue funding short and even longer-term overseas US missionary work. In her book *Living Faithfully in an Unjust World*, Melissa Caldwell (2017, 139–47) documents vocal opposition to evangelism or missionary activity among progressive Christian volunteers in Moscow aid organizations, whom she describes as "pluralistic, and even resolutely secular" (7). I rarely if ever witnessed such opposition among Lutheran laypeople involved in the aid endeavor. To the contrary, it seemed that laypeople tacitly endorsed the possibility that aid would operate as a way of spreading the Gospel message, potentially in Malagasy clinics (see chapter 5). It was *who* was doing the evangelism that seemed to matter the most; Malagasy pastors were approved of as evangelists by both ELCA Lutherans and their conservative Lutheran brethren. Thus, even though the style of worship introduced by Gabriel fit more with conservative and charismatic US Lutheran denominations, his presence also confirmed liberal Lutheran tenets of cultural exchange as a cornerstone of equitable, postcolonial relationships between national churches.

The laypeople who attended the Malagasy-led healing services overlapped only slightly with those who were regular volunteers at IHM or Malagasy Partnership. Connections abounded, however, between the healing services and the medical aid organizations, showing their interrelationship in a cultural field of faith-based therapeutic activity spread across distinct sites in Minneapolis–St. Paul. Pastor Gabriel is a long-time friend of Gene's and an occasional volunteer at Malagasy Partnership who attended the group's annual volunteer picnic with me at Gene's house in August 2005 and participated in sea-container packing sessions at the warehouse. Walter, the Norwegian American missionary who initiated the healing services, was friends with several figures in the medical NGOs who were retired Madagascar missionaries or their children, including Gene, Lois, Janet, and the former SALFA director Dr. Fosse and his wife Rose. Through their mutual ties to SALFA, Dr. Fosse knew Pastor Gabriel personally in Madagascar prior to Gabriel's move to Minneapolis–St. Paul for seminary training, as did other missionaries. All these Euro-American missionaries and their children knew one another, at least as acquaintances.

Through this tangle of connections, both medical aid organizations continued to have strong ties to SALFA in Madagascar, even as IHM broadened its scope since the late 1980s to send medical supplies to hospitals in many other world regions. As I described previously, the agencies were formed by Madagascar missionaries and SALFA doctors who experienced shortages of medical supplies in their clinics during the Malagasy economic crisis and structural adjustment reforms of the late 1970s and early 1980s. Though the *fifohazana* dates to 1894 and was marginalized for most of the twentieth century by mission churches, the Malagasy Lutheran Church worked in the late 1970s to bring the *fifohazana* and its *toby* (Malagasy, healing camps) under the biomedical services and evangelism arms of the church. As the *fifohazana* gained national prominence in Madagascar in the 1970s as an "indigenous" Christian movement (Rich 2008; Keller 2005, 55), this institutional arrangement had the effect of making the *fifohazana* known for its collaborative approach to biomedicine, more so than comparable African Initiated Churches in South Africa according to one revivalist (Rakotojoelinandrasana 2002). Pastor Gabriel participated in these cultural transformations since he spent years practicing medicine in Malagasy Lutheran clinics prior to coming to the United States for his seminary education. Therefore, Gabriel, a Merina Malagasy pastor in his fifties, was a culturally significant figure to lead healing services in Minneapolis–St. Paul because he was perceived as someone who could speak authoritatively about both a biomedical approach to the body and the Christian healing paradigm.

Malagasy Evangelism of Americans in Minneapolis

Cultural exchanges like the Minneapolis healing services are not isolated incidents but constitute part of what some scholars call "reverse mission" as members of African Initiated Churches evangelize European and US Christians (Kwakye-Nuako 2006; Olupona and Gemignani 2007; Bongmba 2007; Rice 2009). Indeed, Gabriel told me he considered himself a missionary to the people of Minneapolis; he identified the evangelical "commission" of Matthew 28—where Jesus calls on followers to spread the Gospel message—as the most influential scripture in his life. As a self-described descendant of three generations of Lutheran Christians, Gabriel said that he grew up in a household where church involvement—in Sunday school, confirmation, and InterVarsity Christian Fellowship—always was central if not assumed. Gabriel and his fourteen siblings (ten brothers and four sisters) moved frequently in his youth to live in several highland villages with his parents. It was in their hometown of Betafo, however, that his great-grandfather, a Malagasy Lutheran pastor, first met the Norwegian Lutheran missionaries John Engh and Nils Nilsen, who had been stationed there since 1866.[6] When he first mentioned this, Gabriel said so with a smile and indicated that it was a striking, even fated, historical tie between us: Nilsen was my great-great-grandfather, a fact I had never before mentioned to Gabriel. Knowing that I was a non-Christian, Gabriel sometimes seemed amused that he was now in the position to evangelize this wayward descendant of Nilsen. He often told me, after listening to me explain my research countless times, that I should "try Jesus in [my] life as a working hypothesis."

Gabriel's US seminary education in the early 2000s built on a long and distinguished career in medicine in Madagascar. He emphasized that, even prior to his seminary training, he had never separated his faith from his ostensibly secular work. He held positions in Christian hospital settings for twelve years and participated in the Malagasy branch of the International Hospital Christian Fellowship. He also formed a clinic in the *Soixante sept* hectare of Antananarivo, an area known to be one of the city's poorest neighborhoods, where he taught employees to be "disciples of Jesus" and preach the Gospel to patients and other doctors. Gabriel had also been a trained *mpiandry* (Malagasy, shepherd or lay preacher) in the *fifohazana* since 1976. Although he tried to obtain a position in the Malagasy Lutheran Church after seminary, Gabriel admitted that personal disputes and what he haltingly called "jealousies" among the church leadership prevented him from acquiring the position he hoped for. Even in the United States, Gabriel struggled to find a permanent, full-time post and settled for part-time positions that offered

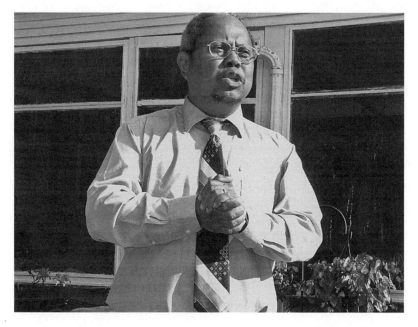

FIGURE 2.4. Pastor Gabriel leading a special outdoor service at the St. Paul house church.

no health-care benefits for his family. In the small house church he led
weekly in St. Paul, which I participated in for eighteen months, Gabriel
several times asked for prayer for these personal hardships.[7] At the same
time, he often would assure the participants by saying, "Jesus is our insurance," a statement that interestingly suggested he understood the risk
of ill health to be something partly mitigated by the work of prayer and
his faith. I spent time with Gabriel, his wife, and two of his four children
in many of the religious organizations in which they participated, as well
as in some of the clinical settings where Gabriel formerly worked as a
medical doctor in Madagascar. After years apart while he was in seminary, Gabriel's wife Inès, also a trained *mpiandry* since 1976 and an ordained minister in the Church of Jesus Christ of Madagascar, joined him
in 2004 in the Twin Cities with two of their four children.[8]

Sanctifying the Body, Uniting Biomedicine and Prayer Healing

During 2005–6, Gabriel led both healing services and an addiction
counseling and support group with a biblical basis at the suburban Minneapolis church Good Shepherd Lutheran. The church, a 1960s A-frame
construction, was situated alongside a busy divided highway lined with
fast-food restaurants and quick oil-change shops that had sprung up
since it was built. Gabriel's post at Good Shepherd drew upon his training in substance abuse counseling at Hazelden, a nationally known drug
addiction treatment center in Minnesota (in 1987), and his work for the
Malagasy Lutheran health care department on chemical dependency
in Madagascar (1982–86, 1988–94). I participated in healing services at
Good Shepherd in 2006 as a field researcher and draw upon my first-
hand experiences in this section. Gabriel's healing ministry, as he called
it, involved monthly services at the suburban church, which took a holistic approach to treating "emotional, relational, physical, and spiritual
problems" with prayer, the casting out of demons, and anointing with
oil. Though Gabriel rarely drew attention to their Malagasy origins, the
services' holistic approach stems partly from Malagasy cultural understandings that regard illness as something theoretically caused as much
by broken social relationships and by external agents, such as evil spirits
in the *fifohazana*, as by biomedically isolated pathogens understood as
internal to the body (Sharp 1993, 1999).

Gabriel's healing services at Good Shepherd were primarily attended by Euro-American laypeople.[9] The healing services nurtured

bodily dispositions that were not historically part of the traditional US Lutheran liturgy or the contemporary ELCA but are certainly common across charismatic Christian movements. Through sung worship, prayer, and sermons, Gabriel taught laypeople to see their own bodies and bodily states as vessels or conduits for the Holy Spirit. Each service opened with a period of sung worship, during which time a young man led the congregation in song on an acoustic guitar and the hymn lyrics were projected on a white screen behind the altar. The hymns drew attention to the embodiment of Jesus through the Holy Spirit, comparing in sung lyrics the Spirit to the "air that I breathe," a romantic beau fanning the "flames within my soul," a "shield about me," and "Your holy presence living in me." At strategic moments before and after the opening message, sermon, and hymns, Pastor Gabriel signaled to a group of eight trained healer-preachers whom he called "shepherds," building on the cultural role of *mpiandry* (Malagasy, shepherds) or lay preachers in the *fifohazana*. Working in pairs, the shepherds spread out in four small circles across the front of the altar where they stood ready to pray with any congregants who requested their counsel. When the service transitioned from Gabriel's sermon to the period of healing, soft classical music began playing over the loudspeaker system; people gradually moved forward from their pews individually or with others; and they prayed and talked quietly with the shepherds, often in tearful exchanges, at the front of the sanctuary for nearly twenty minutes.

Gabriel's services also established body-based approaches to prayer healing as legitimate components of Lutheran worship. In his sermons, he defined Christian healing in relation to two problems: that of biomedicine and that of what he called "magic." First, in a way that suggested he sensed Lutheran laypeople may be unfamiliar with prayer healing, Gabriel verified the legitimacy of Christian healing by contrasting it with magic and assured the congregants that the healing services were not spurious "magical meetings." Second, he urged those present to "give [their] burdens" to Jesus in prayer, but cautioned that prayer healing may not occur like a medical cure, through "one shot of prayer." Rather, it was necessary to develop a long-term "relationship with Jesus, the living and healing God" for healing to take place. When Gabriel contrasted "magical meetings" with Christian healing services, he laid claim to the rationality and modernity of healing practices as well as the ease of their reconciliation with biomedical science. Gabriel thus made Christian healing techniques and their primary agent, the Holy Spirit, fully *present* within the services in two discrete senses: as something embodied and known by the congregants and as something fully modern, reliable, and perhaps comparable to science. Even though they unfolded on different time scales, individual participants were encouraged to ideally embody these diverse approaches to healing and medicine, recognizing the healing power of God while embracing the modern advances of biomedicine.

The healing services thus established a multilayered dialogue between biomedicine and Christian prayer healing, in which prayer healing in particular could be understood through the familiar and authoritative cultural lens of biomedical techniques. In a personal testimonial during the August 2006 service, one tall Euro-American woman in her sixties explained to the Good Shepherd congregants that their prayers for her daughter's breast cancer remission had worked; as proof, she stated simply, "The scan is clear this week." In this reversal of cause and effect, the outcome (clear scan) became the action of the Holy Spirit: a "clear" vision that operated in the healing service as a sign of Christian healing power. Moreover, Gabriel routinely told the congregants that their participation in the healing services should not preclude them from taking prescribed medicines, a point also written in the program, since "Jesus might also use medicines to heal." Drawing upon his experience as a medical doctor, Gabriel recounted how he hung a sign in his office during his twelve years of practicing medicine in Madagascar that further clarified the relationship of biomedical authority and divine authority, as translated in English: "I treat, but Jesus heals."[10] Healing through Jesus was thus a higher-order activity that ultimately dictated the extent and success of biomedical treatment. Yet Gabriel simultaneously relied on biomedical imagery, especially the "shot of prayer," to impart to laypeople the rationality and mechanisms of Christian healing.

Conjuring Border Crossings through Biotechnologies

Gabriel's use of the syringe as a rhetorical device not only speaks to the authoritative cultural position of biomedicine but also links his services to the broader set of faith-based activities in Minneapolis–St. Paul oriented around the global provision of biomedical supplies. Syringes occupy a particularly significant social and historical role in global biomedical practice. Sarah Hodges (2008, 20–21) notes that syringes, and injections in particular, share a metonymic relationship with the "biomedical therapeutic encounter" between patient and practitioner. As a result of widespread immunization programs instituted in many world regions since the 1950s, Hodges points out that the syringe, as opposed to respiratory tubing or a surgical suture, "is an item with which people have personal histories" (2008, 20). Syringes, therefore, are among the most ubiquitous but also the most individually known medical supplies, something that gives them special relevance as rhetorical tools. Gabriel built on such personal associations to associate Christian healing practices with the efficacy of modern medicine.[11]

Syringes or "shots" are also objects that draw attention to what Klassen (2011, xiii) calls the "mysteries of transmission" central to bodily healing. They conjure awareness of the movement of fluid medicine across bodily boundaries, just as the Holy Spirit conceivably traverses the body's inner workings to effect healing. In addition to Gabriel's rhetorical efforts to visualize spirit agents not previously embodied in Lutheran services, this imagery of border crossing is culturally significant because of the social visibility of biomedical technologies as objects that mediate or link Lutherans in diverse world regions, thus traversing the boundaries of national church bodies as well. With Gabriel as their guide, Euro-American laypeople at Good Shepherd, some of whom have ties to the medical aid NGOs, may have been prompted to consider how US aid circulations, which do include hundreds of syringes, are received in Malagasy Lutheran clinics. Through the prevalent historical imagery of Madagascar among Minnesotan Lutherans (see chapter 1), it is possible to see that Gabriel himself operated as a border crosser traversing sovereign bodies in the healing services, while also linking past and present in complex ways. His services thus mapped and tacitly evoked a variety of bodies—individual congregants' bodies, the ailing bodies of their loved ones, Jesus's wounded body, and national church bodies— and allowed laypeople to reflect on the seen and unseen border crossings between them. In the broader US framework of cultural exchange between Lutheran national churches, described in chapter 1, Gabriel culturally authenticates some of these ties in the global church, even as he emphasized the transhistorical, biblical basis of the healing services.

The Minnesota healing services show how certain religious practices, in addition to medical aid itself, have been circulated through contemporary relationships between churches in the United States and Africa. Indeed, in the Minnesota-Madagascar aid alliance, Malagasy-introduced *fifohazana* practices form an important, reciprocal flow of cultural understandings of medicine and healing. Such exchanges, I suggest, are an equally significant component of therapeutic initiatives linking Lutherans in Madagascar and the United States, since they ignite the body as a site of Lutheran religious activity and shape biospiritual imaginaries of Malagasy Lutheran medicine. Moreover, cultural exchanges importantly create a space for the valuing and recognition of theological knowledge derived from transdenominational, charismatic, and Pentecostal African Christian movements, echoing a widespread notion among US evangelicals that the "center of gravity in the Christian world has shifted inexorably southward" (Jenkins 2002, 2). For instance, in 2002, after a trip to southwest Madagascar with two other retired missionaries, the charismatic Lutheran pastor Walter was interviewed by a reporter in the local Lutheran newspaper in Minneapolis–St. Paul and was quoted as saying, "American churches need renewal badly. We can learn much from the *fifohazana* in Madagascar." Walter's comments built on his and other Madagascar missionaries' pride in the fact that, in 2002, the self-identified evangelical president of Madagascar, Marc Ravalomanana, himself a supporter of the *fifohazana*, had just been elected and installed through the protest of *mpiandry* in the capital city (Keller 2005, 56).[12]

Cultural exchanges like the healing services, however, can also contribute to a variety of cultural processes that mark and reproduce the difference of Malagasy Christian practices, possibly engendering "new forms of subjectification" for Malagasy pastors in particular (Johnson 2007, 39). For pastors like Gabriel, their expertise is primarily defined through activities of bodily healing rather than equally important practices of Bible study and textual exegesis (Keller 2005). This offers a skewed view of Malagasy Christianities and could echo colonialist associations of African religions with bodily practice. Moreover, Americans like Walter have described African Christian healing practices as those that can energize US Lutheran congregations characterized by waning participation. In the case of the healing services, such a framing risks placing Malagasy Christians in the role of providing a service to European and US churches. Even as the healing services positively regard Malagasy Christian healing approaches and contribute directly to Lutheran therapeutic initiatives, some of their value in this social and historical context may derive from their cultural otherness, as it is subtly marked through the services themselves. As Klassen (2011, 175) points out, the otherness of non-European Christian traditions have long formed part of the self-conception of Euro-American Christian communities. Thus, although the sites of interaction between Malagasy and Americans have shifted from Madagascar to the United States, it is important to recognize that discourses and practices of cultural exchange may draw upon a deeper history of conceptualizing the US body through encounters with foreign ways. Together, these often subtle cultural subtexts warrant attention as they show on a micropolitical scale how Christian therapeutic initiatives feature and rework power inequalities between Christians in the United States and in sub-Saharan Africa.

Conclusions

I have argued in this chapter that biospiritual imaginaries constitute central components of the medical relief endeavor. As social formations differently known and actively made through a variety of embodied activities, including healing services and medical aid labor, biospiritual imaginaries affectively tie US volunteers to a global therapeutic community with seen and unseen dimensions. Individual US congregants do not necessarily experience the same biospiritual imaginaries, in that they interpret the global significance of Christian medical care through various life experiences, denominational affiliations, and sites of religious participation. These variations cohere around a central focus, however, on the moral value of biomedicine, its global appeal, and the compatibility of Christian healing and biomedicine. As Pamela Klassen (2011) has argued, North American liberal Protestants of many stripes have since the late nineteenth century found inspiration, rather than conflict, in biomedicine's scientific modernity, building hospitals and medical research facilities and globally propagating the social gospel through foreign medical mission work. These interlinkages between North American liberal Protestants and the globalization of medicine are thus not at all new, nor are the socially recognized compatibilities between religious healing and biomedical science.

What is distinctive about the Minnesota-Madagascar aid program is the use of biomedicine and medicalized healing as a collaborative space of global engagement among both liberal and conservative branches of Lutheranism. In the context of acrimonious Lutheran sectarian conflicts in Minneapolis–St. Paul, medicine appears a neutral terrain among those variously oriented toward global social justice, alliance-building across Christian churches, and evangelism through Christian healing.

In contrast to mid-twentieth-century US Lutheran programs to support foreign mission work in Madagascar, which focused on orphanages, seminaries, and churches, medical clinics currently take primacy over other kinds of Malagasy Lutheran institutions through which such ties could conceivably be built. Furthermore, it is now through African Christians' reciprocal influence on Americans on US soil, particularly Merina Malagasy evangelists like Gabriel, that US Lutherans are culturally endowing a range of embodied activities with transnational religious significance. Among US Lutherans, this has resulted, I argue, in a heightened focus on embodied ways of knowing for imagining ties with Christians elsewhere. Thus, multiple bodies, whether the medicalized patient body or the body of the global church; body parts, such as hands; and even the techno-scientific instruments circulated as aid between the United States and Madagascar have been harnessed in rhetorically imagining and embodying these connective (and disconnective) bonds in Minneapolis–St. Paul.

Yet among the US Lutherans I know in Minneapolis–St. Paul, the individual's physical body exists amid a rather crowded field of different bodies that culturally compete for attention and sometimes contradict each other. These include the medicalized patient body, the aid recipient's suffering body, the wounded body of Jesus, the holistic body-soul of prayer healing, and the Christian doctor's expert hands. Bodily sensations, body parts, and embodied experiences are a busy intersection of slippages and points of partial overlap between diverse and contradictory views of the body politic of global Christianity. Among laypeople, the dominant discourses of Lutheran medical aid, which celebrate biomedical knowledge and biomedical success, also feature several disjunctures that become subtly apparent within the aid organizations. Lesser acknowledged bodies—the ailing bodies of volunteers and their families, a desired holism of body-soul in Gabriel's services, and reductively racialized bodies of the colonial encounter—erupt in the aid organizations and other spaces of faith-based medicine, creating cultural dissonance for the medical aid project. Analyzing the broader field of Malagasy and US therapeutic activities reveals a cultural ambivalence with biomedical practice and biomedical commerce. Malagasy Lutherans and US Lutherans propagate biomedical approaches to healing yet, through their own faith-based medical activities, can be understood as articulating limits to biomedical success.

The transnational popularity of therapeutic Christian practices, such as the forms of medicalized care, caregiving, and religious healing I have described in this chapter, shares a relationship with neoliberal policies that have increasingly made health care provision the domain of religious communities and other privatized entities. As Andrea Muehlebach (2012, chapter 3) has argued, local aid organizations frequently assume public services previously regulated at the regional or national level, forming a "welfare community" in place of the "welfare state." Within the Minneapolis-based religious landscape I have described, US Lutherans and their Malagasy coreligionists are interpreting through the body what it means to be humane and compassionate in this neoliberal context (Haskell 1985). Among US Lutherans and Malagasy Lutherans, biospiritual imaginaries foster understandings of aid and its effects that transcend individual bodily limits, yet, as I have shown, individual Christians keep returning, circling back as it were, to these bodily boundaries. In the next chapter, I extend this focus on the relationship of humanitarian care and neoliberalism to explore how Lutheran medical relief critiques, yet also contributes to, the inequalities of global medical commerce.

CHAPTER THREE

Redeeming Medical Waste, Making Medical Relief

After my first walk through the IHM headquarters, I struggled to render in my field notes a realization lurking at the corners of the experience: in several ways, I had not only walked through a warehouse in northwest Minneapolis but toured the excess of institutionalized US biomedicine, along with the global travel circuits through which it re-acquires value. Within the aid warehouse, these pasts and futures, absences and presences, seen and unseen partners coalesce and inter-mingle through the medical discards and the dynamic cultural work of sorting them. Atop wall-to-wall warehouse shelves rest shrink-wrapped pallets of labeled and scanned medical supplies, mummified for inter-national transport. Between these oversized plastic bubbles are strewn the assorted detritus of institutionalized medicine, awaiting sorting and shipping: tubs and stacks of IV needles, respiratory tubing, cauteriz-ing tools, hospital beds, scales, tubing, catheters, blood bank contain-ers, bandages, surgical scissors, gloves, and much more. These supplies find their way to the NGOs through US volunteer workers and other do-nors who collect them from local hospitals, private clinics, and doctors' offices in Minneapolis–St. Paul and the Upper Midwest. Volunteers then bring these medical donations to the NGOs' warehouses in an industrial area of northern Minneapolis, a small manufacturing corridor of auto parts dealers and welding shops.

Scholars have long argued that waste flows are an integral part of consumption practices, revealing how persons and institutions differ-ently relate to things and relate to other persons through the things they dispose and keep (Frow 2003). Disposal in relatively wealthy societies often sparks global flows and markets of secondhand goods, such as used clothing in Zambia (Hansen 1999, 2000) and e-waste in China (Tong and Wang 2012). Furthermore, large-scale disposal techniques, whether through landfills or dumps, spur industrious and sometimes illicit recovery, reuse, and recycling efforts the world over (Alexander and Reno 2012). Together, these "redemptive economies" (Hawkins and Muecke 2003, xi), or efforts to infuse new value in discarded goods, have become a significant focus of scholars interested in the interconnected margins of so-called formal and informal economic activities and the wide-ranging productive strategies individuals employ to get by in advanced capitalist societies marked by entrenched inequality. The global circulation of medical waste, however, is a less familiar subject within these studies of waste economies, which often have focused on slightly more accessible consumer goods or materials like cloth, electronics, and building supplies. Yet, in North America, the US medical establishment is second only to the fast-food industry in the volume of municipal solid waste it produces annually (Collier 2011, 1245), expelling garbage that a variety of groups seize and sift through, often before it even makes it to the landfill.[1] This is precisely the position of the two medical relief NGOs, which "recover" mostly unused US medical discards and then ship them to clinics in Madagascar and elsewhere.

Medical aid organizations can thus be conceived as "conversionary sites" at the crossroads of different ways of valuing medical discards, concurrently understood as institutional waste products, charitable donations, sacred gifts, potential commodities, relational tokens, and aid forms. Drawing from my eighteen months as a laborer inside the Minneapolis aid warehouses, I uncover in this chapter how aid workers, who perform waste work as a central task, negotiate and produce these multiple forms of value in their activities with medical discards. Though as volunteers they do not accrue the negative social stigma of laborers working with discards for a living (Reno 2016), their work is, in ways similar to other waste workers, a cultural activity of value regeneration and specifically one that focuses on repurposing discards (Boarder Giles 2014; Resnick 2016). Cast-offs almost always bear a latent potential to be exchanged and revalued, even if they have been temporarily "deactivated" as commodities, which enables them to be pressed into a new use (Kopytoff 1986, 76). I use the term *workers* or *laborers* to highlight how, even though most are unpaid volunteers, they perform work with waste forms that does contribute to the formal economy. Furthermore, as described in the previous chapter, they often value their labor as a special kind of socially productive religious and moral work, rather than a form of volunteerism per se. Although US aid workers certainly do not face the danger common to waste work in open-air landfills, such as that performed by *catadores* in Brazilian garbage dumps (Millar 2012), they do share with other waste workers concerns over the moral status of the discards they handle and how it may reflect negatively upon their personhood, both in a collective sense and as individual Christians. I suggest US aid workers' moral disquiet reveals their awareness of their inability to *fully* and *completely* remake hospital waste into suitable aid and results in a variety of ritual activities that seek to morally redeem the medical materials.

In what follows, I first examine how disposal is economically productive for institutionalized biomedicine in the United States and trace how, in contradictory ways, international aid facilitates a globalized landscape of inequality in biomedical resources. In the subsequent sections, I explore the foundational paradox underlying the US supply of medical technologies to Lutherans in Madagascar: How do US Lutherans affirm their moral relationship with their foreign brethren through material things deemed by some to be institutional discards, ultimately cast off because of their nonusefulness or obsolescence in the US hospital setting? In rather unusual ways, aid workers bring medical discards, often presumed to be inert, fixed, scientific, and secular objects, into a Christian ritual framework, socially reconstituting them in the process. I suggest US aid workers attempt to resolve the ethical dilemmas surrounding medical waste by muting the past institutional life of the medical technologies, placing the materials they collect into a social calculus of "useful" and "junk" supplies and associating this classification system with a divinely sanctioned gift economy involving blessings and sins. What is interesting about ritual activities surrounding hospital waste is that, even as medical discards accrue sacred and ethical value in a ritual framework, their value continues to be derived, at least partly, from their market value as manufactured tools that need to meet a basic clinical standard. It is this tension between the ethical and sacred value of the medical discards—congealed through acts that acknowledge the relational exchange with aid partners in Madagascar and elsewhere— and the discards' potential use value or usefulness that creates ongoing moral anxiety for US aid workers. I therefore recast the notion of "redemptive economies" in this chapter, a term that has been developed by scholars to refer mainly to economic processes surrounding waste forms but not their religious dimensions to illuminate the *mutually reinforcing* religious and economic dimensions of such practices in a Christian context.

Some additional notes on the notion of value are necessary before moving forward. As David Graeber (2001) has cogently argued, value has had several distinct meanings in anthropological discourse, from the salient difference of Saussurean linguistics to worthy social values in the plural, such as liberty and equality (see also Robbins 2013), to economic value. Following Marx, economic value can be glossed as use value (utility) and exchange value, or value determined through establishing commensurability in exchange, sometimes through other exchanged goods but more often through price (money). In this chapter, I leave room for activities of valuing that are not strictly capitalist, understood in a limited sense as exchange value and use value, yet continually intersect in the aid warehouses with the capitalist valuations of things (as commodities, or things with potential exchange value). I use the term *value*, then, in mainly the first and the third senses described above (i.e., value as socially organized salient difference and economic value), though I occasionally distinguish them from the "higher" worthy values of being compassionate and equitable, which undergird the aid organizations' ethical platform. I trace activities of valuation and devaluation (e.g., in its sacred, ethical, and market forms) as they emerge through the labor process in the aid warehouse. Such activities center on medical discards and result in an ongoing and selective "transvaluation from the activity to the object" (Eiss and Pederson 2002 cited in Lambek 2013, 142), and vice versa.

I am interested in not only how capitalist, ethical, and sacred values coexist in the aid warehouses but also how, through situated moments of social recognition, they reverberate in people's labor activities, sometimes harmonizing together and other times creating discord through their difference. These moments reveal the contradictory position of the NGOs at the intersection of global medical commerce and global religious communities. My account endeavors to capture how aid workers themselves negotiate what Jane Guyer (2004, 27) calls "asymmetrical" value conversions in which there is a gap of commensurability or equivalence, sometimes sparked by the commingling of multiple valuation scales. I see the work of revaluing medical discards—and the disjoints these activities bring to light—as part of the Minnesotan agencies' overall effort to repurpose discards and make them into new things, in this case medical relief objects. Before turning my attention to these valuation activities, however, I first address how medical materials enter the Minneapolis NGOs and how they acquire value through being converted from medical property to charitable donations. By exploring the acquisition of discarded medical technologies, I highlight the unlikely alliance between faith-based humanitarian initiatives and the property regimes in biomedicine that make their operations possible.

Hospital Waste and the Medical Property Regime

Most recent studies examining property debates in biomedical practice and biomedical science have focused on the problematic social attributes of human bodily materials like tissue, organs, and DNA sequences. These forms defy traditional property divisions of persons and things and raise numerous questions about whether they constitute things fully separable from persons (see Parry and Gere 2006; Sharp 2006). Despite scientific work to make such forms into "biotechnological artifacts," or separable objects, some research shows that organ recipients forge intimate ties with traces of the persons from which donated organs were harvested, making organs difficult to categorize through property models (Sharp 2006). Others have pointed out that DNA sequences, for example, bear little resemblance to the "donated parts" of the human body once the research scientists, technicians, funding bodies, and institutions involved in reinventing them have "mobilized new claims in, or to, them" (Parry and Gere 2006, 153). I examine a biomedical form less analyzed in the scholarly literature on property and biomedicine: hospital waste. The divisibility of these objects from persons and from clinical practice is seemingly a given from the medical institution's point of view. Indeed, the object status of biomedical discards goes hand in hand with their ability to be expelled from the medical institution as waste forms.

Yet I suggest that, in different ways, biomedical discards bear qualities that more informally unsettle or call attention to the regulative limitations of property ownership. Their form often bears strong ties to their itineraries through the medical system and sometimes also to human bodies, particularly in the case of more "personal" objects like eyeglasses or bed pads, which prompt different kinds of interaction than things used only in clinical encounters (e.g., respiratory tubing and syringes). Many medical discards, in ways distinct from the tissue samples and cell lines discussed by Parry and Gere (2006, 140), "unsettle the binaries on which so many regulatory regimes rely for clarity." Because traces of other persons and former institutional lives remain unsettled or unresolved by the mere transfer of property rights, medical discards carry signs of what we might consider unresolved pasts, whether in the form of manufacturer expiration dates, institutional insignias or more rarely, bodily fluids. In the subsequent sections of this chapter, I explore how aid workers work to refine the material and moral qualities of the medical discards that signal such unresolved pasts.

Here, I explain how the disposal of hospital waste creates economic value for US biomedicine and furthers a multifaceted medical property regime. Legal scholar Carol M. Rose (2004) uses the term *property regime* to refer to "the dominant set of shared understandings about property in a given political economy" (Verdery and Humphrey 2004, 19), enacted through a variety of interwoven regulative practices. My use of the term *medical property regime* on subsequent pages is meant to highlight how, rather than possessing, the acts of disposal and ownership transfer can be economically productive for institutions like hospitals. Relinquishment is thus equally constitutive of the category of medical property through clarifying and maintaining a separation from what is *not* property. These property transfers reinforce a broader set of practices, such as limiting medical risk, which ensure medical profitability.

Hospital Waste as a Polyvalent, Contested Category

Several basic questions surround the hospital waste that Malagasy Partnership and IHM ship to Madagascar and elsewhere: How do the agencies receive so many clinical materials without ostensibly paying for them? Why are these things discarded by US hospitals, and why can't they be put to use somewhere else in the United States? For US biomedical institutions, appropriate disposal of medical materials is an adherence to the germ theory of disease and hygienic measures for the prevention and isolation of infection, and for this reason a legal obligation. Through the disposal process, medical discards occupy multiple statuses simultaneously, and this makes the terms used to describe them imprecise but also particularly revealing. Calling them "hospital waste" presumes the hospital's institutional perspective on such materials, which anticipates the materials' eradication from the hospital setting in assigning the waste classification. Hospital waste also must be distinguished from medical waste, which usually refers to biohazardous materials contaminated with bodily fluids and used "sharps" like scalpels and needles, all materials that hospitals in the United States are legally required to discard separately. Hodges (2008) alternates between calling the combined category of hospital waste and medical waste "biotrash" and "medical garbage," which she describes as the material remnants of the clinical encounter between patients and practitioners, including used syringes, plastic tubing, blood bags, pharmaceuticals and pharmaceutical containers, and even human tissues and fluids. The materials handled by IHM and Malagasy Partnership have participated to various degrees in the clinical encounter described by Hodges (2008), with many traveling through the medical institution while remaining fully unused. The IHM operations manager, Mark, once pointed out to me the crucial difference between recovered supplies and reused supplies, making the argument that many IHM supplies were in fact never previously used in the biomedical institution (see also Rosenblatt and Silverman 1992, 1443). Many of these medical supplies can be sent overseas only because they cannot be used in US hospitals because of insurance regulations.

Materials are donated to Malagasy Partnership and IHM from hospitals and clinics in Minneapolis–St. Paul and the surrounding region for one or more of five central reasons. The items may be "short-dated" and close to reaching their manufacturer expiration dates with about three or four months of existent "shelf life." Furthermore, a new product vendor may have been chosen for a piece of equipment, making the former one outdated or superfluous (even if completely new). Further, a surplus of a particular medical item could result from a change in medical procedures at the hospital and the materials they require. If more than the requisite number of supplies has been opened for a given procedure, an operating room situation that Rosenblatt, Chavez et al. (1997, 478) call "over-preparedness," they generally may not be assigned to another procedure at a hospital even if they have not been used. Finally, some items may remain unopened and unused but are no longer considered sterile as judged by the manufacturer's expiration date on the packaging. On the rare occasions when they accept expired medical supplies, the Minneapolis agencies do so with the understanding that the item may be resterilized at the receiving hospital. Sterility is not required of all medical supplies and corresponds to sterile and nonsterile zones of the medicalized body (e.g., blood versus skin, respectively) that determine the appropriate preparation of medical items for a given procedure.

Even as these disposal practices regulate US biomedicine, considerable debate exists among North American medical communities about reusing medical supplies *within* North American clinics, especially single-use devices. Many clinicians recognize that manufactured supplies are increasingly geared toward disposability, which ultimately raises health care costs and compounds environmental waste. Though medical supplies may be labeled for one-time use, some argue that they can actually be resterilized and reused without jeopardizing patient safety. One 2008 study found that 28 percent of Canadian acute-care hospitals had adopted reuse policies for such single-use devices (Canadian Agency for Drugs and Technologies in Health 2008). Others suggest that, ethically, patients should give their consent to this reprocessing practice so that they understand the potential risks of receiving care with reused (though resterilized) materials, labeling this practice a kind of "hidden rationing" on the part of the hospital (Collier 2011, 1245). Reuse used to be the norm and not the exception, with medical items made of glass, metal, or rubber. Thus, this argument for patient consent whenever reusing single-use devices—which implies heightened risk—may serve to ultimately reinforce the medical manufacturing industry's commercial aims. It also demonstrates a focus on liability concerns within the medical community, in that patient consent would presumably absolve the hospital of responsibility for the risks associated with the reuse of single-use devices.

This debate among North American practitioners mainly concerns single-use devices and not those originally designed for resterilization. The two Lutheran agencies in my research acquire mostly single-use devices that have never before been used, as well as items designed for resterilization, though it is possible single-use devices will be reused in the receiving clinic. What is important to take away from this debate is the understanding that disposal and the category of hospital waste in North American medical establishments is a contested process rather than only a straightforward matter of compliance. Some North American clinicians, patients, and environmental activists readily apprehend single-use devices as part of the waste and rising costs of the medical industry. They try to curb additional waste in North American medical settings, even while insurance regulations clearly limit their ability to do so.

Medical Risk and Its Relationship to Global Medical Relief

It is perhaps hard to overestimate the importance of risk as the engine that drives the medical relief endeavor. Insurance industry assessments imply that the presence of expired medical supplies or those close to reaching their expiration dates increases the risk of legal liability for the medical center and for individual health care workers (Rosenblatt and Silverman 1992, 1441). In receiving a donation, the faith-based nonprofits assume this liability on behalf of the medical institution. Therefore, materials may be deemed unsuitable for US biomedical institutions as a result of the "legal and political climate" (Rosenblatt and Silverman 1992, 1442) that surrounds biomedicine. Those materials may still be used for "safe, effective patient care," as Rosenblatt and Silverman (1992, 1442) note in their discussion of the recovery program for unused surgical supplies at Yale–New Haven Hospital in Connecticut. The safety of the donated medical supplies of course depends on a number of factors, such as the kind of supply, whether it was originally designed for one-time use, its age and appropriateness for a given procedure, and any previous use in the clinical setting. It is clear nevertheless that insurance requirements often prohibit supplies' use in the United States no matter how well they may meet a basic standard of care.

Though the monitoring of medical risk is among the most pronounced in the United States, it forms part of a transnational medical-legal regime with an uneven but far reach. In her discussion of the "biomedical waste recovery industry" in Chennai, India, Sarah Hodges (2008, 13) attributes its growth more to the influence of transnational insurers than the Indian juridical system designed to enforce certain methods of medical waste disposal. She notes, "Global insurers thus regulate medical commerce as well as attempt to maintain levels of acceptable risk: both financial and epidemiological. If these new regimes of regulation do anything at all, they create conditions for enterprising illicit, informal economies of waste" (13). IHM and Malagasy Partnership clearly participate in such waste economies. As I describe further below, both straddle formal and informal economic activities by enabling the materials' disposal or temporary removal from formal, monetized market exchange.

The notion of risk has been analyzed extensively as an outgrowth of modern life, a way of conceptualizing the dangers of technology, environmental destruction, and large-scale institutional processes such as financial investment that indelibly affect individuals in direct and indirect ways. Risk also operates as a tool of governance through its ability to manage and contain uncertainty and vulnerability among a populace, fostering in the process new modes of self-governance through risk avoidance (Giddens 1990, 1991; Beck 1992). Other scholars point out that, rather than viewing risk only negatively, many market processes rely on the management and transformation of risk as a means of generating profit (Zaloom 2004; Ho 2009). Caitlin Zaloom (2004, 365) describes financial futures markets where "aggressive risk-taking" bears the twin possibility of immense profits and peril and thus plays an integral role in financial speculators' displays of self-mastery. Although the rejection rather than embrace of excessive risk is emphasized in US medicine, conceptualizing risk here, as in Zaloom's (2004, 367) work, as a lynchpin in the "creation and conservation of economic goods" helps us see *both* its negative and its productive dimensions.

Medical risk is commonly understood to be something that opposes value generation in the medical setting by, for instance, increasing malpractice insurance premiums or legal liability (financial) and fostering a potentially hazardous environment for patients (epidemiological). I follow Hodges (2008) and others, however, in pointing out that medical risk, in both its financial and its epidemiological forms, critically underpins medical commerce, thereby producing rather than merely diminishing economic value. By expunging hospital waste through the various means described above, medical-supply manufacturers infuse the medical system with new technologies and instruments, maintaining robust medical commerce. Agencies like Malagasy Partnership and IHM participate in this medical marketplace by serving as a largely hidden "conduit of disposal" (Hetherington 2004, 165) for US biomedical surplus. Shipping these medical materials elsewhere, but not allowing their use in the United States, creates value for the medical-supply manufacturing industry and the medical establishment, including medical insurers, hospitals, and health care workers keeping medical risk at acceptable or low levels, and the companies for which they work. Individual health care workers do not necessarily benefit financially from such policies, though they may have a financial incentive from their employers to maintain low levels of medical risk and, thereby, keep insurance premiums manageable. When we look at medical risk as part of an economically productive process, we can trace an uneven, dendritic flow of resources into various branches of the US biomedical establishment when they comply with this medical-legal regime.

Taking on so much medical risk has, perhaps unsurprisingly, placed the NGOs themselves in an awkward and ill-defined position relative to the global insurance industry. The IHM executive director, Curt, once explained to me that no major insurance companies, besides Lloyd's of London, would insure the organization because of the excessive liability (risk) it assumed in acquiring discarded medical materials. Because the agency could not pay the high premiums required by Lloyd's of London, Curt characterized this insurance regime as an obstacle to the NGO's wish to make "something good" from biomedical waste but elided the NGO's reliance on the very same legal regime that makes its operation possible. When bringing together these points, it is possible to see how practices of medical disposal intertwine medical-legal risk and humanitarian engagement. At a fundamental level, the NGOs facilitate the expulsion of risk from the clinical setting, which maintains medical profitability; both NGOs absorb the risk, which, from an insurance perspective, makes them uninsurable. The NGOs, in turn, attempt to nullify the risk of US medical discards by emphasizing their use value for overseas partners. What I describe later in the chapter is that this process is by no means seamless or resolved. Rather, aid workers endeavor to abrogate this distribution of social "bads" through valuation activities that include prayer over the discards.

The US disposal process creates value for the biomedical establishment through the supplies' absence or removal, and the donated medical supplies take on new economic value when received by the Malagasy Lutheran health care department (SALFA) in Antananarivo. As a health care network providing administrative assistance to each medical center, SALFA accrues a portion of the funds for its operation by charging a small service fee for the medical supplies it distributes to each clinic. In effect, medical materials donated or recovered from hospitals and ostensibly removed from the biomedical-supply trade in the United States (i.e., valued as "gifts-in-kind" for taxation but not priced for direct sale) construct a small subsidiary market in Madagascar for SALFA. With devaluation of the Malagasy *ariary*, SALFA cannot always purchase medical items directly from multinational biomedical suppliers. The donated medical supplies from the United States carry the potential of economic value for SALFA. Such redistributed goods channel recent biomedical tools into the country while enabling SALFA to create a market that propels its operation. It is interesting to note that many donors in Minnesota are unaware that the medical supplies become revalued monetarily once they arrive in Madagascar. (See figures 3.1 and 3.2.) In addition, the value in *ariary* placed upon each item is not referred to by SALFA as the selling price but rather as a service fee. Each medical center within the SALFA network pays this service fee when it requests a medical item and the collected money finances the central operation. The term *service fee* endeavors to avoid the possible misinterpretation that the organization may be financially profiting in any way from the donations. Even as both NGOs turn institutionalized waste into life-saving technologies, this situation arises from a deeply unequal global medicine in which US donations to foreign clinics spur biomedical commerce and SALFA's inability to resell such items upholds the medical property regime. Medical relief facilitates a globally uneven distribution of "bads" in the form of medical risk, even as those involved in the relief endeavor seek to reframe such liabilities as opportunities for making more equitable the distribution of global medical resources.

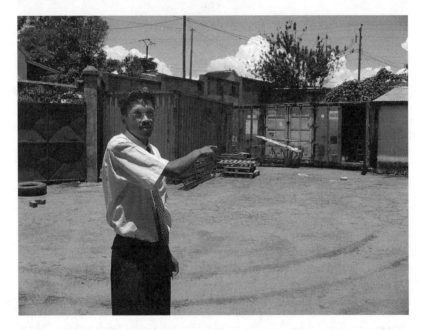

FIGURE 3.1. Clement, the SALFA liaison to Malagasy Partnership and IHM, showing the area on the outskirts of Antananarivo where medical supplies are sorted and stored in old sea containers, called by some Minneapolis aid workers "container city."

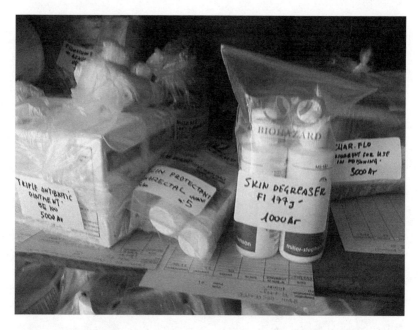

FIGURE 3.2. Bags of skin degreaser and triple antibiotic ointment sit inside one sea container in Tana's "container city," awaiting transfer to a SALFA medical center. The bag of triple antibiotic ointment has been assigned a service fee of 7,000 *ariary* or approximately US$2.55.

Revisiting Medical Disposal as a Multifaceted Economic Transaction

If we return our focus to the disposal process, we can better appreciate, then, that disposal is a multifaceted property transaction for the biomedical institution that both devalues supplies as active property of the medical center and revalues the materials as charitable donations. In addition, multiple transfers of value underpin the movement of supplies between the medical institution and the NGO and perhaps overdetermine the transition as a shift in their value. From a legal and business standpoint, the revaluation of donated items according to their "fair market price" is a central part of the transaction, for it offers hospitals a monetary figure that may be claimed as a tax deduction. Nonprofit organizations are legally prohibited in the United States from valuing their donors' gifts-in-kind, although they must do so for their own financial records.[2] The transfer of ownership, signaled by paper documentation, gives the hospital the legal ability to revalue items monetarily that were otherwise designated as waste. Sarah Hodges (2008) suggests that hospitals also find valuable the paper trail documenting such transfers, which verify that the hospital has followed insurance regulations mandated by the state. Such adherence also makes the hospital eligible for continued accreditation, auditing processes, and high accreditation ratings, all commodity forms interlinked with appropriate waste disposal. Although conceived legally in the United States as nonprofits, then, organizations like IHM and Malagasy Partnership play an integral role in property transfers that ultimately reconstitute the materials' exchange value. In other words, they enable the profitable exchange of different forms of capital (i.e., commodities and credits). (See figure 3.3 for an illustration of these value conversions.)

The hospital and business contacts made through repeated donations are also economic forms transferred with the medical donations and just as valuable for the medical aid organizations as the medical supplies, if not more so. In the September 2005 monthly volunteer meeting, the IHM executive director, Curt, a Lutheran pastor and social worker, voiced his opinion that IHM should accept a large donation of unsorted supplies (approximately fourteen pallets of stethoscopes, blood pressure cuffs, and hospital gowns) from the St. Paul Area Service Guild in order to receive access to their "network links" of cash and medical supply donors. Because the guild was closing down its warehouse, its network links were "up for grabs," Curt said, and would give IHM a stronger "network of feeders."

Gene also once told me how his fifteen-year relationship with a large

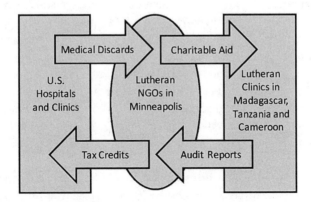

FIGURE 3.3. Value conversions in global medical relief.

Minneapolis linen supply service, which he visited weekly, gave Malagasy Partnership favored status and the best pick of discarded linens among competing agencies. Malagasy Partnership obtained from the linen service bed pads, surgical gowns, and even valuable bedsheets. When the economy was better, Gene told me one evening in 2006 as we sorted linens, the company discarded bed pads and surgical gowns after twenty washings (something that was actually tracked on the reverse side of each cloth), no matter what their condition. It was considered more costly for the company to hire someone to inspect the linens than to just stop using them after twenty washings. At the time, this policy had been reversed and the linens were in circulation until an employee deemed them too worn for hospital use. As a result, the quality of the donations was not as high. I had noticed as I was folding bed pads, for instance, that some of the blue cloth was ripped or demonstrated the tell-tale signs of having been caught in an industrial dryer, which mangled the blue plastic fabric. As Gene spoke to me, he spotted a rip in one of the bed pads. He said that the bed pad, although in poor condition, could be sliced in half, and the cotton backing could be used in the bottom of a bassinette, like the one to our left that was being packed securely in a wooden frame by two other volunteers.

Each of these examples indicates that supply acquisitions, from the perspective of the aid agency, are multifaceted economic negotiations where value may be organized through a series of transactions subsidiary to the actual exchange of medical materials or even the formal paperwork signaling ownership transfer. From the perspective of the donor, too, medical donations accrue value in a number of ways beyond the mere assurance of a tax credit. Donations often are made on the hospital's or supplier's terms, meaning that NGOs must be willing to accept whatever a hospital or medical relief agency is willing to give, as was the case with the St. Paul Service Guild and the linen service. NGOs must provide the volunteer labor to sort through donations to determine what items may be useful and even what items are actually contained in donated boxes. IHM held a series of what the volunteer coordinator Dagmar called "sorting marathons" in spring 2006 to sift through the forty-cubic-foot sea container of medical supplies it received from the Service Guild. In this way, medical suppliers and hospitals reduce labor costs involved with the disposal of supplies. In addition, hospitals and medical relief organizations decrease the cost of disposal itself. If NGOs subsequently find certain supplies unusable, they must assume the financial responsibility for their disposal. To better understand how supplies enter the NGOs and continue their itinerary to overseas clinics, I turn now to the practice of sorting, a crucial juncture in determining and negotiating value.

Converting Medical Discards into Useful Things

Converting medical discards into objects other than hospital waste is a social and moral practice that entails "fixing propriety" in things, a second sense-meaning of property relations originally discussed by John Locke (see Verdery and Humphrey 2004, 5). Rather than focusing on the transfer of property rights as an event that makes the medical supplies the NGOs' valued possessions, I see the labor of handling, sorting, and classifying the medical materials, or "fixing propriety" in them, as an equally important process that endeavors to refine the material and moral qualities of the medical donations. Because the medical donations are highly heterogeneous in composition (Rosenblatt, Ariyan, et al. 1996, 630), however, volunteer workers, myself included, were continually asking questions, seeking advice, making temporary classifications, and reorganizing the supplies. Classifications were routinely overturned, items reordered, new materials arrived, and some things appeared unclassifiable (e.g., stray tubes). The medical supplies were not understood plainly or with fixity as those that could be used and those that could not, but rather most supplies existed in a state of flux as they moved through the warehouses. Therefore, I will illustrate in the next two sections the multiple ways in which volunteer laborers work to establish ethical relations with their foreign Lutheran brethren by negotiating, establishing, and debating the usefulness of medical supplies in the sorting process that took place in the two warehouses.

Sorting: A Crucial Juncture in Determining Use Value and Usefulness

If we examine the sorting process more closely, we can see that placing an item in a biomedical classification is a first step in establishing its eventual institutional use—an act of reinstitutionalizing the medical discard—but not a practice that fully secures its usefulness. In most cases, the act of sorting compartmentalized the supplies into predetermined biomedical categories. At IHM, more than twenty labeled plastic bins, such as "respiratory" and "anesthesiology," existed in the sorting room, a long rectangular space with handmade wooden sorting tables surrounded by shelving units. At Malagasy Partnership, volunteers consulted Gene when they sorted materials, because he was the only health care worker among them, and he would tell them that a surgical dressing, for instance, should be classified as "sterile dressings" rather than "surgical supplies." Uncertainty still existed, though, about whether the classified items would be requested by an overseas clinic. The possibility also remained that the medical relief would not find a use value in the overseas clinic, because of the different circumstances of biomedical practice or the ill fit of the supplied goods, and the items would be thrown away.

Moreover, even as some volunteers threw things away at IHM to avoid sending nonuseful things overseas, others retrieved items from the trash bin to bring them home, giving them a use outside the NGOs' official circuits of usefulness. Maude, a monthly volunteer appearing to be in her seventies, joined Harriet and me in the IHM sorting room one September afternoon. Maude observed a thin, clear plastic rectangular container with an attached cover that had been placed in the trash bag in the sorting room. "It's a shame to throw this away," she said as she gingerly picked the plastic tub out of the trash. Harriet nodded, observing the container as Maude rotated it in her hand. Maude said she could use the container "for small things" at home and placed it beside her handbag on the floor. Many of the IHM volunteers share Maude's concern with the moral implications of "waste" and "wastefulness," something that both draws them to IHM's work but also is constructed in the very experience of sorting, salvaging, and packing used and donated medical supplies (Reno 2009).

Another way aid workers approached the ethical issues surrounding use was by suggesting that what made something useful was the anticipated duration of its use in the receiving clinic. Value was negotiated in this way through the recognition of particular qualities in things that nurtured specific futures. As we sifted through medical materials in the IHM sorting room one afternoon, Lois, a former missionary, described having once opened a box in Madagascar shipped from a US congregant only to discover that it looked as though the person had overturned their "household junk drawer" into the carton. For Lois, the overturned junk drawer served as the negative image of thoughtful giving against which she organized her volunteer work at IHM. On several occasions she refused to package disposable supplies. A Baptist missionary couple stopped at IHM in October 2005 to pick up two duffle bags worth of supplies for an orphanage they operated in the Philippines. Gesturing toward a box of facial tissues as we located items for the orphanage, Lois remarked, "I don't like to send anything out that's just gonna be thrown away." A substantial number of items in the warehouse were made for one-time use, although they were sometimes used beyond that in a clinic short on supplies. It was important to Lois that anything coming from IHM could be used more than once and *useful* in the long term, not something that could turn to waste shortly after it arrived and be placed back in the social category (waste, trash) from which IHM attempted to recover it. Lois did not draw attention explicitly to the religious significance of waste work but it is worth pointing out that her commitment to extending usefulness echoes salvationist discourses. Making things last and extending their productive life is socially entangled with, though not necessarily equivalent to, other acts of renewal and redemption (see Alexander and Reno 2012; Graeber 2012). Some productive ambiguity exists, therefore, between the religious principles shaping Lois's lifelong work and sorting practices that offer opportunities to confirm or reflect on those values.

Lois's approach to usefulness challenges the idea, often attributed to a generalized, churchgoing US public against which volunteers in the two nonprofits defined themselves, that any charitable donation, no matter its quality or kind, is a moral good. Lois questioned giving things simply to reduce one's own waste and its moral entailments, symbolized by the household junk drawer, but she also wanted giving to extend the life and usefulness of an object, thereby limiting or delaying the waste of others. This stance partly communicated the notion that US aid workers should take responsibility for the disposal of nonuseful things, and the quality of their actions more generally, rather than passing on their culpability to others. Moreover, Lois conveyed an overarching value in fostering the durability, and long-term commitment, of the transnational ties that she and others created through the exchange of medical materials. For Lois, this practice could also be linked to the kinship relations she maintained through working as an IHM volunteer: at age seventy-nine, she saw her work as a way of "staying connected" to Madagascar at a time when travel was becoming difficult for her, but also a project that could benefit her own family who remained in southern Madagascar. One of her sons, a US-trained engineer-turned-Bible translator, mar-

ried a Tandroy Malagasy woman, and they lived together with their son
in the town of Tsiombe. Lois's son and family maintained ties with the
Lutheran medical clinics in the southern region, which received monetary aid from IHM, and occasionally journeyed to the regional center
of Tolagnaro–Ft. Dauphin for special care, supplies, and visits with travelers to the area. Indeed, this is how I met Lois's son, daughter-in-law,
and niece, when I visited with them in Tolagnaro–Ft. Dauphin in 2005
and brought them a gift from Lois. Although we can see how Lois pro-
motes multiple kinds of relations through her sorting work, her direct
connection to people who frequented Malagasy Lutheran clinics was exceptional. For most IHM volunteers, the supplies' destinations and the
people who would be receiving them were not differentiated but rather
organized in a more general category of "brothers and sisters in Christ."

Talk of use and usefulness, along with sorting the supplies for eventual institutional use, can be seen as acts that revalue the materials
rather than only referring to their value. These valuation processes overlap with, but are not equivalent to, capitalist notions of use value. We can
take "use" in this case as not merely part of a "utilitarian calculus," as
Frow (2003, 32) himself opposes, but a locally elaborated scale of value
with ethical dimensions. Because the medical supplies are discards with
no ostensible use value when they enter the aid warehouse, "use" becomes a clear indicator or trope of value generation among aid workers. Frow (2003, 26) points out that the cultural category of waste shares
an interrelationship with use, though the two are often contrasted. Aid
workers in both agencies tended to label behavior wasteful when it involved throwing things away as a result of obsolescence, excess, sheer
convenience, or the "veneration of newness" (Strasser 1999, 5). Some
linked the waste of things to the improper stewardship of relations, as
in the notion of the "throwaway society" (Strasser 1999, 13), a term I
heard occasionally. These terms impart a concern with the stewardship
of things as part of a broader moral and ethical practice.[3] Agency leaders supported the ethical project of "giving intelligently," in the words
of the IHM executive director, in which *refining* use as a category and
distinguishing appropriate from inappropriate use as Lois had done was
readily encouraged. We can see that, following Frow, refining use simultaneously distinguishes the discards from one another, complicating the
generic category of waste. As indicated by Lois and Maude, aid workers
have various understandings of appropriate use, which emerge through
the material process of handling the medical discards. In the aid ware-

houses, these different, subjectively assessed standards of use affected individual and collective efforts to secure blessings from God for aid labor. As I describe below, they electrified collective prayers with productive uncertainty.

Valuing Medical Discards through Prayer

Establishing a use for discarded medical materials linked the circulation of medical relief to a broader moral economy involving divine blessings, which operated as a kind of return on the transmission of a useful object to foreign Lutheran physicians. IHM brochures commonly promised donors and volunteers blessings in return for their work: "God bless your effort to serve Him by helping the hands that heal!" During the Christmas luncheon for volunteers in 2005, Curt told those seated that they were the "life and blood" of IHM and "make gifts of [them]selves" to the agency; the chair of the IHM board of directors concluded the program by wishing "blessings" to the listening volunteers. In narrating his exasperation at not knowing what to do with a school group arriving at the warehouse, Mark commented to me one afternoon that he worried he sometimes forgot to see the volunteers as "blessings from God." In one sense, this language of blessing placed the warehouse operation in a divinely orchestrated gift economy: volunteers could be blessings to the agency by giving their labor, much as they could receive blessings in return for their work.

Prayer played a central role in securing these returns. After suddenly acquiring the adjacent warehouse in 2005, which enabled the agency to double its physical space, IHM volunteers commonly referred to the warehouse expansion as an "answer to prayer." In the May–June 2006 IHM newsletter, Dagmar described the warehouse acquisition as a "tremendous blessing." These observable "returns" for prayer and obedience reinforced the idea that the IHM operation was divinely "blessed" in the general sense or woven into a sanctioned gift economy. But they also served to heighten volunteers' efforts to continue this cycle by securing "blessings" in return for their work and attempting to ensure that the medical supplies operated as "blessings" in the recipients' lives. Anthropologist Susan Harding (2000, 122) calls these reciprocal exchanges a "gospel economy." Harding (2000) points out that giving is in fact constitutive of Christianity, and, through specific linguistic and interpretive framings, gifts may signify obedience to God and may ultimately be given to God, even though they may be designated for particular worldly purposes.

The best example of how volunteers asked for divine blessing for the medical supplies occurred during special container-packing sessions when the final preparations were made to ship materials overseas. At both agencies, just before the doors of the transatlantic sea containers were shut, volunteers formed a ritual prayer circle that faced the cardboard cartons of the shipment. The placement and timing of the prayer is significant because it indicates how the prayer text suffuses the container with requested blessings just before it leaves the physical presence of the volunteers. The container doors were typically shut only after the prayer had ended. For example, in August 2005 IHM volunteers gathered in the warehouse before a container destined for a hospital in northern Cameroon. When the final box had been shoved into the metal frame, the operations manager Mark suggested that everyone "gather in prayer for the container." Mark began the prayer, asking that the container "be blessed," that it have a safe journey, that Cameroonian customs officers "be kind" and perhaps not charge as many tariffs as for the previous container, and that "God bless the work" of medical doctors in Cameroon. In one packing session at Malagasy Partnership, I observed a comparable request just before the container's doors had been closed. One middle-aged engineer and regular volunteer, Theo, led a prayer circle for the container. His college-aged daughter asked that the things in the container "bless and acclaim You." In his turn of talk, Theo prayed that "the Lord would bless each item in the container" and that the items would "be a blessing for and through You, Lord."

Prayers for the supplies to be blessings can be viewed as valuation activities that intersect in complex ways with discourses of usefulness. Although it appeared to be a matter of faithfulness to trust that the medical materials would be turned into blessings (or useful things) after spoken prayers, it was also the volunteers' moral responsibility to demonstrate their faith by acquiring and selecting useful things. The possibility thus remained that the supplies might not have been sorted and selected with the volunteers' most rigorous attempts to prioritize the requests of overseas clinicians. As an ad hoc process, sorting left open to question whose measures of usefulness were correct. In addition, for volunteers, it often was unclear exactly how the supplies that they handled would be used in the foreign clinics where they were sent. The geopolitical distance between the Minneapolis NGOs and foreign clinics in Madagascar, Tanzania, and Cameroon further mystified the use relations of the medical materials but simultaneously contributed to the overall awareness among volunteers that the NGOs were linked to broader landscapes of divine activity. From this perspective, prayer was a value-adding activity that helped to secure the potential for a supply, as Theo put it, to "be a blessing for and through You, Lord." We can see, therefore, that spoken prayers endeavor to reduce several distinct forms of uncertainty encircling the medical materials, such as their eventual use and the impact of their reception, as well as how they will shape the relationship between US Lutheran volunteers and Lutheran clinicians in foreign hospitals.

Scholars have observed that prayer is a particular kind of valuing activity, though valuing can conceivably emerge from any act and be objectified in things (Lambek 2013, 148). In fact, ritual objects imbued with spiritual potency served as the template for Karl Marx's famous but pejorative term "commodity fetishism," which refers to the talismanlike quality of exchange value powerfully congealed in a commodity form. Christianity of course problematizes the fetishization of things, prohibiting the direct worship of images and arguing that things are never a complete manifestation of the divine, convictions that became a hallmark of Christian modernity (Keane 2007). In practice, however, things can become signs of divine agency or a relationship with the divine, and these dividing lines between fetish and token are often carefully articulated through prayer language. Lambek (2013, 148) points out that performative language like prayer often conflates means and ends, as it "accomplishes itself in the enactment." Although prayer is commonly (mis)taken to be an immaterial, even transparent form of reflection, prayer gives material shape to the spoken desires of religious supplicants, constituting a material act in itself, and often has observable material effects for believers (Keane 1997). Through these qualities, volunteer workers like Theo enlisted God in valuing the supplies as divine gifts (blessings), implying a positive transformation of their usefulness while distancing them from their discard status. It is important to note that aid workers also fashioned themselves as obedient through such prayer talk, concretizing the divine relationship, and worked to secure blessings from God in exchange for thoughtfully secured goods. Though Lambek (2013, 154) traces examples where ritual acts "decommoditize value," in this case, ritual prayer diminishes the predominance of exchange value but does not necessarily decommoditize value. Part of the medical supplies' congealed value comes from their latent usefulness, implicated in prayer talk, and that still derives at least partly from market logics of supply and demand.

By ascertaining usefulness, volunteer workers in both agencies participate in material practices that revalue discards, engaging them in further valuation through ritual prayers. Despite the extensive effort of sorting and reordering the supplies at both warehouses, however, some piles of stuff existed that no one knew what to do with, and these supplies sat in abeyance on the edges of countertops, in bags, or on utility tables (see Hetherington 2004, 166). At IHM, the difficulty of establishing use can be attributed to the global scope of the agency's aid program and its efforts to standardize the relief operation to fit numerous world regions. Several times, Harriet, a longtime volunteer and retired missionary nurse, expressed frustration and uncertainty about whether her own medical training was applicable to the many places where IHM sent supplies. She was trained to practice medicine at one hospital in northern Cameroon, adjusting her practice to that setting for thirty-six years, but she had retired and left Cameroon permanently some sixteen years earlier. IHM's use of retired medical professionals as arbiters in the sorting process resulted in situations where they indicated some unease or hesitation about making blanket judgments concerning the appropriateness of certain medical technologies for the range of foreign Lutheran clinics with ties to IHM.

Signaling small rejections of broader efforts to standardize aid responses, the unease of people like Harriet in making final judgments about a medical item's usefulness contributed to the growing pile of odds and ends that had no clear use. Harriet's refusal to categorize certain medical supplies and her decision to leave them in abeyance could be seen as part of an ethical practice of sending only useful aid overseas. By contrast, aid workers frequently referred to nonuseful supplies as "junk" forms that vacated medical-supply processing of the potential for receiving blessings. By looking at things deemed "junk" medical supplies, we can see how the very materiality of the hospital discards limited the NGOs' ability to infuse new value into discarded things and to create charitable donations from them. As we will see, the category of junk further links the medical relief endeavor to a set of Christian moral categories governing individual behavior. These regulate Christian aid giving through a moral framework that *personalizes* the moral repercussions of unethical aid, implying negative effects for individual aid workers rather than only for the agency as a religious community.

Sinfulness and Junk Medical Supplies

I have argued thus far that Lutheran aid workers engage in a variety of practices that dissociate hospital waste forms from their discard status. One subtle yet significant refinement to this practice, however, can be seen through a pointed statement hand written in marker on a whiteboard hanging in the IHM warehouse: "Junk for Jesus is still junk." The sign advises the volunteers that sending junk items overseas, even with the aim that they be used to do the healing work of Jesus, doesn't obviate the fact that these items are "still junk." In other words, certain medical materials have immutable junk qualities that empty them of their potential for securing blessings and simultaneously verify their nonusefulness. The scrawled reminder implies that it is necessary for volunteers to create waste themselves, throwing things away that are not useful for foreign practitioners. Furthermore, the statement "Junk for Jesus is still junk" suggests that medical practitioners in Tanzania, Madagascar, and Cameroon are not necessarily the only or final recipients of the medical relief but instead Jesus forms one predominant exchange partner ("Junk *for* Jesus") or, in the least, a form of divinity implicated in all human relationships, including aid partnerships.[4]

This sign and other, related discourses socialize a model of ethical aid in both agencies through a broader Christian framework of giving: Aid workers were taught to distinguish the "intelligent giving" of professional aid work from a more self-referential exchange aimed only at reaping individual rewards through one's personal relationship with Jesus. Limiting or abolishing self-interested action is arguably a long-established moral and theological ideal in many forms of Christian compassionate giving. What is unique here is the way the NGOs have sutured ethical standards common in the broader aid industry to a refined Christian model of giving, now accompanied by culturally distinct moral understandings. These convictions inject the aid endeavor with new forms of moral discipline and moral surveillance.

Technical Exchange for Christian Healthcare
(TECH) and a Moral Landscape of Aid

I came to realize shortly after beginning my fieldwork that the warehouse sign at IHM ("Junk for Jesus is still junk") originated in the language and policies of Technical Exchange for Christian Healthcare, namely the widely used TECH axiom "No junk for Jesus." Malagasy Partnership and IHM constitute part of a network of more than one hundred US-based Christian medical aid organizations, which has been known collectively since 1990 as Technical Exchange for Christian Healthcare or TECH. IHM was one of the first five organizations, with the North Carolina–based organization Samaritan's Purse (run by Billy Graham's son Franklin) and the Michigan-based agency that became International Aid, to join TECH. IHM assisted TECH with becoming a 501c3 organization, filing the paperwork in the state of Minnesota. Over time, the IHM operations manager Mark has observed what he called an "evolution" in TECH organizations that began as supply procurement agencies like IHM. Many have become more specialized over the years, focusing on the procurement and refurbishment of one medical item. The leaders of these organizations have "felt called to focus on a few items and *do it well*," Mark emphasized in a conversation one day. He listed several that came to mind: Hope Haven acquires wheelchairs and mobility support; an agency in Erie, Pennsylvania, called Chosen, which stands for Christian Hospitals Overseas Secure Equipment Needs, obtains surgical tables and sterilizers; Worldwide Lab collects laboratory supplies; Patterson Dental specializes in dental equipment; and Gleaning for the World simply gleans medical supplies for other agencies but does not ship materials abroad itself. These agencies aim to professionalize Christian aid provision, uniting a religiously-based moral discourse on usefulness with common evaluation standards from the broader aid world.

IHM and Malagasy Partnership cooperate regularly with other TECH organizations, sometimes drawing from fellow agencies' unique specializations. For instance, a Lutheran doctor in Tanzania with whom IHM works requested six surgical lights out of a larger aggregate donation that arrived at IHM in 2006. Since the lights required electrical modifications to make them appropriate for the Tanzanian hospital, Mark sent them to Chosen, a TECH member affiliated with the United Methodist Church. Chosen completes surgical light repair as a free service to Christian medical suppliers like IHM. Chosen initially received, sorted, and sent all medical supplies abroad (like IHM and Malagasy Partnership), but over time the organization came to specialize in the repair of surgical lights and tables. This was mostly because Chosen's location of Erie, Pennsylvania, had been the regional home of AMSCO (now Steris), a surgical equipment manufacturer.[5] Many of the agency's volunteers are retired AMSCO employees with specific skillsets not found elsewhere. Chosen acquires its funding from the fees it tacks onto repaired equipment that it sells. TECH agencies like Chosen capitalize on unique localized labor markets in various regions of the United States, gesturing to another way their work complexly combines formal and informal economic activities.

TECH organizations also pool their vast resources by swapping actual medical materials needed in the clinics they serve overseas. When his Malagasy liaison Clement requested gauze in March 2006, Gene posted a notice on the TECH website that he was seeking "4×4s" or four-inch by four-inch square gauze; he received many offers, and then shipments, of gauze in response. Since I planned to attend the April 2006 TECH meeting in Kingsport, Tennessee, Gene instructed me to thank the TECH members who had supplied these items. I was also told by Gene to ask TECH members for a series of items that Malagasy Partnership still needed at the time for its next shipment: multivitamins for adults and for children, sutures, dental needles, sterile and examination gloves, ultrasounds, pulse oximeters, fetal dopplers, and blood transfusion bags. Many of these materials later arrived at the warehouse, as Gene followed up on correspondence with TECH supply contacts I made during the three-day meeting. In short, TECH organizations across the United States support one another and form a crisscrossing web of equipment, global contacts, shipping circuits, technical expertise, and diverse denominational histories.

What binds these diverse agencies together is their agreement to follow the TECH "statement of faith," which is derived from the Nicene Creed, and to abide by a nine-point list of "quality standards" for donations, both of which form preconditions for membership. Member organizations conceptualize themselves not only as provisioning aid but as receiving it as well. In accordance with the TECH quality standards, one board member and employee of Samaritan's Purse in North Carolina proudly revealed at the TECH annual meeting that he turns down as much as 50 percent of the donations he is offered by biomedical institutions because of their poor quality. I saw a similar process at work with Gene at Malagasy Partnership, who often checked with the SALFA liaison Clement about the usefulness of an unknown supply before accepting a large donation (see chapter 6).

At IHM, these issues came to a head with the large unsorted donation from the St. Paul Service Guild, mentioned earlier in the chapter, which the executive director Curt wanted to accept to gain access to the Guild's "network links" of donors. Mark argued in the September 2005 meeting that IHM should *not* accept the Service Guild's unsorted materials; he had visited the guild's warehouse a year earlier and found the supplies there "not useful," though he admitted eagerly "eying" a few valuable sutures. In taking this stance, Mark was following the TECH ethical platform that only a small percentage of donations were useful and that rejecting poor-quality donations was what distinguished TECH members from less ethical agencies. In the debate over the St. Paul Service Guild, Mark eventually acquiesced, but held his ground on rejecting most of the items. During the subsequent three months, IHM held a series of "sorting marathons" in which a considerable percentage of the donation was thrown away. This disagreement shows how agency leaders, with their distinct roles, may see the organizations' goals in rather different ways at any one time. Although Curt was focused on building networks and future financial support, Mark felt his task was to uphold donation quality. At the TECH conference, the presenters instructed the members that they should send not just needed medical equipment but particular models that could be easily or inexpensively repaired, that used the appropriate voltage, and that could be retrofitted to use other power sources if electricity was unavailable. TECH thus defined quality aid as things that were needed by overseas partner institutions as well as items that *sustained* overseas institutions independent of the international biomedical market.

As an umbrella organization, TECH demonstrates certain qualities of denominationalism, yet it does not take the place of the churches that TECH members attend individually. Although some TECH organizations operate in conjunction with large US Protestant churches, others began as the independent efforts of people who took short-term mission trips and perceived shortages of supplies in overseas clinics, vowing to work to remedy the situation upon their return to the United States. At the April 2006 meeting that I attended, one board member who sends medical equipment to Central America asked me about my research during a coffee break between sessions. I described it as best as I could, including a somewhat naive comment about how I saw TECH as a "social movement." He disagreed with my characterization and told me that the notion of a social movement was "man's construct." Sensing perhaps that my language did not reflect a Christian witness, he continued on. "A personal relationship with Jesus—that's it," he said. "People here see heaven as more real than the fact that your hair is red and mine is white. It's truly more real to them. They would rather die than deny the existence of Christ here. It's *all* about Christ here." His witness constructed the reality of heaven and the personal relationship with Christ as a presence in our interaction ("It's *all* about Christ here"), as well as what ultimately inspired TECH. To talk of religion or social movements, therefore, would in his view be to secularize the pursuits of TECH members and ignore the "personal relationship with Jesus" that motivated each participant. TECH therefore aims to professionalize but not *secularize* its aid provision techniques, maintaining a strong focus on the spiritual basis of its work.

TECH holds two conferences per year where members come together for worship and to share resources with one another. Conference sessions strikingly showcase TECH's unique sacralization of the technical specificity, medical know-how, and everyday labor of medical relief operations. Conference participants often weave their involvement with TECH into a deeply spiritual testimony that becomes part of the conference format. Although he was unable to attend the year I went, Mark described the TECH conference to me before I left Minneapolis as a "spirit-rich environment" and a place for "fellowshipping." At the April 2006 meeting, each agency was invited to provide a five-minute update on its activities during the previous year. Meeting in a hotel conference center sandwiched within the rolling hills of eastern Tennessee, the agency representatives who were present repeatedly portrayed God as an active collaborator in their organizations and diminished their own agency in the procurement of medical technologies. "God gives you exactly what you need," one woman who was preparing a shipment for Honduras witnessed to the attendants. Still another woman explained that her laboratory equipment agency benefited in the last year when "God expanded the operation to pathology." Another man who directed an organization in the Washington, DC, area strikingly told the seated audience, "TECH is the body of Christ for me." Although no one else named the redemptive value of TECH quite this pointedly and poetically, TECH leaders drew attention to the spiritual foundation of medical aid by handing out circular stickers with the phrase "No junk for Jesus" that the participants wore on their clothes throughout the three-day meeting. The stickers signaled the participants' pledge to follow the TECH quality standards, as well as the TECH affirmation of faith.

In their personal testimonies and organizational rhetoric, TECH members voice a contemporary Christian discourse that positions Jesus as a personal friend and mentor, an active participant in one's daily life, rather than a distant figure or icon of salvation. The adages "Junk for Jesus is still junk" and "No junk for Jesus" share a relationship with other popular sayings, such as the precept "What would Jesus do?" (WWJD) that appeared primarily in the early 1990s on US Christian consumer goods that could be worn on the body. Many of the most popular aphorisms, such as "No junk for Jesus," imagine Jesus as not only an everyday consultant but also as the recipient or object of worldly giving. One young woman who volunteered infrequently at IHM paraphrased for me a favorite quotable that she attributed to Mother Teresa: "Would you send your used clothing to Jesus? Then don't send it to someone else, either."[6] These sayings convey a contemporary reworking of language from the North American ecumenical social gospel movement of the late nineteenth and early twentieth centuries. The popular maxim WWJD stems from the social gospel writing of the Reverend Charles M. Sheldon. When it was first published in 1897, Sheldon's novel *In His Steps: What Would Jesus Do?* addressed the problems of unemployment, corruption, and homelessness by marrying the Christian social gospel with the political language of the Progressive movement (Butler, Wacker & Balmer 2000, 317; Smith 2007, 193). Since Sheldon did not take a particular theological perspective in his novel, his work was not associated with the contentious debates in Protestantism at the time, such as that between fundamentalism and modern biblical criticism. As a result, the mass-mediated language of *In His Steps*, Smith (2007, 194) suggests, has been especially "appropriable" by later generations of Christian writers and clergy. I would suggest it is not only because of theological neutrality that such sayings hold importance in contemporary Christian discourse. In pithy yet strikingly effective ways, they follow evangelical efforts to resituate Jesus in a variety of moral problems of everyday life, reconfirming one's religious commitment in the process.

   Although TECH leaders publicly affirmed Jesus's role in their work, they were strikingly critical at the meeting of nonmember Christian agencies that have ended up sending what they called junk overseas. Commonly referenced junk materials included spare parts for medical equipment, undesirable items (silk surgical sutures), and machines without appropriate technical support or electrical wiring. In leveling their assertions about the unethical practice of circulating junk, TECH leaders made the broader argument that nonmember agencies engage in a kind of hypocrisy and damage the reputation of TECH members with secular humanitarian agencies and non-Christians. But they did not only label such practices "unethical." They repeatedly characterized them through a language of sin, rooting aid provision in a Christian moral framework. Sinfulness occurs when aid providers make an insufficient effort to match medical supplies with the expressed needs of aid recipients. In this framework, sending nonuseful things is akin to sending junk medical supplies overseas. In their testimonies, some TECH members even witnessed that they were "sinning" by "sending junk" overseas prior to their TECH involvement, evoking the transformation of the self characteristic of the testimony genre. I find especially notable how TECH members use the moral weight of sin to indicate that unethical aid is a form of disobedience to God. TECH infuses waste recovery efforts with an evangelical discourse that emphasizes the redemption found through an individual relationship with Jesus and personal accountability for one's actions. Through their moral scrutiny and even censure of contemporary aid approaches through a discourse of sin, TECH members suggest that they see their work as an enchanted landscape on which small battles between human sin and divine justice play out in a variety of decisions involving medical technologies.

Sinfulness and Moral Discourses of "Junk Aid"

Some IHM volunteers, like TECH leaders, explicitly connected junk medical supplies with human sinfulness. In a conversation one afternoon, Richard, a retired engineer and regular IHM volunteer who repaired equipment, likened storing junk in the warehouse to "keeping sin in you and not freeing it up." He added that the storage of junk was something that "kept [people] from receiving blessing." Richard's language attended to the way junk functions as a detrimental force, not merely a series of stationary, nonuseful commodity forms, but a social act that shapes the relationship between people working in the organization and God. Junk supplies blocked the blessing a person might receive for acquiring and storing items to send overseas. By linking junk analogously to sin kept inside the human body, Richard implied that the full effects of junk medical supplies may be obscured from view or unseen by volunteer laborers yet continue to be powerful nonetheless. It is interesting that, in Richard's estimation, the medical supplies that remained at the warehouse, without a certain purpose or destination, were already junk because of their nonusefulness. To hold items in abeyance would only verify their junk quality because their usefulness had not been readily identified. In some ways, it was the very ambiguity of their position in the circulation of medical supplies that had made them into junk. Because IHM draws volunteers from many Lutheran denominations, including those that assert the literal inerrancy of the Bible, those that embrace the charismatic gifts of the Spirit, and those that emphasize a social justice theology, not all volunteers used a language of sinfulness as Richard did to describe morally dubious aid practices. Nevertheless, IHM's and Malagasy Partnership's long-standing affiliation with TECH resulted in a situation where the moral censure of donor-centric aid provision was woven into the broader discourse of aid giving within the agencies.

This broader moral discourse was socially endorsed through a number of practices in which volunteers participated collectively. One way of specifying that the warehouse supplies were not junk was to designate them as divinely "called" things. At Malagasy Partnership, Gene stipulated on several occasions that the medical supplies packaged within the warehouse had been "called" by God and were not merely "sent" by a hospital, a pivotal distinction. On one snowy February evening in 2006, before the group prayer circle that concluded the evening's work session, Gene narrated the story of his interaction with a company that supplies the medical industry with Hemocue finger sticks, which are used to obtain blood samples for tests. Each small test kit (*cuvette*) costs about US$1.25, Gene explained, which makes it difficult for SALFA to stock all its clinics with an adequate number of kits. Gene emailed the manufacturing company to ask about the price and tacked on what he called a short description of Malagasy Partnership. A woman at the company replied by writing "that's a really neat organization" and offered the agency two boxes of two hundred finger sticks as a donation. Gene paused and then summarized plainly: "So God brought the Hemocues." On another occasion, also just before the evening prayer circle, Gene explained that he had recently received a list of "laboratory needs" from SALFA. Bulky laboratory equipment, however, had often posed a shipping problem because of its high freight costs. Gene scanned the Internet to locate a piece of equipment SALFA requested, and he happened to find a doctor on the neighboring island of Mauritius who was selling it. After being contacted by Gene, the man offered to ship the equipment for free to Madagascar, since he planned to send other materials there. Gene concluded with a tone of awe, "Just how God put that to-gether." Although both stories incorporated details about Gene's efforts to find suitable medical materials for SALFA, he diminished his own role and amplified the surprise and gift of the donations.

Gene reinforced the idea that the medical supplies were "called" rather than simply sent through elaborate stories that he would tell about each medical item. One evening two families from Gene's church, total-ing nine people, suddenly arrived at the warehouse during a regular work session. Gene provided the families with a brief tour and then brought all the volunteers together in the middle of the warehouse for introduc-tions and a short prayer session. As we crowded together in the few open spaces within the warehouse, Gene pointed out to the guests how "God has kept the warehouse busy" during the past few weeks. He gestured around us in a circle, saying that each large carton or crate facing us "has a story attached to it." Gene turned around, drawing our attention to the back of the warehouse. In front of a bulging pile of boxes that filled the space from ceiling to floor were a number of boxes that originally car-ried frozen french fries. They contained some 5,400 pairs of eyeglasses, Gene said, noting that they came to the warehouse through his response to a posting on the TECH website. Pointing still further in the arc he drew around us with his finger, Gene placed our attention on a stack of crutches atop another cardboard box on the second level of shelving. They would be sent to Madagascar, he said, for polio patients. By attach-ing stories to the supplies, Gene implicitly denuded the previous lives of the medical materials in the biomedical institution and accentuated their divinely orchestrated role in the aid program. Moreover, the stories played an instructional and interpretive role, since they included telling details about the ailments and programs for which they would be "used."

At IHM, perhaps because of the higher volume of medical materi-als, leaders like Mark did not often *singularize* each donation (Kopytoff 1986) and place it within a divinely orchestrated gift economy as Gene had done. In fact, Mark once explained that the most valued, godly di-rected supplies were often *not* visible at IHM because they had already been sent abroad. Moving a box to a warehouse shelf one morning, I found Mark there with a small metal cart, collecting items for a shipment to the Lutheran hospital in Ndolage, Tanzania. Practitioners at Ndolage had requested thousands of sutures for that week's shipment. I asked Mark whether IHM would actually supply all those sutures. Not at all, he said. The requested number is a hoped-for goal, which IHM is not

obliged to produce but "makes every effort to do so." Flipping through
the pages of the medical-supply tables in Ndolage's "needs list," Mark
pointed to orthopedic supplies. The requested numbers were in the single, or at most double, digits: for instance, five leg braces had been requested. Orthopedic supplies are present in high volume in the warehouse, Mark explained, but infrequently move in and out of the space:
they're simply not in high demand. Sutures, syringes, dressings, and bandages *are* in high demand but constitute a very small part of the overall
volume in the warehouse. In Mark's space calculus, built clearly on market notions of supply and demand, what can be seen in the warehouse
at any one time may simply be what is infrequently needed by overseas
medical practitioners.

At the time, I found this interesting because I often heard IHM volunteers speak positively of the *fullness* of the warehouse shelves; the
stacks of cardboard boxes and overflowing bins were taken as signs that
God had *provided*. Mark certainly didn't dissuade volunteers from this
view or completely denounce it himself, for in at least one group prayer
I heard him thank God for "providing" for the warehouse. For Mark,
though, market principles of supply and demand made certain supplies
less useful *and* less valuable, producing a graded scale of usefulness and
reinforcing a moral association between stasis and sinfulness. Like Richard mentioned earlier, to hold items in abeyance in the warehouse might
only be to verify their junk quality. In this calculation, medical discards
that circulated outside the warehouse gained value through mutually
reinforcing market and nonmarket valuations: market demand, the expressed needs of overseas clinicians, and godly provision. Though Mark
rarely expressed this aesthetic calculus, except to roving anthropologists,
it points to the agencies' diverse ways of conceptualizing the relationship
of "use" and "junk," as well as the different ways of perceiving godly direction among variously positioned workers.

In sum, although the aid agencies draw from broader, well-established
forms of Christian moral discipline, their work interestingly uses such
moral categories to regulate and refashion medical relief as a distinctly
evangelical Christian endeavor. The category of junk brings the potential
for moral backsliding into each aid transaction. Junk medical supplies
effuse the negative values and personal moral implications of nonusefulness, noncirculation, lack of care, and even sinfulness in medical-
supply acquisition. The sinfulness of junk medical supplies is an "absent
presence" that forms a crucial part of the two operations (Hethering-

ton 2004, 163). By representing the possibility of sin within each and every medical-supply transaction, medical aid workers coconstruct the religious value of nonjunk forms, make useful discards into embodiments of divine agency, and underscore their work of pursuing moral relations with Lutherans overseas. The discourse on the sinfulness of junk medical supplies indicates that the NGOs are not only identifying usefulness as a positive moral relationship between persons through things. They also extend and tie the process of medical relief to moral categories that establish negative values in these commodity exchanges. Moreover, through adherence to the TECH standards, the Lutheran agencies indicate that they are putting into place a category shift: waste forms are things to be redeemed (Hawkins and Muecke 2003) but only under certain circumstances. Differentiating among kinds of waste forms and practices and perceiving waste as a productive process are all central components of this ethical endeavor.

Conclusions

I have argued in this chapter that the medical relief endeavor stems from the aid agencies' reliance on medical property transfers and their active role in producing capital (tax credits) by assuming ownership of the trash of the medical industry. With each medical-supply acquisition, the organizations participate in a series of value conversions between two property regimes, medical property and charitable donation, and thereby rely on the medical system's categorization of the supplies as hospital waste in order to produce new uses for these things. The agencies' moral endeavor of supplying useful and needed things to their overseas partners entails a rigorous insistence that the medical materials are precisely *not* waste and a social distancing from the hospitals' classificatory scheme. In determining the usefulness of medical donations, the NGOs momentarily silence the hospital classification that resulted in their acquisition. Even this process, however, is plagued by further uncertainties: Will foreign Lutheran clinicians realize the supplies' use value identified by US Lutheran aid workers? The crisis in the materials' ontological status is produced by the NGOs' complex position at the intersection of several economies: the medical-supply industry, hospital adherence to theories of practitioner and patient risk, the moral economy of historical relations with Lutherans in former mission sites, and the "informal" economic channels of nongovernmental organizations. I suggest, therefore, that working with the medical supplies, assessing their usefulness or nonusefulness, and accentuating their potential use value is an ongoing and unresolved practice focused on building moral relationships with foreign Lutheran doctors while emptying medical discards of their relations to the US hospital system.

By sorting the medical materials and assessing their usefulness, Minneapolis aid workers socially negotiate, reject, and absorb the distributions of "goods" (property rights, charitable donations, biomedical tools, gifts, blessings) and "bads" (risks, liabilities, sins) evidenced in circulating medical technologies (Hayden 2004, 118; see also Verdery and Humphrey 2004). The religious practices of blessing and prayer are not completely separate pursuits from the circulation of medical technologies, nor merely attached to them, but for Americans play a prominent role in morally redeeming medical discards as social forms suitable for transnational aid. In making this argument, I have benefited from a growing body of scholarship that refutes popular views opposing religious and economic activities. I follow Simon Coleman (2004, 437) in arguing that such depictions mistakenly advance "narrowly secular assumptions about the autonomy of the economic sphere in Western social life." As Coleman (424) points out, these assumptions gain traction through a series of other related contrasts between short-term individual strategy and long-term relational moral responsibility and obligation; (secular) material returns and (sacred) nonmaterial forms of transcendence; and "religious hucksterism" involving money and more trustworthy dealings by religious leaders in the nonmarket realm. By focusing instead on processes of valuation and devaluation, I have pointed out that different kinds of economies play a role in regulating the transnational circulation of discarded and recovered medical technologies (e.g., the conferral of blessings for forms with identified use values). Indeed, we can see how economies of blessings and sins collude in transforming medical discards into suitable or unsuitable aid forms.

Throughout this chapter, I have sought to make the case that the aid warehouses are a particularly revealing crossroads, or "conversionary site" among disparate value regimes, understood here to include spiritual and ethical values rather than only capitalist exchange value. As the US Lutheran foreign mission movement came to a close, the two US Lutheran NGOs in Minneapolis filled a gap in global engagement vacated by the end of foreign missions and the deprofessionalization of the missionary vocation. NGOs, in particular, operate in the fabric of US Lutheranism as new kinds of converting sites that engage in a variety of transformative and potentially regenerative tasks involving waste forms. I suggest that these sites tie together social processes with spatial and temporal qualities. In significant ways, hospital discards constitute "products of time" or institutional "end products" that aid workers try to make into a new beginning by capturing their redeemable life and pressing them into a social future (Hawkins and Muecke 2003, xiv).

We can see that at the heart of aid workers' practices of salvaging, recovering, and sorting medical materials is also a social recognition of the connections between destruction and renewal. This process simultaneously carries historical, religious, and economic dimensions that ambiguously collude with one another and cannot be easily disentangled. By carving out a new ethical practice through their work with medical discards, Lutheran aid workers and former missionaries engage in a subtle process of converting their own practice and reforming it in relation to the negative image of other possible pasts. A heightened awareness exists that the NGOs occupy a space between multifarious economies, or a "gap moment . . . where value is yet to be decided" (Hawkins and Muecke 2003, xiii). This serves as a powerful synecdoche for the practice of an "economy of redemption" but also for making a break with the problems of a colonial past. In the next chapter, I follow the medical materials into the SALFA offices in Antananarivo, Madagascar, tracing how SALFA administrators engage them in further acts of revaluation. Building on the idea that Christians "convert" and press the value of discards into a variety of social projects, I show how accepting the discards is itself an act of value generation that, for individual SALFA administrators and the collective operation, selectively values ties with foreign donors.

CHAPTER FOUR

Restructuring Value in Antananarivo

Making one's way to SALFA's headquarters, perched high above much of Antananarivo in the neighborhood of Andohalo, requires a slow and circular ascent up several interwoven hills. From the city district of Tsiadana, where I was staying, I walk several blocks through dusty street vendor stalls and hail one of the city's cream-colored taxis. The small taxi slowly climbs the city's steep hills, carefully turning tight bends as shiny sport-utility vehicles and motorcycles speed downhill in the other lane. Hundreds of people, some leaving work briefly and others frequenting street-side market stalls, step precariously between the parked cars and the whizzing traffic. On occasion, as the taxi winds uphill behind minibuses emitting plumes of dark smoke, the taxi momentarily fills with the pungent odor of diesel before the black cloud dissipates in front of my eyes. SALFA's headquarters exist within a four-story brick building nestled on an Andohalo hillside. A pharmacy and clinic reside on the first floor and SALFA's administrative offices are divided between the upper levels and the basement. I spent the bulk of my time in these basement rooms and other SALFA offices, asking questions, tape-recording conversations, or discretely waiting as SALFA administrators answered telephone calls and coordinated tasks with a variety of coworkers who pop briefly into their workspaces.

SALFA is an umbrella organization serving all the medical clinics of the FLM, which total nine regional hospitals and thirty-nine dispensaries located across the island. As an arm of the FLM, SALFA occupies a unique space in the convergence of African Christianities and aid work. It acts as a central coordinating agency for foreign aid and grants, as well as supply and pharmaceutical purchases. SALFA uses preexisting national religious structures for the dissemination of foreign medical aid, taking part in and being transformed by practices of aid patronage and aid accountability common to other African-based NGOs. Yet it is arguably also a religious organization in its own right, propounding a spiritual vision of Christian medicine that is perhaps best encapsulated in the SALFA motto *Izahay mitsabo; Jesosy manasitrana*—"we treat (medically); Jesus heals."

This spiritual platform partly stems from SALFA's close relationship with the *fifohazana*, a charismatic Malagasy revival dating to 1894 that prioritizes holistic Christian healing. Through the efforts of FLM leaders, the revival's twentieth-century Prophetess Nenilava, and other revivalists, the *fifohazana* became part of the FLM in the late 1970s, receiving financial support from its evangelism department even as it nurtured transdenominational connections with other Protestant and Catholic churches in Madagascar. In helping to form SALFA in 1979, Nenilava, an Antaimoro Malagasy woman who lived from 1922 to 1998, made strategic employee placements and through her prophetic visions urged several SALFA employees, now senior staff, to become consecrated *mpiandry* (shepherds or lay preachers). Today, SALFA provides basic medical supplies, pharmaceuticals, some funding, and the assistance of SALFA physicians to the revival's two hundred *toby* (communal healing centers) across the island. Most *toby* are near SALFA dispensaries or district hospitals. Some doctors have suggested to me that *toby* visits cause them some frustration because they can delay patients from receiving necessary biomedical care. In these physicians' estimation, *toby* workers without medical training can erroneously prioritize spiritual treatments in cases where biomedical care is urgently needed. Still, a substantial number of SALFA employees working outside the capital city, including some physicians, are also *mpiandry* and do not appear to perceive a conflict between the *toby* and biomedical treatment.

Organizations like SALFA do not appear very much in the broader literature on African aid and development. Scholars have studied African churches primarily as institutional sites from which both religious and secular NGOs began emerging when structural adjustment reforms in African states favored distributing foreign aid to nonstate entities (Bornstein 2005; Ferguson 2006). Other accounts, such as James Pfeiffer's (2002) writing on faith-healing churches in Chimoio, Mozambique, illuminate how African Independent Churches, often considered to be separate from more established Protestant churches, treat a range of afflictions, including infertility and children's chronic illness, in a context of deepening inequality and the absence of other forms of social support (see also Comaroff 1985; Cole 2010; Piot 2010). Much research focuses on what scholars call Pentecostal-Charismatic Churches and African Independent Churches (see Gifford 1998; Meyer 2004) rather than the established, mainline Protestant churches, formerly considered mission churches. The FLM, however, is a mainline Protestant church that has had a long and often ambivalent relationship with the *fifohazana* movement, arguably a Pentecostal-Charismatic Church or an African Independent Church. The Antananarivo-based SALFA employees on whom I focus in this chapter participate in both the national promotion of institutionalized biomedicine and in charismatic Christian activities of prayer healing drawn from the *fifohazana* and do not perceive these pursuits as opposed or separate. To highlight SALFA's unique religious *and* humanitarian functions, as well as its position within an established church, I trace in this chapter and the next one how employees combine and pursue in their work diverse identifications as foreign aid brokers, administrators, revivalists, and church elites. This phenomenon is echoed across the various sites of the aid endeavor, as those involved in the United States and Madagascar, such as Pastor Gabriel in chapter 2, juggle multiple roles and relations.[1]

In what follows, I begin with a description of SALFA headquarters and an account of how SALFA employees weave US medical discards into SALFA's operations. I continue to approach work with medical discards in this chapter as a kind of "conversionary" work in which transforming discards' value is also a broader social project of shaping pasts and futures. Doing so enables us to better appreciate relief work as a culturally productive activity in which discards play a central, though culturally variable, role. After focusing on the specific activities of revaluing medical materials at the SALFA headquarters, I widen the analytical frame to describe how such valuation activities were disrupted and reoriented during the recent five-year political crisis in Madagascar (2009–13). The chapter gradually broadens its focus to illuminate how SALFA workers position their paid employment within more far-reaching religious and professional networks. I profile three SALFA employees to examine how they selectively foster and activate several distinct sets of affiliative ties, including foreign aid partnerships, congregational membership, public-private health partnerships, and lay involvement in the *fifohazana* movement.

Collectively, these ties can be analyzed as interlinked zones of classed potential and prosperity that play a central role in SALFA administrators' efforts to secure their class status. Scholars have pointed out that many emerging middle-class workers hold jobs as civil servants for the state or as bureaucrats in the development sector and have financial stakes in international aid flows (West 2002; Liechty 2003; Pfeiffer 2004; López and Weinstein 2012). Though global and domestic religious connections are infrequently analyzed as sites of cosmopolitanism and class fashioning (but see Werbner 2009), they should be considered part of an interwoven social landscape in Antananarivo through which SALFA aid workers solidify class-based aspirations. My overall aim in the chapter is to show how SALFA workers leverage foreign connections and other affiliative ties as both professional and personal sources of prosperity.

Revaluing Medical Discards in Antananarivo

As one of the largest not-for-profit systems of its kind in the world, SALFA consolidates medical donations and equipment from foreign donors like its two US NGO partners and also purchases some pharmaceuticals and supplies, tacking on a service fee for these items to each of its forty-eight member clinics. As described in the last chapter, these service fees collectively form a central part of SALFA's budget. When multiplied to account for the thousands of individual relief and discounted supply items that SALFA obtains annually, this small amount, which could be as low as 303 Malagasy *ariary* or US$0.11 for a single suture (ordinarily US$2–4 each), helps fund the central operation. In turn, individual SALFA clinics acquire these items from SALFA headquarters at a discount. Rather than spending an unsustainable portion of their hospital's budget on equipment and supplies, they can reserve revenue for basic operational expenses, such as staff salaries and building upkeep. Through this system of donations, individual clinics additionally conserve a greater portion of revenue derived from patient visits.

As private medical clinics, SALFA facilities charge patients 1,000–3,000 *ariary* per visit (or US$0.37 to $1.12), which varies by region and location, thereby passing on some operational costs to the patients. The costs are unquestionably prohibitive for many (e.g., Harper 2002, 165). SALFA clinics sometimes waive fees entirely, however, drawing from special foreign-funded grants for those unable to pay. I was also told of cases in which, in lieu of cash, rural SALFA clinics in southern Madagascar ac-

cepted payment for services in the form of zebu cattle. The SALFA structure is based on a nested system of revenue generation linking SALFA
headquarters and individual clinics. This model varies substantially in
practice, with some operational funds coming from donated relief items
and some from discounted, purchased supplies. The calculus depends
fully on what the US NGOs and other relief donation agencies send, as
well as whether individual SALFA clinics need and request those items.
Though medical discards play a significant role in SALFA's operation,
I explore in this section how SALFA employees in Antananarivo handle discards and infuse them with new value. Building on my analysis of
Americans' work with medical waste, described extensively in the previous chapter, my aim is to illuminate significant cultural differences in how
Malagasy Lutherans approach the aid program's trade in medical castoffs.

Comparing Malagasy and American Work with Medical Discards

Two basement rooms in SALFA's Andohalo headquarters are where
most of the donated medical materials from the United States and
elsewhere—items like syringes, sodium chloride solution, and catheters—
reside before being sent to individual SALFA clinics across the island.
SALFA also operates a dusty storage facility outside Antananarivo composed of decommissioned shipping containers filled with back stock such
as medical linens, orthopedic padding, and antiseptic solution for sur-
geries (see figures 3.1 and 3.2). By the time they reach Antananarivo
by truck, though, the medical materials have already been in Madagascar for a considerable period of time. The supplies begin their journey
in the eastern port city of Toamasina, where the shipping container arrives from the United States aboard a transatlantic ocean freighter. A
SALFA worker named Jeannine, stationed in Toamasina, handles the
government customs clearance for the shipping container. She attempts
to pay the customs fees and expedite the paperwork to get the container
released in a reasonable amount of time from Malagasy customs agents,
which is no small feat. In the meantime, security guards stand watch over
the container, a labor cost SALFA must absorb. This prevents the container's contents from falling into the port's lively black-market trade, a
risk that confirms the discards' potential economic value. Jeannine often
sends word by email to Malagasy Partnership when the container arrives,
because she is the first point of contact with the relief aid in Madagascar.
    The supply rooms inside SALFA headquarters in Andohalo are

where donated materials, as well as those purchased from medical and pharmaceutical discounters like the International Dispensary Association in the Netherlands, are assigned a small service fee in *ariary* to help fund SALFA. In many senses, this is the space in which the value of the medical supplies is further reconstituted, where values are selectively muted, amplified, or highlighted as part of the social process of reworking discarded materials. Although SALFA does not reinstate the supplies' full exchange value on the international market (what US donors call their "fair market price"), as mentioned earlier, it reignites their economic value by attaching a price that each clinic will pay. This economic value, marked on the items themselves, stands metonymically for the broader market worth of the medical supplies. The SALFA service fee resembles Guyer's (2004, 113) description of price, referring to fuel sales in Nigeria under Abacha's regime, as an aggregate open to "combination and permutation under crisis conditions." Yet, by charging only a portion of the supplies' actual market value, SALFA creates a small subsidiary market for its forty-eight medical clinics, which enables them to

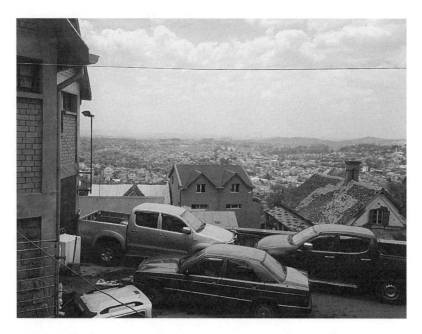

FIGURE 4.1. The SALFA parking lot with aid program cars, showing the view of Antananarivo from the hills of Andohalo.

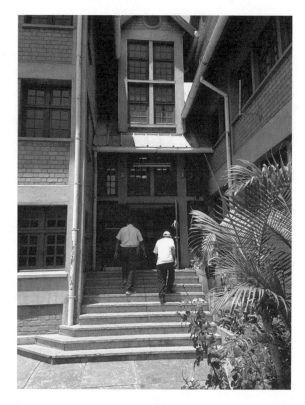

FIGURE 4.2. The main entrance to the SALFA headquarters building in Andohalo.

acquire materials many of them would otherwise not be able to afford. Occurring on a different scale from the international medical market, this microeconomic market simulates a kind of global medical commerce that does not otherwise exist, a more equitable form of medical-supply resourcing in which clinics can conceivably acquire the medical supplies necessary to serve their patients. Creating a donor-supported supply chain helps SALFA erect a firewall, so to speak, between its member clinics and the pricing mechanisms of global medical commerce. It prevents them from being bankrupted by the costs of equipment and basic medical materials or simply from losing the ability to access them.

Several differences are noteworthy when comparing the SALFA revaluation of the medical materials with US handling of the medical discards. In the initial SALFA processing of the donated medical materials, their sacred value as emblems and emissaries of the religiously motivated medical aid partnership are on the whole downplayed while their potential economic and clinical values are amplified. It is certainly the case that individual Malagasy Lutheran physicians may later view donated supplies as significant in religious or spiritual acts of biomedical healing. Although clinics treat patients regardless of religious affiliation, doctors in SALFA clinics are required to be committed Christians, and a substantial number are involved in the charismatic *fifohazana* movement, which focuses on healing as an important spiritual event. In my experience, however, employees at SALFA headquarters do not endow the individual medical discards with blessings or overtly call attention to their complex itineraries as evidence of a divine hand as do US aid workers.[2] In Antananarivo, the most immediate revaluation of the medical discards is clearly an economic one. Second, a process of clinical revaluation of the medical materials unfolds in conversations with individual Malagasy physicians at SALFA clinics across Madagascar in the months and years after receiving particular materials from the US NGOs. Most Minnesotan volunteers understand financial need as a general issue motivating the aid relationship, but they are largely unaware that the medical materials are economically revalued when they arrive in Madagascar.

These differences reveal how medical waste flows can absorb and be placed in the service of a diverse range of cultural and economic projects. At a deeper level, medical waste items exemplify the scholarly observation that material things linked to global commodity chains are continually reworked and even constitute different things across those sites (Thomas 1991; Keane 2003; Henare et al. 2007). They attain cultural meaningfulness and value from within diverse assemblages of knowledge, institutional protocols, expertise, and individual labor practices (Ong and Collier 2005). In drawing this contrast between American and Malagasy practices of valuing medical waste, I do not mean to imply a false separation between sacred and economic value, or between market and nonmarket realms of exchange. These are potential qualities of all material exchanges. As scholars have argued, however, such values are variously elaborated, pulled forward, pushed to the background, or muted across a variety of cultural activities, rather than uniformly present, because material things like discards shape and inflect specific social itineraries and contexts (Appadurai 1986; Myers 2001; Miller 2005).

Perhaps most surprising in view of the elaborate American handling of the medical discards, though, is the fact that the SALFA economic revaluation of the materials happens with little fanfare. Single SALFA employees, sometimes with assistants, work in the Andohalo supply room, stacking medical items on shelves, placing them in bags marked with a service fee in *ariary* or attaching to them a piece of paper with a handwritten fee per item. The storage facility on the outskirts of Antananarivo employs a security guard and a manager, whose desk sits inside a decommissioned shipping container. Doctors occasionally stop by the storage facility to acquire items for their SALFA clinics. In both cases, once US materials arrive and they are unpacked from the shipping container, with the exception of specially procured items or medical equipment, they are mixed in with the broader stock of SALFA medical materials, virtually indistinguishable from materials acquired through various other channels (e.g., the International Dispensary Association, other donors, specially purchased items from manufacturers). Clement, the SALFA financial officer and operations manager, determines the service fees to be attached to the medical materials, using a calculus of what individual SALFA clinics can pay, the market price of the supplies, and an evaluation of how many of the items are regularly needed in a clinic. He coordinates the stock and clinic orders with the storage facility manager and the SALFA storeroom clerk.

Unlike the work with discards that transpires in the two US NGOs, the revaluation of the materials at SALFA is not a collective activity in which individual laborers bear witness to their reconstitution as a social and ritual event. Rather, it is a labor process divided into separate components and performed in a variety of SALFA locations. Though SALFA employees work collaboratively on some tasks, such as clinic supply orders, their responsibilities vary considerably and work with medical discards from the United States is only one task among many that they perform. Furthermore, the uniqueness of US-donated items is often quickly lost, with the exception of special donations and large equipment, for discards appear the same as other supplies and SALFA does not maintain a system for tracking each item's origins. What I have described should make it apparent that Malagasy Lutherans do not necessarily value the discards *individually* as special tokens of their relations with the US NGOs. Nor do they predominantly ascribe qualities of sacredness or uniqueness to the individual medical relief items, as do the US laborers. Following the supplies into the SALFA headquarters in Antananarivo illustrates how discards have complex social itineraries that draw from diverse regimes of value. Discards can, of course, be reactivated as commodities even if they have been temporarily classified as having zero value (Kopytoff 1986). In certain respects, the medical discards have come full circle, having been "singularized" or "pulled out of their usual commodity sphere" in the United States, only to be pluralized once again as medical items with a clinical and economic value (Kopytoff 1986, 73–74).

Accepting as an Act of Value Generation

If Malagasy Lutherans do not necessarily value the *individual* discards as significant tokens of their relationship with their US brethren, how do SALFA employees perceive the trade in discards from the United States? If we approach the discard trade as a socially and culturally variable site of value conversion, as I have done in the previous chapter, how do SALFA employees position or put the discards to use in broader projects of value generation? I suggest that, for Malagasy Lutherans in SALFA headquarters, the moral redemption or even clinical value of discarded things matters less than the position of those things in a broader system of aid patronage. This runs counter to what might be expected at first glance: that the medical supplies will be valued first and foremost for their utility in clinics already short on supplies. The heterogeneity of the discards, however, results in a situation where each individual item may not be predictably valuable to Malagasy medical workers. Looking more closely at how SALFA operates reveals how Malagasy Lutherans accept the heterogeneous discards not only to help fund the SALFA operation, but also as an active move to create future value by sustaining ties with the two US NGOs.

Like many medical systems in sub-Saharan Africa, SALFA balances multiple donors, which include both faith-based and secular organizations, multilaterals, and even individual families. It has built a thick web of foreign partnerships so that, should a grant end or funding priorities change, SALFA's medical centers will not be left without support. Though some of its foreign partners changed, of course, between 2000 and the present, in 2014 SALFA had partnerships with no fewer than thirty-three technical and financial donors, including Médecins du Monde, Global Fund, United Nations Population Fund (UNPF), Norwegian Mission Society, European Development Fund, the ELCA, and USAID. The US aid organizations were among its first foreign partners, but SALFA has quickly diversified its donor organizations in order to gain access to different kinds of materials, funding, and technical aid. Though many donors, such as the Global Fund and Lutheran World Federation, support a range of clinical and technical programs, others underwrite specific initiatives. UNPF, for instance, provided funds and computer equipment for a specific pilot project in five medical centers that will collect statistical information on SALFA's patients and clinical procedures. Some donor agencies are small and specialized. They include Hover Aid, an organization that sends doctors and technicians to hard-to-reach rural areas by hovercraft. Other partners, such as the UN's World Food Programme, address issues of community public health. Among its established financial and technical partners, SALFA also hosts six US-based physicians who do volunteer stints in Malagasy clinics, including one who teaches in a Midwest US medical school and has on occasion led teams of US medical school students on rotations in SALFA clinics.

Through my field research in SALFA headquarters, I noticed that Malagasy clinicians and administrators continually drew attention to the future, rather than necessarily present, value of their donor relationships. The SALFA financial officer Clement, for instance, once noted that, as Chinese-manufactured products began to flood the market in Madagascar in the 2000s, secondhand US-made medical supplies emerged as more reliable and durable than their Chinese counterparts. The US medical equipment's value interestingly reinforced his view of the long-term durability of SALFA's US donor ties. When I visited Clement in Antananarivo in October 2014, SALFA had just begun a twelve-month audit program with USAID, which Clement saw as a thinly veiled proving ground. USAID has also visibly expanded its presence in Malagasy organizations since the mid-2000s and he hoped SALFA could convert this time-limited trial into a more sustained and profitable partnership. Adhering to the audit program became, in Clement's eyes, not only a test of SALFA's reliability for big donors, but also a forum in which to prove SALFA's value of those partnerships. The hope for future collaborations here is as much a resource as the US medical discards.

Other SALFA medical workers find they must creatively seize ties with funders to convert one form of support into something more enduring. Dr. Andry is a gregarious and warm Betsileo man with a booming voice that sometimes rivals the volume and stylized enunciation of a pastor. He appears to be in his late fifties, with only a hint of white in his hair. Formerly SALFA's technical director, he now oversees the organization's role in the islandwide *Projet Tuberculose*. SALFA clinics treat thirty-five hundred people with tuberculosis each year, out of the twenty thousand total tuberculosis patients treated annually in Madagascar. When the tuberculosis project's initial funder, the Norwegian Development Authority (NORAD), rescinded its support in 2005–6, the Global Fund stepped in as a new patron. Since 2009, Dr. Andry has served on the fund's Country Coordinating Mechanism, or national overseeing structure. Though Dr. Andry began his career working in SALFA clinics in various regions of the island, his livelihood now depends on large-scale global health patrons like the Global Fund. One day, as I was eating my lunch outside the SALFA building, I could not help noticing Dr. Andry drive up in a shiny, white, late-model pickup truck, a "Fonds Mondial" (Global Fund) placard prominently placed on the driver's door. Program perquisites like trucks, cars, and computers are certainly necessary for the tuberculosis project, which requires Dr. Andry to do regular clinic visits across Madagascar. But they also enable local liaisons like him to turn their often fleeting attachment with these projects into something longer-lasting.

What I have described so far may give the impression that it is the policies and priorities of the global health patrons on which SALFA relies that determine its current approach to foreign funders. This is partly true, but it overlooks the active role Malagasy aid workers play in selectively valuing those relationships and aid resources. SALFA's ties with the two US NGOs stretches back to its inception in 1979, before it developed relationships with large global health donors. My Malagasy informants, however, characterized SALFA's more-than-twenty-five-year partnership with the two US NGOs as a set of ties nurtured for what they *could* produce rather than necessarily for the valuable things that they *did* produce. I would suggest that this approach underscores a Malagasy cultural emphasis placed on valuing foreign ties as resources that bear future potential, or as relationships with conditional value.

Clement, Dr. Andry, and another SALFA informant, Mr. Rajoanary, each separately observed that the sea containers they received from the United States in the early 1980s were not initially dedicated solely to SALFA's medical needs but were partitioned for US missionary families still living in Madagascar and Malagasy living in the United States who wanted to send things home. This arrangement changed by the late 1980s with the departure of most US missionary families. Many of the supplies sent through the aid partnership were clinically and economically useful for SALFA, particularly medical equipment and basic supplies like syringes and gloves. Containers still included things that could not be used, however—or at least not immediately—requiring a storage facility in Antananarivo. The storage facility itself underscores this view of the supplies' stored or anticipated—though not necessarily current—value. Even if Malagasy clinicians *did* later find some medical materials to be discards, the broader ties of which they were a part imbued the transaction with value. It was the future market value and anticipated use of other supplies, as well as the potential for support provided through these ties, that made the connections valuable, rather than only what was contained in any particular shipping container.

Further evidence to support this interpretation of the way SALFA employees view the value of the supplies is their long-standing awareness that the medical discards are often not procured to meet Malagasy clinical needs but are acquired by the US NGOs on the basis of convenience and availability. One day Clement and I were talking in his office about the tax credits US hospitals and manufacturers accrue when they make a donation to one of the two US NGOs. He asked me when I had pieced together this commodity chain, and I described how it had gradually become clear in 2006 when I was working at the US NGOs. With a flicker of delight, Clement said that it was an incident in 1991 that had revealed this aspect of the aid program to him. SALFA had received some expired drugs from Malagasy Partnership, which were, as he put it, still viable and of better quality than what was available within Madagascar. The World Health Organization, however, along with several prominent aid organizations and multilaterals as signatories (including the Churches' Action for Health of the World Council of Churches), issued guidelines in 1990 that discouraged agencies from sending expired drugs as medical aid or even those within a year of their expiration date.[3]

When SALFA continued to receive some expired medicines in subsequent shipments after 1990, Clement asked Gene, the Malagasy Partnership founder, and the other agency leaders why this was the case. In Clement's recollection, they made the arrangement because a large manufacturer had wanted to donate the medications.[4] This incident impressed upon Clement that the power of the US NGOs to control the flow of resources was limited. It made even clearer to him how difficult it was for Malagasy Lutherans to set aid priorities even if their US partners actually desired to send only things that they needed. Gene himself observed to me that, because of global inequalities in institutionalized medicine, items that are the highest priority in Madagascar, such as syringes, blood pressure cuffs, and bandages, were often the most infrequently received by Malagasy Partnership, because they were also in high demand in US hospitals. Having been purchased for the "highly capitalized" environment of US institutional medicine (Livingston 2012, 66), the majority of Malagasy Partnership donations, Gene said, are appropriate mainly for SALFA's surgical centers, located mostly in Malagasy cities. In short, the organizations did not necessarily set their own aid priorities. Often those priorities were set by large manufacturers or hospitals that, for reasons of convenience, may wish to make a sizable donation. Incidents like this underscored the idea among SALFA administrators that the discard trade brought them a heterogeneous set of materials that were not always of immediate value for Malagasy Lutherans.

By accepting and revaluing the discards, Malagasy Lutherans contribute to the broader set of medical commerce transactions that Clement and I discussed (and which I outlined in the previous chapter). Such transactions enable US hospitals to revalue medical discards as charitable donations and, perhaps above all, absorb risk deemed undesirable for US health care institutions. Malagasy Partnership and IHM export not only medical goods but also financial and epidemiological risk, a social "bad" (Hayden 2004, 118). This uneven global distribution of risk maintains a two-tier structure of global medicine that upholds a form of cosmopolitan or prestige medicine in the United States and its legal regime (DelVecchio Good 2001, 396). Risk is an object of active reduction in US health care, but, through this medical-legal regime, Malagasy institutionalized medicine is less explicitly characterized as an inherently risky proposition or practice in which patient risk is normalized. Elizabeth Povinelli (2006, 32) refers to this as the geophysical distribution of ordinary and exceptional life, death, bodies, and illnesses: a form of "biosocial spacing" based on profoundly unequal presuppositions about intentional and unintentional harms. Together, the medical commerce transactions I have described create a global topography of medicine characterized by inequality in medical resources and unequal access to prestige or cosmopolitan medicine, even as the aid program seeks to address such inequalities. Part of what I have suggested here, however, is that, as with US aid workers, the value of these transactions is often understood by Malagasy Lutherans in other ways, that is, not merely through the dominant market or biosocial perspective.

I observed that part of making hospital waste from the United States valuable is negotiating incongruities between the present economic and clinical value of those discarded goods and the future potential value of their US aid relationship. Malagasy Lutherans in Antananarivo work across, and attempt to reconcile, these two incongruous time scales as they value US medical discards. Although they recognize some medical donations as clinically and economically useful, they also contend with a number of items that are not immediately useful or economically profitable. By storing them and forestalling their movement back into the social category of trash, SALFA employees retain a connection with the US donor organizations. They position value itself in this process as not merely something that adheres in, or refers primarily to, the medical discards, as in common market notions of use value or exchange value (discussed in the previous chapter). Instead, value also manifests through cultural understandings and mechanisms of conditional *value in relationships*, negotiated in this case through the collective lot of medical discards.

Malagasy Lutherans regularly face the entrenched hierarchies of value in global medical resourcing, which results in SALFA being given institutional castoffs and things deemed past or obsolete for US medicine. What I have suggested is that, in this deeply unequal context, SALFA employees partly seize value for their operation in slowing institutional cycles of use and disposal and holding medical waste in abeyance. This points to an active Malagasy form of value generation that challenges common portraits of Africans in the receiving "shadows" of international aid flows (Ferguson 2006), while also appreciating the challenging and intricate work performed at the margins of global medical commerce. Cultural activities of valuing are often a nexus of intersecting valuation scales with different time orientations (Munn 1992; Frow 2003; Guyer 2004), and individual actors frequently must make sense of their competing demands, persuasiveness, and shortcomings. Specifically, as Malagasy aid workers organize value in accepting medical waste flows, they are intricately working through temporal incongruities between the present value of those things and the future potential of their value as it may be later realized.

Cultural Views of Faith-Based Aid as Interdependency

Examining the circulation of medical discards from the United States to Madagascar unveils a revealing set of contrasts in how discards are valued and positioned in broader projects of social reproduction. The

Malagasy aid workers in my research consistently positioned the circulated discards as a sometimes-valuable commodity chain, situated within a potentially much more valuable foreign partnership. Although US aid workers tended to emphasize the value of their aid relations through the value of the things they handle, Malagasy administrators tended to view value as a function of the perpetuation of ties with foreign NGOs. I choose to interpret these views not as dichotomous because, in fact, qualities of each pervade the other but rather as a differently placed cultural emphasis. The differential value of medical discards—and the various ways value itself is culturally apprehended—stems partly from Malagasy and Americans' unequal positions in global medical commerce and also from their distinct ways of recognizing their historical relations with each other.

In making this argument, I do not wish to minimize the precariousness of medical resources in Malagasy clinics that underpins the aid relationship. Indeed, in the wake of political upheaval, the devaluation of the *ariary*, and other effects of structural adjustment programs, Malagasy Lutheran clinics are certainly in a position in which they have little choice but to look to foreign ties to sustain their operations. What we see in the SALFA headquarters is echoed across many clinics in sub-Saharan Africa, where the evisceration of state services demanded by structural adjustment programs compels health care systems to rely heavily on foreign donations and private partnerships (Pfeiffer 2003; Ferguson 2006; Crane 2013). As with the health care workers in Mozambique that Pfeiffer describes, Malagasy Lutherans must creatively maintain ties in a broader system of health care featuring "fragmentation caused by disjointed aid projects" (2003, 734). Although we can see how SALFA, like other African health care NGOs, participates in an "aid-specific patronage system" (732), I have chosen to take the perspective of SALFA employees here to show the maintenance and valuation of such ties as an active cultural practice that is variously organized across social and historical settings.

This approach follows other recent scholarship on humanitarian aid that has been unsettling the notion that the act of receiving aid is necessarily a passive, dependent, or subordinate practice, as receiving aid has been frequently generalized in relation to giving aid. Recent work emphasizes the need for contextualizing aid in historically and culturally variable systems of interdependency (James 2010; Scherz 2014; Klaits 2017). In Frederick Klaits's (2010) ethnography of caregiving in

Gaborone, Botswana, church members regarded aid giving during the HIV–AIDS pandemic as a practice of compassionate love. Klaits argues that Baitshepi church members led by the charismatic MmaMaipelo perceive *tumelo* (faith) as a moral exercise of maintaining and nurturing interdependence with others in times of suffering. In China Scherz's (2014) work, Ugandan Catholic nuns pursue aid giving for children orphaned by HIV–AIDS as a social relationship specific to historically established systems of Bugandan patronage. Scherz has pointed out that analyses of humanitarian aid and development frequently assume an inherent "poison" in the charitable gift. That is, by making a one-size-fits-all cultural argument that systems of dependency are inherently negative or subordinating, commentators on humanitarian aid may overlook how historically shaped systems of patronage can lead people to view interdependence positively, or at least as a relationship with forms of cultural flexibility for both parties. Such is the case in Scherz's Ugandan research, where patrons have historically competed for clients and where a plurality of patronage opportunities afforded clients considerable cultural maneuver, as they were thought to actively "join and leave a chief" (Scherz 2014, 21). Scherz has argued that relations with God are often positioned by Ugandan Christians as a related form of patronage, as God protects and provides for Christian believers.

Moreover, in her studies among Sakalava in the Analalava region of Madagascar's northwest coast, anthropologist Gillian Feeley-Harnik (1986, 1991) has argued that people forge interdependencies with various "masters," which can include "their own ancestors or those of their neighbors, merchants and government functionaries and royalty" (1991, 157). Although the specific cultural practices of Sakalava villagers are in many ways different from that of SALFA's mostly Merina Protestant staff in Antananarivo, SALFA employees similarly identify distinct yet interlinked sources of power and prosperity that they nurture. These include their individual congregations, Bible study groups, office networks, paid employment, and the SALFA-endorsed web of foreign Christian and multilateral donor connections. A common thread running through these activities is an emphasis on God as one who protects and provides, one to whom credit is ultimately due for health, security, and advantageous connections with others. Prevalent Malagasy Christian theologies of healing and medicine, which shape SALFA's operations and underpin all prayer healing among the *mpiandry* on SALFA's staff, repeatedly portray God as the provider of health and well-being. As Malagasy Lutheran theologian Péri Rasolondraibe (1998, 140) asserts in a discussion of the *fifohazana*'s treatment methods, Malagasy Christians primarily attribute the ultimate success of healing, including medical treatment, to "God's healing power," because God is understood as advising "doctors in their diagnoses and [blessing] the medicine prescribed." Reflecting this understanding, the healing treatments pursued by revivalists, which include prayer healing and exorcism, are referred to as "the work of support and strengthening or empowering" (*asa sy fampaherezana*), which seeks to access and channel divine power.

In line with this broader cultural notion that God is a powerful source of prosperity in Christians' lives, some SALFA workers make it explicitly clear that, to them, it is ultimately God who is the patron of their aid partnership with aid workers in the United States. From this perspective, Americans act merely as vessels or instruments of divine agency, a position amply supported by IHM promotional language. Though it is clear to all parties that the US NGOs supply SALFA with medical relief items and financial support, SALFA employees and NGO volunteers alike continually and deliberately emphasize God's role as provider in the aid program. I sometimes observed that, in their correspondence with the US NGOs, Malagasy Lutherans would assert that it was US aid workers who had *received* a gift in the aid partnership, not the reverse. In a December 2005 message to Malagasy Partnership volunteers, Clement wrote, "Thank you for bringing love and life to the patients whom you do not always see but whom God gives to you to [take] care of." Here, Clement subtly reminds his US partners that they are beholden to God. He suggests that US aid workers should recognize Malagasy patients and clinics not as the recipients of US gifts, but rather as a special gift from God *to* US aid workers. This makes US aid workers themselves into clients and receivers of gifts for which they must be grateful to God. I address the limits of this dual subjectivity posed through accountability work in chapter 6. It is important, however, not to view this perspective as merely rhetorical window dressing on an inherently unequal relationship of dependency, but rather as a more multifaceted system of patronage or interdependency in which both Americans and Malagasy can exist as clients. Pointing to God as a patron of US aid workers is a potent reminder of the diverse and shifting positions from which power and authority are organized in faith-based aid.

Perspectives on SALFA as a Church Organization in Transition

Like many other Malagasy organizations, SALFA underwent significant hardship after the 2009 coup d'état in Madagascar and its five-year
aftermath. During those years, the coup government established a transitional regime and foreign multilaterals increasingly halted foreign aid
to Madagascar to protest the postponement of democratic elections. In
2009 Andry Rajoelina, a thirty-five-year-old local radio disk jockey and
entrepreneur who was then the mayor of Antananarivo, gained enough
military and popular support after months of increasingly public criticism of the current government to overthrow President Marc Ravalomanana (2002–9). National elections were finally held in Madagascar in
late 2013, and a new president, Hery Rajaonarimampianina, whom many
view as a Rajoelina supporter, was elected. The five-year political crisis had taken a severe toll, however, on the national health care system
and other public services because of diplomatic and economic aid sanctions that were leveled against Rajoelina's regime. In 2010 government
expenditure on health care fell 30 percent from its 2009 level, a process
that continued in 2011–12 and resulted in the closure of many community health centers ("Health-Madagascar" 2012).

These sanctions affected part of SALFA's programs, but certainly
not all of them, because many multilaterals and NGOs (including Malagasy Partnership and IHM) continued to send humanitarian aid, which
is allocated separately from long-term economic and development assistance. Nonetheless, the coup significantly weakened SALFA's financial
viability in these years, and Clement referred to 2009–11 in particular as
a time of "crisis." The coup government charged exorbitant customs fees
for shipping containers in these years, partly to refill government coffers emptied by the suspension of foreign aid, which had constituted up
to 40 percent of the government's budget before the 2009 coup (Rabary
2014). The customs fees made it difficult for SALFA employees to collect shipping containers in Toamasina in order to import the donated
medicines and supplies that made its operation viable. As a time that
saw the agency come close to collapse, the 2009–14 period emerged in
my 2014 conversations with SALFA employees as a pivotal, transitional
era for them.

SALFA Administrators and Middle-Classness

SALFA administrators' efforts to develop and nurture a range of affiliative ties can be seen in this somewhat precarious economic and political context not only as efforts to sustain the organization, but also as attempts to maintain and secure their social status. As bureaucrats in a church-based organization, SALFA employees' salaries do not afford lifestyles of free-wheeling consumerism nor—with their reliance on foreign grants, the devaluation of the Malagasy *ariary*, and support for kin—do their salaries keep them from periods of debilitating economic insecurity. When combined with their relatively stable professional jobs, however, other practices do work toward socially communicating and securing for them a kind of middle-classness. As social scientists have argued, class is not based simply on fixed indicators like household income or parental (historically, the father's) occupation. Rather, as Liechty (2003, 15–16) terms it, class identity is a "constantly renegotiated cultural space—a space of ideas, values, goods, practices, and embodied behaviors."

Forms of class distinction thus emerged quietly, but persistently, in my interactions with SALFA administrator elites. They are avid consumers of various media, such as international television programs, websites, and social media like Facebook, with several "friending" me online within a day or two of our first meeting. Most have lived briefly in or traveled to cities such as London, Minneapolis–St. Paul, and Paris or have been visiting dignitaries to churches in Papua New Guinea, Malaysia, and Norway. All have college educations, which they have leveraged for professional positions in SALFA and other aid organizations. Many are fully trilingual in Malagasy, French, and English. These personal and professional qualities arguably fashion them as cosmopolitans, in the sense of being people who build and wield symbolic and political resources through their influential, though also limited, role in global capital flows and global religious communities (Hannerz 2004; Werbner 2009; Theodossopoulos and Kirtsoglou 2013). As I will show in the next section, SALFA employees shore up social capital through a nexus of religious and humanitarian affiliations, such as their ties to Nenilava, foreign aid agencies, leadership positions in Antananarivo congregations, and public-private health partnerships. These forms of social capital arguably help SALFA administrators maintain their social status as middle-class cosmopolitans, and they provide further opportunities to secure economic resources, as I explore in the next chapter (Bourdieu 1983).

Three Employee Profiles

In this section, I profile three SALFA employees, each of whom has pursued different job responsibilities at SALFA that afford distinct views of the organization. Their different perspectives reinforce the basic idea that aid organizations do not espouse uniform missions but, in practice, often exhibit radically different notions among their employees about the goals and functioning of the organization (just as I argued in chapters 2 and 3 for the US NGOs). These various points of view, including different opinions about SALFA's "crisis" of 2009–11, emerge from and reinforce the employees' distinctive biographies, personal experiences, and roles within the organization. Through these profiles, it is possible to see individual SALFA employees as multidimensional actors, that is, as revivalists, church members, children, parents, spouses, and aid workers. Indeed, sometimes the events they narrate take on religious overtones, their tellers emphasizing spirituality in remembering times of personal difficulty and challenged faith. At other times, overt, recognizable texts of spiritual testimony fade to the background as SALFA workers construct themselves as administrative professionals fluent in the bureaucratic discourse of the medical aid world, itself an economic resource (Irvine 1989; Sodikoff 2012, 88).

I conceptualize SALFA employees' narratives within these profiles as *valuation activities* that substantiate ties of interdependency with a range of sources of authority and prosperity. SALFA workers' stories loop through the sources of strength and prosperity in their lives—their families, foreign partnerships, church congregations, paid employment, connections to Nenilava, and public-private health initiatives—but also position these relationships as interdependencies that can sap vitality and result in personal trials, hardship, and jealousy from others. Narrative reflection enables SALFA employees to link valuation scales, that is, to revisit the terms and disempowering dimensions of various affiliative ties, such as those to the SALFA workplace or to foreign aid partners, and to recast them in a broader valuation framework of connection to God through life's trials (Ochs and Capps 2001, 242–43). Narrative acts, in turn, shape the subjectivity of SALFA workers in multifaceted ways, drawing from the diverse areas of their religious and professional networks in a kaleidoscopic fashion. In the following profiles, I use different naming conventions for each person that reflect my different degrees of social intimacy and familiarity with them.

I. CLEMENT   The financial officer Clement is a tall Merina man who appears to be in his fifties and exudes friendliness and warmth. He has a balanced manner, wanting to work problems over from many sides and seek alternative perspectives. Since I first met him in 2005, his black hair has become mottled with white, something he attributes to SALFA's "painful" crisis in 2009–11, which paralleled Madagascar's 2009 coup. Atop a bookcase behind the desk in Clement's Antananarivo office stands an International Dispensary Association calendar bearing the English-language tagline "Making health care affordable." Beside it is a handmade plaque that reads *"Jehovah otoroy ny lalan' ny didinao aho,"* from Psalms 119:33 ("God's way is my command" in English).[5]

Clement was born in Antananarivo but spent part of his childhood in Asoanala in southern Madagascar, where his parents were public school teachers. Their assignment in Asoanala lasted only a few years, however, and Clement mainly grew up in the highland town of Antsirabe, his parents' hometown. At eighteen, Clement moved to the capital and completed his military service, which, in his parents' tradition, involved working as a schoolteacher in rural communities. He then went to the university, where he was admitted to study economics, though he had harbored dreams of becoming a doctor. After obtaining his bachelor's degree, Clement ran out of money and, with four sisters and three brothers, knew he could not expect any additional financial support from his parents. At twenty-two, he took a job at the Banky Fampandrosoana ny Varotra bank headquarters in Antananarivo but left the job after two months because he found the work boring. After someone asked whether he might want to work for the church—something he seriously considered after watching the struggles of his parents in public service—he visited SALFA headquarters with a curriculum vitae, where he was interviewed by Dr. Fosse, a Madagascar-born US missionary doctor. Displaying his trademark precision, Clement told me he was hired at SALFA on October 31, 1987. He began by reorganizing the medical stockroom and for the next fifteen years worked his way through the office hierarchy to become chief financial officer in 2002.

Clement and I talked about SALFA on multiple occasions. Drawing on his twenty-seven years with the organization, Clement described how he saw SALFA develop and the central role he played in this process. After only one year as a stockroom clerk, he was put in charge of organizing SALFA's much larger medical surplus system, with responsibility for nurturing relationships with foreign medical donor organizations like Malagasy Partnership and IHM. He served in that capacity for twelve years until he was abruptly let go during a dispute between SALFA and the FLM in 2000.

The dispute stemmed from the fact that Dr. Fosse, the Norwegian American missionary physician who was SALFA director at that time, had wanted to leave Madagascar and fully hand leadership of the organization over to Malagasy nationals. Indeed, he had been trying to do so since SALFA was formed in 1979 and had begun to line up several technicians and administrators to prepare for his departure. He found funds to sustain SALFA in his absence, for his salary had been paid by the ELCA, and identified someone as a good candidate for the director position. After months of informal negotiations, he submitted his successor's name for approval to the FLM board. Dr. Fosse, Clement, and other SALFA employees were keenly aware at the time that SALFA needed a good technical and administrative team to move forward; otherwise it could fail as an organization.

The church leaders, however, refused Dr. Fosse's suggested replacement. Dr. Fosse asked Clement—although the FLM had technically fired him—to continue managing SALFA's funds and to stay on at the SALFA office. When Dr. Fosse finally left Madagascar, the FLM replaced him. Clement and Dr. Fosse viewed this appointee as unqualified. After only a year in the position, the new director was suspected of embezzling funds and was forced to resign. The ELCA temporarily suspended its relationship with the FLM while an audit was performed. In 2002 the church appointed a new director, Mr. Rajoanary, who had worked with SALFA and the FLM for more than twenty years. Clement became the financial officer.

This incident seemed to me astonishing enough, but Clement went on to describe SALFA as a workplace that has been plagued by dissension since 2002. In 2008, a long-simmering conflict he had with Mr. Rajoanary picked up steam. The conflict stemmed from their differing perspectives on the future of SALFA, which appear to have hinged on a cluster of issues, but especially on the degree to which SALFA should either espouse more of a business model (Mr. Rajoanary) or continue with an updated version of its long-standing nonprofit revolving fund structure (Clement).[6] The issues seem to have been exacerbated by the fact that both Clement and Mr. Rajoanary claimed expertise in finances and accounting, with Mr. Rajoanary having served as FLM treasurer before being appointed director of SALFA.

Nonetheless, the conflict was broader than one between the two men. It came to divide the body of SALFA employees. Clement described SALFA as steeped in conflict in those years, though it wasn't entirely clear whether he meant that Mr. Rajoanary had nurtured a divisive workplace through his managerial style, whether other employees contributed to the factionalism of the administrative and philosophical conflict, or a combination. Clement attempted to resign three times during this period, but people came forward each time to push him to withdraw his resignation. The conflict ended when the former director, Mr. Rajoanary, resigned in 2010. Since then, SALFA has recommitted itself as a not-for-profit organization with a revolving fund and has taken part in a variety of audit programs (including the USAID program mentioned earlier) for self-evaluation in communication, finance, and human resources.

All this made Clement's twenty-seven years with SALFA somewhat remarkable to me. It would be difficult for anyone to last through such personal and protracted workplace turmoil. It was also hard for me to imagine Clement in these acrimonious conflicts. I have known him as reserved, warm, quietly humorous, and even-tempered. Perhaps even more surprising was the fact that, unprompted, Clement suggested I speak with Mr. Rajoanary and promptly dialed him up. Clement said that Mr. Rajoanary had a different perspective on SALFA that would be valuable to my research. Perhaps sensing my surprise at this gesture, he assured me that he has had to try to let go of their past conflict. What emerged across these conversations was that Clement espoused a kind of faith *in* SALFA. The organization and its struggles operated as a test of faith for him, or something that bolstered Clement's own commitment to God. During the conflict with Mr. Rajoanary, he prayed regularly and read the Bible with a group of friends. He found strength in his leadership role in his home congregation, the Ambatovanaky church in Andohalo, where he is a deacon.

As a third-generation Lutheran, Clement said his parents provided a strong example of faith. His mother taught him to pray for others and his parents formed part of a small church group in Antsirabe. They and other congregants attempted to do neighborhood improvement projects in their town quarter. Watching his parents repeatedly challenged to enact change in their neighborhood, he said, prepared him for the struggles he would face at SALFA. He said he believes that SALFA came through the 2009–11 crisis because of God's protection. He feels God was watching over him and SALFA during this difficult period and ensured that SALFA would not dissolve because of its spiritual importance. By this, Clement seemed to imply that SALFA was formed with important ties to the *fifohazana* and the Prophetess Nenilava. He also seemed to suggest that SALFA has a kind of spiritual role in the movement, a unique purpose of providing holistic medical care that combines Christian spiritual counsel and biomedicine. Some of the workplace conflicts that Clement described thus began to look slightly more like a spiritual testimony or witness to me, and some of our conversations took on a confessional tone. Tracing God's role in shaping SALFA's path through this period of turmoil enables Clement to understand his position within a much larger spiritual plan to which he must relinquish control.

Clement and his wife have been married since 1992 and they have three children. Two of their sons are now in college and their youngest, a ten-year-old girl, is still in school. One son is currently in medical school, and another is studying communications and marketing. Clement and I brainstormed lists of the various directions where these areas of study could lead, because he was interested in what I have seen among university students in the United States. Clement was understandably apprehensive that his sons would not find employment unless they chose occupations carefully. Spending time with his family outside SALFA, I saw his relationship with his sons as close and congenial. When I accompanied them to church services at Ambatovanaky, his sons—dressed in slacks, shirts, and ties—kept watch over their younger cousins in the adjacent pew. Whispering across the pew during breaks in the almost three-hour service, they quietly pressed me for information about US television, especially the drama *Bones* that features a physical anthropologist. Clement looked on with a mixture of bemusement and pride.

As a middle-class college graduate and administrator in Antananarivo, Clement clearly has resources at his disposal that few Malagasy do. It was clear that, perhaps because of a class-inflected sensibility of achievement and success, he invests considerable energy to help his children build more secure paths forward. This characteristic seems to parallel his future-oriented approach to SALFA. When taken together, it is possible to see how SALFA workers like Clement actively negotiate for themselves and their children a precarious middle-class space, which inflects and reinforces their position amid Malagasy political and ethnic hierarchies as well as transnational NGO networks. Many SALFA employees take combating inequality in Malagasy access to health care as their professional aim, building on the Prophetess Nenilava's teachings about the spiritual value of aid to the poor. Yet, amid sustained economic insecurity in Antananarivo, SALFA employees and their children also seemed understandably ambivalent, both enchanted by and critical of overt markers of class difference.

II. JOSETTE R.   Josette runs a relatively new IHM in-country office in Antananarivo and supervises an IHM-funded project called AVIA (Antanosy Villages Integrated Actions). Located in Andohalo near SALFA headquarters, Josette's highly organized office is a large, high-ceiled room with a modern design and new-looking furniture. It features a conference room table, Josette's desk, and several bookcases. "IHM Tana" (Tana is short for Antananarivo) stickers mark each item, to identify the NGO's property (see figure 4.3). Long curtains frame the room's tall windows, and potted plants brighten the space. On a wall under the clock hangs a set of carved wooden letters vertically spelling out *Velona Jesosy* (Jesus lives). Josette is a petite woman who appears to be in her late fifties. She seems reserved, speaking quietly and slowly at first, but she gradually warms to particular subjects, especially the Good News of the Gospel (*vaovao mahafaly*), a subject about which she is clearly passionate.

Josette is a consecrated *mpiandry* in the *fifohazana* whose family has had close ties with the revival. The Prophetess Nenilava actually knew Josette's parents but worked particularly closely with Josette's aunt (the sister of Josette's mother). When Josette finished a sociology degree at the University of Antananarivo in 1983, her mother asked Nenilava to help Josette find a job. After some prayer, Nenilava sent Josette to the headquarters SALFA had established in Antananarivo in 1979, where Josette was hired as an assistant. Josette became unhappy with her low pay, however, and after several unsuccessful attempts at procuring a raise, she quit. Thinking she had turned away a job given to her by Jesus, Josette's mother became angry with her. Josette worked part-time jobs for several months, but then SALFA administrators offered her the salary she had desired. Summing up the lesson of the story, Josette said she

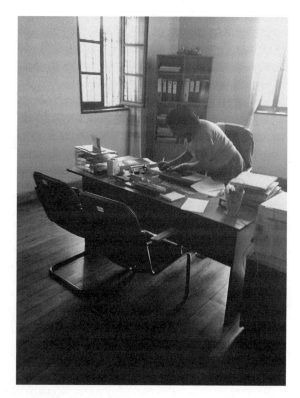

FIGURE 4.3. Josette in her Andohalo office.

has learned step by step that Jesus's calling for her involves working for the health department of the FLM.

Like other SALFA employees, Josette's spiritual testimony clearly positions her paid work in a broader context of Christian service and obedience to God. Narratives like Josette's also illuminate how she turned social connections with the revival, and especially Nenilava, into a sustained professional career with SALFA and now IHM. Thus, in her reflection on her work experiences, several interlocking spheres of affiliation and prosperity became visible, as she has sought material and spiritual benefits from paid employment, foreign aid partnerships, former missionaries, and lay involvement in the *fifohazana* movement.

For most of the seventeen years she spent with SALFA, Josette's work has focused on community health care in rural areas. She spent about 40 percent of her time in SALFA's Antananarivo headquarters, and she devoted the remaining 60 percent of her time to visiting seven primary health care teams scattered across the island. Each team included a nurse, a nutritionist, and a driver and spent time visiting outlying villages, training locals to be representative health workers. The program aimed to sensitize villagers, mainly women, to fundamental aspects of preventive medicine. Specific subjects included teaching people to boil water before drinking it, in order to improve the water supply; encouraging breastfeeding for infants under the age of two; showing caretakers how to introduce infants to solid foods at six months of age; and providing educational workshops on the symptoms and treatments of common illnesses (including diarrhea, cough, fever, malaria, malnourishment, and worms).

Josette's current work with the AVIA program is quite similar to her role as a community health care worker for SALFA. Based in Tolagnaro–Ft. Dauphin, the IHM-sponsored Antanosy project employs seven full-time workers and entails six spokes of action: clean water, nutrition, agriculture, women's literacy, evangelism, and hygiene and sanitation. The key difference between community health care and AVIA, Josette said, is that AVIA emphasizes integrated actions across all these domains, supporting a more expansive view of what constitutes health. I asked Josette how evangelism was woven into the program. Biblical lessons, she said, are used in the women's literacy program. Participants are encouraged to come to local church services, where the first text they read is often a hymnal. Field teams also often teach the children to sing hymns and introduce them to the figure of Jesus. Josette admitted that some parents have gotten angry with AVIA workers for influencing their children in this way. As Josette put it, such people say they worship only what they see, not what is invisible.

For Josette, a clear demarcation exists between the veneration of the ancestors and Christianity. To be fully Christian, she implied that one must renounce the ways of the ancestors, a position common in the *fifohazana* movement in which Josette has been involved. Throughout Madagascar, Josette said, as in the small southeast villages where AVIA works, many venerate the ancestors (*razana*). She identified this as a problem and it became clear that she opposes certain practices of venerating ancestors, such as the famous *famadihana* (turning of the dead) ritual practiced in the highlands. At one point, much to my surprise, she said that being Christian is more important to her than being Malagasy. She explained that her first priority was to find salvation individually and to be right before God. After that, she embraces being Malagasy.

Josette fittingly describes the IHM-SALFA-FLM partnership as spiritual and religious. IHM's support, she says, enables the FLM to become "*vaolombelona tsara*" (a good witness). The relationship strengthens IHM's witness in the world as well. For Josette, the relationship is based on the Scriptures and a common love of Christ. Josette was reminded of a Malagasy proverb that she said illustrated IHM's partnership with SALFA: "*Tanana miara, mitondra. Sororoka miara, mizaka. Tongotra miara, mandeha*" (a second hand to accompany, a second shoulder to support, a second foot to walk together). This proverb interestingly conjured the biblical model of accompanying in a Malagasy idiom, and, like Luke 24, implied that individual Christians occupy a shared body on their "walk" toward salvation in the world. Josette added that she perceives IHM more as a continuation of the work of the departed US missionaries, many of whom she knew or met, than of the current ELCA. She pointed to the ELCA's embrace of same-sex marriage and ordination of gay clergy as something that could affect its relationship with the FLM. Signaling her own rejection of the ELCA's welcoming stance toward homosexual unions among both congregants and clergy, she said she sees IHM, by comparison, as closely connected to the basis of the Scriptures rather than embracing a lot of "new ideas."[7]

Josette has done extensive work for IHM since she opened its Antananarivo office in 2009. It took her some five months to formally register IHM as an NGO operating in Madagascar. She completed numerous documents for the local government and the ministries of health and foreign affairs and proudly showed me the stamped authorization document that grants IHM its status as an NGO in Madagascar. In her work now, she supervises the seven AVIA workers in Tolagnaro–Ft. Dauphin, often by phone, email, and Skype. She attends FLM and SALFA meetings on IHM's behalf, giving the agency a voice and a pair of eyes on the ground in Antananarivo. She prepares quarterly reports for IHM and sends a copy to the Ministry of Health to verify IHM's NGO status. A large part of her work is calling her Tolagnaro–Ft. Dauphin team, as well as other SALFA and FLM contacts, and cajoling them to supply the information she needs.

IHM and AVIA board members have made several visits to the Antananarivo office, sometimes spending multiple days with the organization. From what she has seen, Josette told me she perceives the IHM-SALFA-FLM relationship as one that champions the values of "self-reliance" and "sustainability," she said, using the English-language terms common to the broader aid world. Keeping in mind that Josette is an IHM employee, I had initially wondered whether she might not feel comfortable saying anything critical about the organization. I assured her that I would protect her privacy and not report anything she said to IHM or the ELCA. But she insisted she had nothing to hide and would even be content if I used her real name in my writing. (I have chosen not to do so.)

III. MR. RAJOANARY   When I first arrived at the SALFA building one morning, a little after 8:30, Albert Rajoanary was talking with a small cluster of SALFA employees, leaning over the front steps with one knee thrust forward in animated conversation. A few minutes later, when he stepped into the building, he spotted me sitting on a bench and apologized for keeping me waiting, though it was still well before our 9 o'clock appointment. He summoned over an older man, a porter casually dressed in a "Stop SIDA" (AIDS) T-shirt and slacks, and asked him to take his black leather valise to his fourth-floor office. Mr. Rajoanary excused himself for a few minutes to check in with the first-floor clinic before returning to collect me and walk the three flights of stairs to the top level.

Mr. Rajoanary's office is a long rectangular space stuffed with piles of papers, bookcases, devotional objects, mementos from overseas travel, and assorted signs and motivational posters in English and Malagasy. A wall of windows partly faces another wing of the SALFA building. The windows' only open curtain panel, at the far left edge of the office, offered glimpses of the building's expansive views of the city below. As I glanced around the room, I saw a framed photograph of a group of travelers mounted on an ornamental mat and encircled with Chinese characters, a commendation for short-term mission work in Malaysia, a small wooden carving featuring the words "Papua New Guinea" in hand-painted black letters, and a posted paper that read in English type "I am a leader, not a boss."

Mr. Rajoanary is a distinguished-looking man who appears to be in his late fifties or early sixties. He seems serious in conversation, pausing briefly sometimes before continuing with long stretches of pointed observations. His observations are often pitched in a way that shows he is

accustomed to explaining SALFA's complex operational needs to a wide
range of constituents—funders, collaborators, and coworkers. He is precise in his ideas and critiques of SALFA, betraying an immense, bird's-
eye view of the system gained from his nearly thirty years of experience.
Mr. Rajoanary often smiles warmly, seeking to build a connection and
make sure I understand what he is trying to say. Toward the end of a
long morning together, for instance, he even remarks that he appreci-
ates the opportunity to talk about SALFA. Since 2010, when he resigned
from his former position as SALFA director, something we broach only
obliquely, he says he has not been asked for advice or input from any of
the current SALFA leaders.

Mr. Rajoanary was born in Tolagnaro–Ft. Dauphin in southeast Madagascar into a family of seven children. His father, a policeman, died in
1970 when he was still fairly young. Albert had to find a job to help support his mother and siblings. From 1971 to 1980, he worked in a local
government office in Tolagnaro–Ft. Dauphin. But he also had extensive
contact with the Prophetess Nenilava of the *fifohazana* movement, which
indelibly shaped his life after 1979. One of his two sisters lived in Paris
for a short time in the mid-1970s, studying finance. In 1976 Nenilava was
in Paris visiting one of her "spiritual sons," a term referring both to children she fostered for struggling parents and those she mentored spiritually. Through her connections among Malagasy expatriates in Paris,
Mr. Rajoanary's sister met Nenilava and even arranged for the prophetess to stay with her while she was in Paris. When Nenilava was leaving
France, Mr. Rajoanary's sister gave Nenilava a T-shirt to take home to
her brother. Back in Madagascar, Nenilava called Albert and, because
she could not read or write, asked for his help with some reports and correspondence. Mr. Rajoanary had just finished his bachelor's degree in
1979. Unsure of whether he wanted to work for Nenilava, he hesitated
for three years before agreeing to do so. He now laughs at this, knowing
what a significant figure she became for Malagasy Christians.

In 1981 Nenilava had a vision that Dr. Fosse was having difficulties
establishing SALFA. She told Albert to go to him and ask whether he
needed help. Mr. Rajoanary traveled to Isoraka, a neighborhood of Antananarivo where Dr. Fosse was staying in housing run by the ALC-ELCA.
Mr. Rajoanary was already familiar with Dr. Fosse and SALFA because
he worked with youth organizations that supported the Ankaramalaza
toby and, even at that time, they were already procuring some medicines
from SALFA for the *toby*. Dr. Fosse, he recounted, was extremely sur-

prised that Nenilava knew about his difficulties and he hired Albert with Nenilava's endorsement. Albert became his main administrative coordinator while Dr. Fosse retained a focus on clinical and medical needs.

At the same time, in 1981, Albert became a consecrated *mpiandry* in the revival movement. As she has with many other revivalists, Nenilava played a key role as a matchmaker for Albert and his wife, something he said reflects the biblical idea that a spouse is a gift from God. Albert and his wife have now been married for thirty years and have four children who are all members of the FLM. In 1983 his wife also became a *mpiandry*. From 1986 to 2004, Albert was the treasurer of the FLM and a SALFA administrator. He directed SALFA from 2004 to 2010. He is currently the director of Salama (Malagasy for healthy or well), a Malagasy NGO that procures large amounts of drugs and sells them at a reduced price to Malagasy clinics. SALFA allows him to retain an office in its headquarters, though, perhaps in a nod to his years of service to the church.

Mr. Rajoanary's perspective on SALFA is clearly shaped by a free-market ideology, yet he does not come across as an ideologue. There is a quality of pragmatism to what he says, for much of his perspective is built on the idea that SALFA never operates outside the global market. He quickly pointed to many overlooked dimensions of SALFA's operation, as well as its relationship with foreign donors. Between 1980 and 1981, he worked half-time with Dr. Fosse. They used Catholic Relief Services to transport medicines into Madagascar, which Albert would collect at the international airport in Ivato (Antananarivo). But in 1982, Catholic Relief Services asked to separate its activities from SALFA's. As a medical missionary, the ELCA paid for Dr. Fosse's salary, housing, and equipment needs until his final retirement in 2004 (after many failed attempts to retire, blocked by the FLM). When Mr. Rajoanary took over as SALFA director in 2004, SALFA had to come up with a director's salary for the first time.

Moreover, until 2006, SALFA had a monopoly on foreign medicine and medical-supply acquisitions for its network, using the International Dispensary Association in the Netherlands as well as donations from Malagasy Partnership, IHM, and elsewhere. According to Mr. Rajoanary, however, all that changed in 2006, when the government-sponsored and government-subsidized NGO Salama, which receives funds from the World Bank, UNICEF, UNPF, and Global Fund, began to organize purchasing power at the scale of the clients they represented. They were increasingly able to make large-scale drug orders for generic medicines with manufacturers in China and India, negotiating a low price based on volume. From Mr. Rajoanary's description, Salama may also have begun to quietly poach clients from the SALFA network. Individual clinics and hospitals in Ambohibao, Mahajanga, Tamatave, and elsewhere began to buy directly from Salama, rather than order through SALFA. The reason he gave for this was that they could get the supplies cheaper from Salama. With no rule against SALFA centers buying from external sellers, more medical centers may do the same.

Albert showed me the bottom-line calculations, scratching out the numbers on a used envelope in front of him. SALFA would add a service fee to procured medicines, which could be as much as 25 percent of the original price. Then, sometimes, individual clinics like Manambaro would add 15 percent to help fund their own operations and handling of the medicine. This results in a 40 percent markup for individual patients, potentially making those medicines offered at SALFA clinics unaffordable. In this scenario, either patients would not be able to afford the medicine in places like Manambaro (where there is no other competition) or, in larger cities, they would try elsewhere, even taking *taxi-be* (city bus) from pharmacy to pharmacy to shop for the best deal. To add to this complexity, SALFA sometimes changed the percentage of how much they charged as the service fee, in proportion to whether the clinic could afford it. Sometimes, with clinics unable to afford the service fee, foreign grants or designated monies for rural clinics were used to subsidize the cost of medications.

By comparison, because of the volume it purchases, Salama charges only a 5 percent processing fee to clinics and hospitals. It does not charge for the distribution and delivery of the medicines and maintains six offices across the island in Antananarivo, Antsiranana, Fianarantsoa, Mahajanga, Toamasina, and Toliara. Besides this, Salama has the staff to do quality-control checks of medicines, something that SALFA currently does not have the expertise or ability to do. In what sounded slightly like a business meeting pitch, Mr. Rajoanary emphasized that Salama could meet 80 percent of Malagasy clinics' needs locally, without requiring separate infusions of foreign currency or bargaining individually on the international market. Indeed, although it was clear Mr. Rajoanary is partial to Salama as a more cost-effective method for the delivery of medicine than SALFA, I could easily see how it was smart to organize the purchasing power of hundreds of clinics in Madagascar, bringing together government-run and private medical facilities, to make medicines more accessible.

Mr. Rajoanary eventually focused more on the way SALFA is currently involved in numerous internationally funded aid projects aimed at specific diseases like tuberculosis. As it stands now, the thrust in aid is toward high-profile, multilateral disease prevention programs, and IHM forms only a specialized part of SALFA training and community-health initiatives. Unfortunately, these programs bypass the centralized SALFA structure. Many of them, such as Dr. Andry's national tuberculosis prevention program, facilitate the government-endorsed NGO mandates with which SALFA complies, and which benefit SALFA patients. But SALFA itself is not compensated for overhead costs for using SALFA facilities, administrative coordination, and office space. Mr. Rajoanary gestured toward his window, mentioning the cars and trucks wedged like puzzle pieces in the small SALFA parking lot. These are all program cars, acquired through specialized grant programs on tuberculosis, HIV–AIDS, malaria, and family planning. Sometimes officials get to keep these cars after the programs end but, like computers, cell phones, and other project equipment, they do not become SALFA property (and therefore do not contribute to its structural or financial viability).

This medical aid system has grown since 1990, Mr. Rajoanary said, when funding agencies wanted to work with local NGOs on specific health initiatives. SALFA became a natural outlet for these projects because it has a health care network stretching across the island. But the NGOs in charge of the funding were setting the priorities and SALFA did not have control over the projects. The other problem with these programs is that they run time-dependent projects with clear end dates and various strategies, rather than offer long-term, consistent forms of structural support. Furthermore, sometimes SALFA ends up sandwiched between the regional church synods, where programs are administered in local health clinics, and the NGO funding the project. SALFA must supply the NGO with reports attesting to the program's clinical outcomes and budget. Some of the synod leaders misunderstand SALFA's role, though, and insist they be compensated for supplying budgets and reports. They see the cars in the SALFA lot during visits to Antananarivo, Mr. Rajoanary said, and experience some jealousy, pointing out that they are not being compensated for their work as they think all people in SALFA headquarters have been.

Though he had many criticisms and concerns about SALFA's current structure, Mr. Rajoanary still saw a future for the organization. He suggested that SALFA should abandon the practice of using a revolving fund and instead seek funds from other sources, purchasing medicines through Salama. He wanted SALFA to focus on administering and evaluating SALFA clinics across the island, improving their technical and clinical capabilities. It was clear to me that Mr. Rajoanary felt some of his insights had been overlooked during his time as SALFA director. And the rumblings among other SALFA workers about SALFA's crisis in 2009–11 led me to wonder how much Mr. Rajoanary's business interests in Salama overlapped with his work as SALFA director. He once pointed out that Salama was partly built on the model of SALFA. Even if the relationship had been only an indirect one, it could have raised eyebrows as a conflict of interest. Clement framed some of the issues he had with Mr. Rajoanary at that time as philosophical differences, never naming them directly. In either case, Mr. Rajoanary wanted to dismantle something—the cost-sharing structure based on foreign donations—that Clement and Dr. Fosse both thought was the heart of SALFA's operation. The threat of doing so could surely have spelled the end of his time as director. The tension, though, between those who support SALFA's centralized health care system and those who favor a more privatized health care model with subsidized medicines is a real and vibrant issue. Although Mr. Rajoanary said his views were no secret, he never fully explained what led to his resignation, preferring not to discuss it explicitly.

Conclusions

SALFA employees' disagreements over the basic structure of the organization convey more than individual opinions. They signal much broader debates about health care provision in the current global economy. They point to the difficulties of maintaining a centralized health care structure amid market forces that separate clinics from one another, making it seem more advantageous for them to compete independently for the best price of medicines and equipment. The need for antiretroviral medications among the HIV-positive population in Brazil, for example, has created a new role for an activist state that aligns private and public agencies and seizes control of unpredictable pricing mechanisms to purchase antiretrovirals, producing a form of governance broader than the state government alone (Biehl 2010). Anthropologist João Biehl (2010) argues that this strategy expands, rather than renounces, a market approach to health care, diverging markedly from the less marketized public health care programs of an earlier era.

The 2009–13 economic crisis in Madagascar galvanized debates about such private–public partnerships among SALFA leaders, some of whom believe SALFA clinics should join government-run clinics to achieve greater purchasing power on the open market. Indeed, Salama builds on the model of private–public partnership in order to acquire medicines and supplies from China and India, both of which are manufacturing generics at lower costs, rather than relying mainly on foreign donations or foreign drug clearinghouses like the International Dispensary Association. This supply model, of course, diverges from SALFA's current model, which creates a fixed market solely for private Lutheran clinics. If SALFA completely turned over its role in medical and drug acquisition to Salama, it would place SALFA clinics, along with other private and public clinics in Madagascar, into the flow of market competition. Like the situation in Brazil that Biehl (2010) describes, Salama does not critique the pricing mechanisms of the current global market or the privatization policies shaping Madagascar's current economy. Rather, as Mr. Rajoanary recognized, it situates itself within the free market ideology of global medical manufacturers. It points to price competition as the main reason private and public entities should combine their purchasing power. It is still unclear how Salama will affect SALFA in the future, since these debates continue to roil the organization. But I believe SALFA will end up redefining its priorities to account for the rise of public–private medical-supply partnerships in Madagascar and elsewhere.

Another factor at the heart of this dispute is the difference in the opinions Mr. Rajoanary and Clement hold on how to appropriately value ties to the US NGOs and other donor agencies. Mr. Rajoanary clearly feels that it is time to minimize SALFA's investment in these donor ties, partly because of his own shifting status in relation to some of SALFA's foreign partners. Instead, at least in his professional work, he favors nurturing connections with Chinese and Indian medical manufacturers and the broader community of public and private health workers in Madagascar, a set of ties in which he is clearly invested as the leader of Salama. These connections are not static for either Clement or

Mr. Rajoanary. Instead, they are dynamic spaces of maneuver, reevaluation, and self-positioning. They can be considered part of a broader performance of cosmopolitan middle-classness, in which SALFA administrators leverage a number of sources of authority and classed prosperity, as well as the selves and futures they enable or disallow.

By actively nurturing some ties while playing down or even attenuating others, SALFA administrators navigate the domestic and global professional and religious networks in which SALFA is thoroughly enmeshed as an organization. Combined with their professional qualifications, including their multilingualism, fluency in bureaucratic discourse, college education, and international experience, SALFA administrators' ability to move fluidly across and selectively nurture these cultural spheres and connections attests to, and works to secure, their cosmopolitanism. As I have argued more broadly in this chapter, Malagasy acceptance of the heterogeneous stream of US medical discards should be understood in this light: among SALFA administrators, the acceptance of these materials is an act of value generation in itself, a move they actively choose as a means of creating ties irrespective of the uncertain individual clinical and economic value of the medical discards. Although US aid workers organize the value of their foreign relations by infusing value into medical discards, Malagasy aid workers tend to selectively value activities that make foreign ties endure.

This approach to value possibly also contains a subtle Malagasy critique of the discard trade itself. Anthropologists have long argued that cultural critique, rather than only the spoken or public form of protest sometimes prized as critique in the dominant Western cultural lens, happens in forms that fit local cultural logics and what is possible in a given subject position (Ong 1987). Critique is often registered in a cultural form that affords particular individuals a kind of maneuverability and camouflage lest the critique threaten their livelihood or personal security. Furthermore, critique may not be reflexively recognized as such by the individuals participating in it, but rather may serve a broader social role of acknowledging a specific cultural problem and enabling a form of collective catharsis (Ong 1987). Building on these insights, I suggest that SALFA workers can be perceived as engaging in a form of cultural critique of the discard trade through their refusal to treat the medical materials as valuable objects in themselves. SALFA workers are in a position in which open criticism of the medical relief could sour their relationship with their US partners and possibly close off a valuable foreign partnership. To be clear, SALFA workers do not unilaterally devalue or dismiss the discard trade. Some actively point to the significant role of the medical relief items in maintaining SALFA's central operation and serving a useful therapeutic role in SALFA clinics.

Yet their orientation to the discards tells a slightly different story. By examining SALFA workers' handling of the discards and prioritization of the foreign ties as more significant than the materials themselves, it is possible to see a kind of casual dismissal of the notion that the discard trade serves a primary value for SALFA. SALFA employees make visible their long-running awareness that the medical relief is not necessarily geared to Malagasy clinical needs but came about through a complex system of global commerce in which they and their US brethren play specific roles. Furthermore, by shifting attention from the waste forms to the ultimate focus of the aid partnership, SALFA administrators shore up their own classed professional aims as aid administrators and create distance from forms of devaluation often linked to waste flows (Reno 2016). In the next chapter, I examine how individual Merina and Betsileo administrators and clinicians have emerged as aid partners to the two US NGOs, gaining special access to medical aid resources and shaping an aid subjectivity that builds on a notable Malagasy history of Merina-Anglo Protestant alliances.

CHAPTER FIVE

Translating Aid, Brokering Identity

Malagasy Doctors as Precarious Heroes

Neither negotiation nor translation are over or complete, even though both know bounds.
—Nancy Hunt (1999, 23)

Pre•car•i•ous [prəˈkɛriəs] 1. dependent on circumstances beyond one's control, uncertain, unstable, insecure. 2. exposed to or involving danger, perilous, risky.

During October 2005, a SALFA physician and devout Christian in his early fifties, Dr. Rafolo, who was stationed at the Ejeda Lutheran Hospital in southwest Madagascar, visited the United States for two weeks. He had been flown to Minneapolis as the featured keynote speaker for the IHM global health conference, an annual event that had just begun. During Dr. Rafolo's US stay, he met with Malagasy Partnership volunteers at their suburban Minneapolis warehouse. In halting English, he told the dramatic story of having been accidentally punctured by a needle that had been used on a patient with HIV.[1] To combat the onset of HIV, Dr. Rafolo took the emergency prophylaxis available to physicians, but he had also contracted tuberculosis. Malagasy Partnership volunteers, riveted by the story and their appreciation of the risks Dr. Rafolo incurred in his work, asked the Malagasy Partnership leader Gene for updates about his health long after Dr. Rafolo's US visit. In regularly held group prayers, I listened as individual US volunteers entreated God to "lift up," "protect," and "heal" Dr. Rafolo, placing him in the aid program's constellation of named individuals.

This chapter explores the limited yet transformative cultural ties that have developed between a small group of male Merina and Betsileo

Malagasy physicians, including Dr. Rafolo, and US volunteers. I suggest that these Malagasy physicians, who now operate as US aid brokers, embody and navigate a position of precarious heroism in the Minnesota-Madagascar relief endeavor. I use the term *precarious heroism* to draw forward the dynamic, culturally shaped participation structure informing, and affecting, Malagasy physicians' role in the medical aid program. Malagasy physicians' precarity in the aid partnership partly stems from their in-between-ness or middleness (Hunt 1999), as they move among multilayered cultural identities, geographic and professional spaces, and acts of cultural translation. Malagasy doctors like Dr. Rafolo often appear to US colleagues as heroic figures, building on a long Western cultural history of white doctor "hero-figures" that extends to David Livingstone and Albert Schweitzer (Vaughan 1991, 155). Their heroism is culturally constructed, however, through a variety of aid activities, including US visits and narratives of epidemiological and technological risk, rather than given or intrinsic to them. As a participation role with moral, spiritual, and economic dimensions, SALFA physicians' heroism is thus precarious or insecure rather than assured; it is continually made and performed according to the terms and conditions of the Minnesota-Madagascar aid program. Yet, as we will see, contemporary SALFA doctors create spaces of cultural maneuver to access social and economic capital made available through the aid broker role. Current Malagasy doctors, I suggest, build on a historically rooted Malagasy practice of strategic foreign alliances, particularly with Anglo Protestants, in their interactions with the US NGOs.

More than twelve hundred people work across the forty-eight Lutheran medical clinics in the SALFA network today, including more than ninety physicians. What I noticed during my field research, however, was that a small, select group of these Malagasy doctors repeatedly rose to the surface of the aid program as specially qualified brokers or partners of the US NGOs. Through casual interactions with approximately seven Malagasy physician-aid partners, both through the US NGOs and on trips to Madagascar, I came to realize that certain Merina and Betsileo physicians have rendered themselves, and have been crafted by their US colleagues, as culturally elaborated "Malagasy partners." They are known by name, prayed for by US volunteers, correspond with the NGOs, and participate as special guests in global health conferences in Minneapolis–St. Paul. This small group of special aid partners, which include Dr. Gabriel, the physician-turned-evangelist profiled in chapter 2, Dr. Remy, Dr. Rafolo, and Dr. Andry, are predominantly male and Merina or Betsileo, two ethno-regional groups linked to highland Madagascar.[2] It is in the United States, at a remove from Madagascar, that they are primarily regarded as "Malagasy" or "African" rather than "Lutheran," "Merina," or "Betsileo" (or other, more relevant identifiers). Indeed, Malagasy doctors' ethno-regional identification may not be apparent to certain Americans at all, and I draw this into the chapter for the purposes of analysis. Clinic nurses, dockworkers, office staff, and administrators maintain SALFA facilities and transport individual medical relief shipments from the port city of Tamatave to Antananarivo. Yet, with the exception of the SALFA financial administrator Clement, they remain less visible to their US colleagues as aid partners than these SALFA doctors.

In this chapter, I first explore the significant role of Merina and Betsileo Malagasy, particularly Merina Protestant physicians, in forging foreign alliances with Anglo-Protestants in nationalist and anticolonial movements in Madagascar. After sketching the Malagasy historical context that provides resources for the cultural position of Merina and Betsileo aid brokers, I profile a Betsileo physician who has propelled his SALFA connections into a prominent role in a multilateral global health program. Then I show how specific cultural activities with the two US NGOs—narratives of Malagasy doctors as proxy missionaries, accountability documents, and global health conferences—further an aid subjectivity with deeper historical roots in the cultural and religious encounter between Malagasy and Americans. These narratives of Malagasy doctors plot specific participation roles for Americans, as well, and I analyze the cultural and political effects of these various moral relations motivating the contemporary aid program.

Medical aid programs have a range of cultural effects beyond merely their explicitly defined program aims. Specifically, in order to gain access to aid monies or resources, medical aid organizations often compel aid recipients to perform and identify with specific cultural identities through a medical diagnosis, such as being HIV-positive in Côte d'Ivoire, which cements access to antiretroviral medications (Nguyen 2010; see also Biehl 2010). These cultural identifications, whether that of illness sufferer or victim of psychosocial trauma (James 2010), are not assured through the recipients' experiences alone but must be socially established through narrative and testimonial forms recognized as legitimate by aid agencies. Scholars have persuasively demonstrated that aid recipients, while balancing the demands of the reductive cultural roles they perform, also transform and creatively deploy them. Nguyen (2010, 49), for instance, describes how the narrative practices of HIV-positive individuals from Burkina Faso and Côte d'Ivoire feature "gaps, evasions and circumlocutions" that enable them to meet the aid agency–created "market" for narratives about their medical diagnosis while silencing certain personal difficulties.

Fewer medical humanitarian studies examine these issues of self-identification from the perspective of health care professionals affiliated with aid programs. This is particularly true for studies of those working in long-term medical relief or care arrangements (Nguyen 2010, Ticktin 2011), like the participants in my research, rather than short-term medical crises or emergency care, as in *Médecins Sans Frontières (MSF)*. In his ethnography *Life in Crisis*, Peter Redfield (2013) notes that, because of its relative immobility, MSF's large Ugandan national staff of doctors, nurses, cooks, and drivers often appears less "humanitarian" than the smaller MSF expatriate staff, even though the national staff members secure access to forms of social and economic capital through their work. In his writing on long-term medical aid workers in Mozambique, James Pfeiffer (2002, 2004) has described the formation of a class of medical aid professional elites who rely on a patchy field of foreign aid money for their livelihood. Yet, as with aid recipients, the degree to which medical aid workers draw from more deeply rooted cultural roles in their work, shifting and adding to them through interactions with aid providers or aid organizations, remains to be thoroughly explored.

I suggest in this chapter that, rather than an identification borne solely of the aid relationship, the cultural subject position of Merina and Betsileo Protestant aid brokers builds on a Malagasy history of Merina-Anglo Protestant alliances. The current aid alliance between Merina Malagasy and Americans is particularly striking because most now-retired US Lutheran missionaries lived and worked among Mahafaly, Tandroy, and Tanosy Malagasy in southern Madagascar until as late as 2004, rather than among Merina and Betsileo Malagasy in central highland Madagascar. Thus, on the subsequent pages, I examine why certain kinds of aid brokers make more cultural "sense" than others in the Minnesota-Madagascar aid program and trace how the aid broker role itself takes on a distinctive shape through specific cultural practices; it is

compelled into action by the conditions and inequalities of aid while being continually transformed by American and Malagasy understandings
of what it means to broker foreign ties.

Merina-Anglo Protestant Alliances in
Cultural and Historical Perspective

A long and varied history exists in Madagascar of strategic alliances between Merina Malagasy and Anglo Protestants in nationalist and anticolonial movements. Merina and Betsileo elites, in particular, have built
foreign Protestant alliances at distinct moments for their own political goals while actively positioning themselves as national figures, or as
those who act on behalf of and politically represent other people. Although the differences between these historically rooted activities and
the current faith-based aid relationship are many, what is noteworthy in
this comparison is how, like some of their forebears, Merina and Betsileo Malagasy physicians today establish foreign alliances in order to
enhance Malagasy institutions as well as their own individual access to
forms of political and social capital. In addition, as I explore in this section, Merina and Betsileo Protestant elites have long understood themselves as part of a wider, cosmopolitan world that included their travel
to foreign places and their interactions with foreigners living in or traveling to Madagascar. Although aid programs are often characterized as
new social configurations, this Malagasy history suggests the Minnesota-
Madagascar partnership draws upon more enduring Malagasy cultural
practices of making strategic foreign alliances.

Before moving forward, I would like to briefly explain my use in this
chapter of ethnic identifications like Merina and Betsileo. Many scholars
of Madagascar have pointed out that ethnicity is not as significant a form
of identification or affiliation in Malagasy communities as patrilines,
royal dynastic lineages, the distinction between people native to the land
(Malagasy, *tera-tany*) and migrants or strangers (Malagasy, *vahiny*), and
the ancestral connection to land (Feeley-Harnik 1991; Sharp 1993; Cole
1997). In the words of Lesley Sharp (1993, 53), ethnicities are a matter of
"perspective and scale" (see also Cole 1997). From within communities,
people often have at their disposal a variety of more significant identity
distinctions based on the factors named above, and some may not at all

recognize ethnic categories applied in the national census to the regional population where they live (see Eggert 1986 on the ethnonym Mahafaly). Others have traced how ethnonyms like Merina took shape as strategies of political rule among elites in the region called Imerina; in other words, those in the region came to be called Merina as they became political subjects (Larson 1996, 2000; see also Bloch 1986a; Covell 1987, 12; Graeber 2007b). The French seized some of these forms of political rule already established in distinct Merina, Betsileo, Betsimisaraka, and Sakalava communities and created twenty ethnic identities for the populations of Madagascar as part of colonial rule. These ethnic groupings have continued to be used in the Malagasy Republic's census; though some Malagasy individuals do not identify with them, other ethnographies show that such terms hold social resonance as important contemporary identifiers in Malagasy communities (Harper 2002; Sharp 1993).[3] Because of the dynamic, variable, and multifaceted meanings and importance of these ethnonyms, I use the terms Merina and Betsileo advisedly throughout the chapter.

For precisely the matters of "perspective and scale" that Sharp (1993) describes, however, contemporary SALFA doctors' Merina and Betsileo ethnicity can be understood as part of a long and ongoing process of ethno-regional differentiation in Madagascar.[4] Merina elites, for example, have collectively had greater access to forms of institutionalized medicine, higher education, and government and civil service positions in contemporary Madagascar than people of other identified ethno-regional groups (Cole 1997; Sharp 1993, 2002; Keller 2005; Sharp and Kruse 2011). Though Merina royals operated a nascent state prior to colonial occupation in 1896, a privileged position for Merina in an island-wide ethnic hierarchy was also actively nurtured by French colonial policy, which has had an enduring influence in the postcolonial period as well (Andersen 2010).[5] Thus, I am particularly interested here in exploring how male Merina and Betsileo Protestant elites build on a history of ethno-regional differentiation that positions them in particular ways to secure access to foreign ties, a subject that has received substantial attention in Madagascar. As I described in the previous chapter, such forms of Christian identification and affiliation converge in unique ways with ongoing economic marginalization and the effects of market liberalization in Madagascar (Cole 2010; see also Walsh 2003, 2012). This chapter adds to this conversation in Malagasy ethnography and historiography, showing how Merina and Betsileo Protestant elites substantiate access to forms of political and cultural capital through their ties to foreign actors.

Merina and Betsileo Protestant Men and Nationalist Movements

In Malagasy history and historiography, Merina and Betsileo Christian men have frequently emerged as nationalist cultural figures who, at strategic political moments, used foreign alliances to protest French colonial domination. These individuals' Christian networks, stretching across and beyond Madagascar, have been central components of their political organizing and their consolidation of political power. Among the twenty recognized ethnicities in Madagascar, Merina and Betsileo Malagasy have historically demonstrated the highest rates of Protestant Christian affiliation, with even higher overall rates among Merina and Betsileo male elites (Ellis 1985). Although the reasons for their Protestant affiliation are historically and individually variable, Merina and Betsileo Protestant elites have often recognized foreign Christian connections as not merely religious ties but also political resources. This cultural pattern threads through several important nationalist, anticolonial, and postcolonial protest movements in Madagascar.

Among the best-known Merina and Betsileo Protestant political groups is *Vy, Vato, Sakelika* or VVS (Malagasy, Iron, Stone, Branches), considered the first modern nationalist movement. VVS was a secret society of elite Malagasy student intellectuals active between 1913 and 1916. Its members were mainly Merina Protestant pastors, doctors, or doctors-in-training who "sought to adopt Western innovations while . . . retaining a Malagasy cultural identity" (Cole 2010, 98). Though its leaders initially organized at the medical school in Antananarivo, VVS flourished through the new forms of mobility compelled by the colonial state, as traders, officials, and labor migrants congregated along roads and railway networks (Randrianja and Ellis 2009, 164). These pathways provided new communication channels for political organizing, and VVS members like Pastor Ravelojaona (1879–1956) read foreign newspapers, as well, that they used in order to understand French colonial occupation as a broader global phenomenon (164). Scholars of Madagascar have pointed out that nationalism was a foreign construct that Malagasy intellectuals, attuned to the political capital to be gained from foreign networks as older structures of authority crumbled under colonial rule, eventually adapted to the Malagasy political struggle (Randrianja and Ellis 2009). For instance, after attending Protestant schools, Ravelojaona, prior to becoming an influential VVS writer, traveled in Europe in 1904–5 on behalf of a Christian organization with which he was affiliated in Madagascar (Randrianja and Ellis 2009, 278). Ravelojaona's experiences show how foreign Christian connections were part of a wider nexus of foreign ties and foreign concepts utilized by Merina Protestant elites in their efforts to fuse new political alliances under colonial rule.

In their strategic political use of foreign Christian ties, Merina Protestant elites of the VVS built on what was already at that time a Merina Malagasy cultural practice of doing so, which stretched back to the precolonial administration of Merina King Radama I (1810–28; Larson 2000, 222–30). Even though the VVS was largely unsuccessful in achieving its political goals, its underlying cultural foundation—which combined Merina institutions of elite education, such as the Antananarivo medical school; Malagasy nationalism; and strategic Merina-Anglo Protestant foreign alliances—proved far more enduring and politically efficacious. Describing the VVS as one of two poles of Malagasy nationalist protest, Randrianja (2001) argues that, though the VVS was a short-lived secret society, its leaders continued their work through the Malagasy Communist Party and would eventually shape the other, much more violent anticolonial uprising of 1947–48. One VVS leader, Joseph Raseta (1886–1979), a Merina Protestant who was trained as a doctor, became involved in an anticolonial movement and established the Malagasy Communist Party after the VVS disbanded as a result of colonial suppression in 1916 (Randrianja and Ellis 2009, 216). The French colonial response had the unintended effect of binding together the surviving Merina Protestants involved in VVS. Raseta later served as a key figure in the nationalist Mouvement Démocratique de la Rénovation Malgache party and a leader in the anticolonial uprising of 1947–48, after which he was imprisoned in France until Malagasy independence in 1960.[6]

The cultural blueprint of nationalist protest that I have described, which emerges from and often furthers the interests of Merina elites and their institutions, has also surfaced in a reworked form in the postcolonial period. Much more recently, medical school students in Antananarivo, like their VVS forebears, initiated the 1972 protest of neocolonial president Philibert Tsiranana (1960–72), which led to his resignation. Tsiranana's presidency was widely viewed as a continuation of the eco-

nomic and administrative interests of French colonial rule. Following
other African nationalisms sweeping the continent at the time, Tsiranana's detractors championed a program of Malgachisation or nationalism of Malagasy institutions and government offices, including the mandatory use of the Malagasy language in schools (Cole 2010, 38–39; see
also Sharp 2002). In her analysis of the 1972 protest and its aftermath,
Jennifer Cole (2010) points out that these reforms, which unfolded over
the 1970s under the government of Didier Ratsiraka, often favored Merina elites. For example, it was the Merina dialect of the Malagasy language that became the official Malagasy dialect used by the government and taught in schools (Cole 2010, 39). Through the 1972 protest, as
well as other nationalist insurrections, elite Merina and Betsileo interests have often been aligned with and shaped an emerging Malagasy nationalism. The episodes of nationalist protest that I have briefly sketched
thus collectively point to the consolidation of Merina and Betsileo political power and the forms of inequality that this process perpetuates. Indeed, there is an equally long Malagasy history of suspicion and critique
of Merina political rule and Merina use of political resources (see, e.g.,
Feeley-Harnik 1991; Lambek 2002, 67; Cole 2010).[7]

Current SALFA aid brokers thus build on a more enduring Malagasy
cultural history of Merina and Betsileo Protestant alliances with Anglo
Protestants, as well as Merina and Betsileo Protestant elites as nationalist political figures who broker foreign ties. Merina and Betsileo Protestant physicians and administrators can be understood to draw upon
these historically and culturally organized roles, as well as contemporary forms of structural inequality, in their dealings with the US organizations. In sum, I would like to keep in view how the history of Merina-
Anglo Protestant alliances and Merina political power both shapes the
role of foreign broker in the contemporary partnership with US organizations and perpetuates forms of ethnic and gender differentiation in
Malagasy society.

Merina and Betsileo Physicians as Foreign Brokers

Certain Merina and Betsileo doctors often appear as suitable foreign
brokers to the US NGOs today because of their cosmopolitan qualities, attributes that they in turn consolidate through those foreign ties.
As I described in the previous chapter, most SALFA physician–aid brokers have substantial experience with international travel, fluency with

bureaucratic discourse, college educations, and multilingual competence in at least three languages (e.g., Malagasy, French, English). Although these doctors are not financially wealthy, they hold substantial political and cultural capital through their educational and professional achievements as well as their ties to foreign organizations and foreign physicians. One example of a contemporary SALFA foreign broker is a Betsileo physician in his fifties whom I call Dr. Andry. In Dr. Andry's experiences, we can witness how Merina and Betsileo physicians turn access to foreign organizations, such as the US NGOs, into other enduring foreign alliances, catapulting themselves in Dr. Andry's case into well-funded, multilateral disease-prevention programs. Dr. Andry's medical work in rural SALFA clinics in three regions of Madagascar also attests to how SALFA physicians sometimes distinguish themselves from clinic patients.

Dr. Andry's third-floor office in the SALFA building in hilly Andohalo (Antananarivo) has a breathtaking view of the city folding out below like a multicolored quilt. His office is small but furnished with a large elegant-looking walnut-colored desk, several visitors' chairs, a desk chair, and a lightly scuffed laptop computer. Dr. Andry is precise with his words, sometimes pausing to choose them carefully; at other times, he tells an ironic or funny story, pauses for a few beats, and then laughs uproariously, a hearty baritone laugh that fills the office. Dr. Andry's demeanor, including his charismatic personality and his ease and lightness with relative strangers like myself, demonstrates his skill in navigating different spheres of bureaucratic discourse and medical and religious authority.

Dr. Andry was born in Manakara, a southeast town at the end of the East Coast railway line. He is Betsileo and otherwise spent most of his youth in Fianarantsoa (Malagasy, literally, "place of good learning"), where he said education was indeed prized. A Malagasy proverb describes Betsileo as good "second men" (to Merina) because of their hard work and, with only a slight twinkle of humor, Dr. Andry likened himself to a good "second man," showing his awareness of this ethnic hierarchy but also parodying it. Dr. Andry had a career as a SALFA clinician in Manombo, Fianarantsoa, and Mahajanga before earning a master's degree in public health from the University of Antananarivo. Beginning in 1987, he respectively spent three years in Manombo, living among Vezo people in southwest Madagascar; seven years in Fianarantsoa, in the southern part of the central highlands; and two years in

Mahajanga in the northwest, coming to appreciate very different regions and their clinical needs. In 1998 he began to work as SALFA's national tuberculosis coordinator (which he does still today) and as a technical director for SALFA (which he no longer does). He now focuses exclusively on national tuberculosis prevention and, since 2009, he has served on the national overseeing structure for the entire Global Fund–based Madagascar tuberculosis project. About 30 percent of Dr. Andry's job is paperwork, he estimated, about 30 percent is supervising SALFA's tuberculosis centers, and another 30–40 percent is meetings. His work on tuberculosis has taken him to conferences in France, all over the African continent, and to Montreal.

Dr. Andry leverages not only professional connections to bureaucratic aid structures but also ties to a variety of religious organizations in Madagascar. When I asked him whether he views his medical work as spiritual, he quickly pointed out that he is a *mpiandry* (shepherd or lay preacher) in the island's charismatic Christian *fifohazana* movement. What originally piqued his interest in the revival movement and its *toby* (healing camps) was a series of Norwegian Development Authority (NORAD)–sponsored workshops he led between 2003 and 2008 to teach *toby* workers about HIV–AIDS. Inspired by the potential for collaboration between SALFA and the revival, in 2009 he trained to become a *mpiandry* at the famous Soatanana *toby*, which is the 1894 birthplace of the revival. Gradually, Dr. Andry came to see his *mpiandry* work as a spiritual calling. Dr. Andry once met the revival's nationally known Prophetess Nenilava prior to her death in 1998. As a vocal advocate for the spiritual significance of healing and medicine in Malagasy Christianity (see chapter 4), she told him that every doctor must also be a *mpiandry*; though he did not think much of it at the time, he has, quite appropriately, now come to see her words as prophetic. Currently, Dr. Andry spends one day each month at the Ilafy *toby* just ten kilometers outside Antananarivo, counseling patients and laying on hands in prayer healing.

Dr. Andry has been extraordinarily successful in lodging himself at the nexus of a lucrative and powerful global health project. Yet he not only described the significance of foreign alliances for his own professional career but also actively highlighted the value of foreign connections, foreign workers, and foreign supply chains for SALFA clinics. For instance, he observed that some people still refer to the hospitals and clinics in the south, such as those in Manambaro, Ejeda, and Vangaindrano, as the American clinics. Rather than pointing to this perception as a problem, though, Dr. Andry said that he thought the presence and visit of foreign clinicians, whether American or another nationality, could boost SALFA's overall reputation. Under his technical direction, he coordinated several Madagascar visits from a Michigan-based doctor and medical school faculty member, an internist, who has been a long-time SALFA collaborator. This physician, whom I had not met but for whom I arranged supplies while working at Malagasy Partnership, often took with his team specific medical items prepared in advance by Malagasy Partnership. Dr. Andry recalled positively the doctor's visits in 2004 and 2009, when he brought a team of medical residents, with some specializing in family medicine, in pediatrics, and in ultrasound technology. My presence may have partly elicited his positive appraisals of US alliances, but Dr. Andry's comments can also be viewed as ways that he positions foreign connections as cultural and political resources.

Though Dr. Andry has carefully aligned himself with a variety of professional aid structures and Christian networks in Antananarivo, his clinical stories revealed a multifaceted process of collaborating with and yet distinguishing himself from patients, as well as local Malagasy medical specialists like *ombiasa* (ritual healers). Individual Malagasy navigate a pluralistic and hierarchized medical landscape in Madagascar with several treatment options, including healing by Protestant *fifohazana* revivalists, medical doctors, and *ombiasa*. As mentioned in chapter 1, *ombiasa* are local healer-diviners who view illness as something that is caused by spiritual and relational problems, whether an offense to the ancestors or other living people; *ombiasa* employ plant- and animal-based remedies, divinatory readings of the Malagasy *vintana* (astrological calendar), and communication with the ancestors in their treatment techniques.

Because many of his patients in Manombo first sought care from *ombiasa*, Dr. Andry said he developed ways to talk with the local *ombiasa*, whom he called "traditional workers" in French, and trained them in hygiene to address some of the issues he saw in the clinic. Although the *fifohazana* movement, of which Dr. Andry is a part, criticizes all ancestral practices as involving evil spirits or manifestations of Satan, Dr. Andry took a less dismissive and more collaborative approach.[8] In certain respects, he was smart to do so because most Malagasy, particularly in rural areas such as Manombo, seek out their primary care from *ombiasa*. Individuals' preference for *ombiasa* is multifaceted. In addition to the *ombiasa*'s deep understanding of locally shaped elements of illness causation, particularly knowledge of dynamic and shifting multigenerational family relationships, many Malagasy cannot afford the cost of biomedical care and prescribed pharmaceuticals. Further, they must often traverse prohibitively long geographic distances to reach an understaffed and underresourced clinic (Harper 2002; Legrip-Randriambelo and Regnier 2014).

Within Dr. Andry's comments, however, we can also discern the hierarchical relationship that often obtains between *ombiasa* and biomedical doctors. Dr. Andry aimed to teach the *ombiasa* hygienic measures for the prevention of disease but did not necessarily seek to establish a two-way learning process in which he acquired knowledge of the *ombiasa*'s techniques.[9] Several contemporary ethnographers have illustrated the cultural authority accorded to biomedicine, particularly biomedical techniques and pharmaceuticals. Harper (2002, 191–92) tells of a time when her Tanala informant Solo, who was ill with a fever and stomach pain, consulted an *ombiasa*, who treated the ailment with a plant remedy; in her presence, however, Solo's family asked her whether she had aspirin or any other *fanafody vazaha* (Malagasy, biomedicine), as they believed it would improve his condition. Other scholars have observed that some *ombiasa* use recording practices drawn from biomedical institutions, such as prescription pads, thereby incorporating into their own therapeutic treatment the authority associated with these material artifacts (Legrip-Randriambelo and Regnier 2014).

These cultural hierarchies of medicine and medical knowledge were directly evoked in clinical stories that Dr. Andry told and had the further effect of differentiating him from his patients. In one of Dr. Andry's stories, the Manombo clinic's paid leprosy scout had identified a man in a small village outside Manombo whom the scout believed had leprosy. The scout asked the man to go to the Manombo clinic for treatment and the man agreed to do so but insisted he did not have leprosy. Rather, as the man later told Dr. Andry, his physical symptoms could be explained by the fact that someone had cursed him through an act of witchcraft. After performing a series of diagnostic tests, including blood work, Dr. Andry received confirmation that, from a biomedical perspective, the man did indeed have leprosy. Dr. Andry sensed, however, that he would not be able to convince the man that he had leprosy, partly because of the social stigma of such a diagnosis in the local community as well as the witchcraft the man described as a cause of his physical symptoms. In order to get the man to submit to the biomedical treatment regimen that would lessen his symptoms, Dr. Andry instead told him that he had "*bacille d'Hansen*," using a French clinical term for Hansen's disease (also leprosy). Through this linguistic deception, he said with a laugh, he was able to convince the man to be treated for "BH" rather than leprosy.

In this clinical story and others that I heard him tell, Dr. Andry constructs his own expertise and elite position in relation to his patient, who comes across as unfamiliar with biomedicine. By contrast, the listener is invited to share in the doctor's expert knowledge as a coconspirator. Such stories highlight rural–urban and coast–highlands divides in Madagascar that map onto values of modernity versus tradition, as they are cast into and negotiated through bodily experiences. The account omits mention of the patient's consultation with other medical specialists, such as *ombiasa*; the biomedical system's inability to address the illness cause (witchcraft) identified by the patient; and the clinic's possibly prohibitive cost that made the patient's medical visits so infrequent. These gaps, as well as omissions of key details and knowledge in the clinical encounter itself, consolidate the cultural authority of biomedicine and individual medical doctors.

Overall, through Dr. Andry's profile, we can observe several qualities that characterize other physician–aid brokers in the Minnesota-Madagascar aid program. Though Dr. Andry was unusual in his ability to seize a national global health position, particularly one outside the church, he has like others deployed connections in the church hierarchy (such as those with the Prophetess Nenilava), his skill and cosmopolitanism, and his proximity to Antananarivo to secure his status as a recognizable figure in SALFA, and specifically as a foreign broker. In addition, as I described earlier, we see in Dr. Andry's experiences the traces of these aid brokers' ethno-regional differentiation and cosmopolitan self-fashioning. That is, their self-definition as reliable and expert foreign brokers comes partly from how they subtly distinguish themselves from other Malagasy, such as their rural or non-Christian patients. In some ways, Merina and Betsileo Protestant physician–aid brokers align themselves less with their patients, with whom they sometimes perceive quite vast differences in education level, disease etiologies, and spiritual understandings, than with each other and with the foreign Christian organizations with which they are affiliated. Clinical narratives thus perpetuate these ethno-regional divides and forms of differential Merina and Betsileo Protestant expertise and political authority, as they become laden with values of modernity and tradition, cosmopolitanism and parochialism.

Configuring Doctors as Aid Brokers in Three Cultural Activities

In this section I closely study the interactions of US aid workers and Merina and Betsileo aid brokers to trace how these cultural activities establish an emerging aid subjectivity. Together with the Malagasy cultural history described earlier, these cultural activities reveal a multifaceted conversionary process that, in configuring this aid subjectivity, selectively draws forward and reorganizes certain prior cultural practices and subjectivities in the United States and in Madagascar while backgrounding or rejecting others. I explore in this section how different qualities of the aid broker role are socially constructed and evaluated in three cultural activities that today link American and Malagasy aid workers: solicited medical case studies on the use of donated medical technologies, narratives of Malagasy doctors as proxy missionaries, and global health conferences in Minneapolis–St. Paul. What emerges is a view of Malagasy doctors as hybrid figures that combine the qualities of the cultural translator, Malagasy nationalist–foreign broker, humanitarian, and foreign missionary. I consider how Merina and Betsileo physicians eke out spaces of cultural maneuver within this aid subjectivity, which is disproportionately shaped by US aid requirements and understandings.

Accountability Documents and Their Biospiritual Imaginaries

Humanitarian programs vary immensely in the regularity, style, and quality of contact between aid providers and aid recipients. In the absence of substantial face-to-face contact between US and Malagasy aid participants, certain documents, such as medical case studies and clinical narratives on the use of donated supplies, took on heightened cultural significance in Minneapolis–St. Paul as material and linguistic artifacts that brought to life Malagasy clinical spaces and the work of Malagasy clinicians. Through these written accountability documents, increasingly required by the US NGOs (which I discuss in greater detail in the next chapter), SALFA aid brokers rendered themselves and Malagasy clinical spaces selectively visible to US audiences. The accountability documents strengthened connections between US volunteers and Malagasy physician–aid brokers and fashioned specific qualities of their aid subjectivity, specifically their medical heroism. Such documents thus served several roles beyond their express purpose in verifying the receipt and use of US clinical donations.

I. SUTURING SITES   In 2004–5, the Manambaro Lutheran Hospital in southern Madagascar suffered a shortage of surgical sutures. Sutures are small medical items but one of the most expensive overall supplies because so many are needed for each surgical procedure. At US$2–4 each, they constitute a major cost burden for Malagasy clinics; they are also difficult for the NGOs to obtain because they are heavily used in US medical care and hence largely unavailable for donation. Because the Manambaro Hospital had no sutures for several months yet had to continue providing patient care, the hospital consulted with Malagasy and foreign physicians and ended up substituting a tough plastic fishing line instead. The line could be used in ways similar to sutures, was a durable material, and could be sterilized.[10] The plight of the hospital became a rallying point, however, for US NGO leaders, who approached a Pittsburgh-based NGO, Global Links, which deals mainly in international donations of suture material. Global Links donated more than seven thousand sutures to SALFA, approximately sixteen hundred of which I personally carried in a suitcase to Madagascar in 2005.

The Global Links donation was eventually distributed across several of SALFA's surgical centers. As a condition of the aid, Malagasy doctors were required to supply healing and medical stories to Malagasy Partnership about their use of the sutures. Their stories were eventually woven into Global Links promotional materials on the suture donation and read by Malagasy Partnership volunteers in Minneapolis and by Global Links supporters across the United States. For instance, the summer 2005 Global Links newsletter featured a cover story on the seven-thousand-suture donation, titled "Saving Lives in Madagascar." Two photographic images dominated the cover, framed by text describing the scope of the donation. One image shows a white-coated Malagasy doctor, Olivier Ivon, smiling and opening a suture shipment with the aid of an unidentified Malagasy man. The other photo, less prominently displayed than the first, is a sharply cropped image of a woman's bulging abdomen showing successive stitches after a "successful" caesarean section. One of the woman's hands rests gingerly at the top of her stomach, barely visible in the image's corner, her pushed-down blanket and lifted shirt framing the surgical incision line down the abdomen's center. The photo is intimate yet simultaneously strangely disembodied. The caption does not identify the woman by name but notes how "appropriate surgical materials" make a "critical difference in the survival of women and their babies during complicated pregnancies."[11]

At the top of the article, positioned above the text and its accompanying images, is a "report from the field," written by Dr. Benjamin Adrianarijaona at the Vangaindrano Lutheran Hospital. It is worth citing in whole because it exhibits the challenging conditions of practicing medicine in Malagasy Lutheran clinics as well as the soteriological qualities of medical care in which the US audience vicariously participates by reading such accounts.

> A 24-year-old female in difficult labor was brought to Vangaindrano Lutheran Hospital from a village many kilometers away in an extremely weakened condition. The fetus was also in fetal distress. Surgery was performed immediately, at which time the electricity suddenly went out. It was necessary to complete the surgery by flashlight because this hospital is without a generator. Thanks be to God, everything went well with both mother and infant doing well. They were discharged from the hospital after five days of hospitalization. Sutures used: PDS 0, Chromic Gut 3–0, Prolene 3–0. Many thanks to you, Global Links, for helping us out with essential sutures.

This "report from the field" expresses gratitude for the suture donation while enabling readers to appreciate the inspiring and life-saving qualities of the medical care. What comes forward in the account is the doctor's heroism, practicing medicine under difficult conditions; his resourcefulness with limited technology; and, simultaneously, his technological savvy with the donated sutures.

Accountability documents like the Global Links field report contribute to the overall biospiritual imaginary in which US aid participants and Malagasy clinicians participate, which I introduced in chapter 2. Medical anthropologist Claire Wendland (2012b, 116) has described how northern physicians and students who participate in clinical tourism, or short-term medical work, in Malawian hospitals "recaptur[e] an imagined history in which doctors were humanitarian figures, not well-paid technocrats." In Wendland's work, the kind of medical care provided in Malawian clinics, according to foreign clinical tourists, often seemed closer to the "higher purpose" of medicine, rather than the more technologically and bureaucratically shaped job they were accustomed to or being trained in at home (116). This nostalgic temporal framework, applied to Malawian medicine, discursively placed it in a past from which US biomedicine had since advanced. Journeying to do medical work in Malawi was seen by some as a temporal and professional movement enabling them to "refocus" on the "fundamental values" of medicine (116). Wendland insightfully notes that Malawian clinicians serve both as "objects and subjects" in this medical imaginary (118). They ally themselves with foreign visiting clinicians in their work with patients yet also feel as if they are an object of a tourist gaze positioning them in a purportedly more "real," yet temporally past, form of biomedicine (118).

The field reports produced by Malagasy clinicians similarly engender among US readers both a globalized hierarchy of medicine and forms of touristic voyeurism. Though the US aid workers in my research are not participating in clinical tourism, laypeople and clinicians alike envision Malagasy clinical space through accountability reports. Volunteers in the United States can imagine the urgent medical scene that Dr. Adrianarijaona describes, including his surgical work and the limited infrastructure of the operating room. US readers are invited to identify most with the Malagasy clinician's position in the Global Links report, appreciating his medical expertise. The female patient is given only the identifiers of gender and age and is present mostly in the account as a medical case to be "saved" and worked upon. The field report thus sparks forms of connection and disconnection between US aid participants and the Malagasy medical context. Malagasy clinicians become a source of US readers' admiration for their tenacity and expertise yet the Malagasy medical institution and especially Malagasy patients—like the woman in the report—are subject to forms of estrangement.

In her writing on clinical narratives, Mary-Jo DelVecchio Good (2001, 400) observes that these stories, like other narrative forms, employ linguistic strategies that selectively render a "world of the medical imagination." As in the field report quoted above, many complications and uncertainties, also characteristic of the medical context, are omitted from clinical narratives. The therapeutic course is coherently plotted, even though it may not have been so assured. In the field report, we speed through these plot elements to the case's positive "outcome," though it is possible to imagine that the donated sutures were used for procedures where the patient did not fare as well. Countless other details—

portraying for instance the bodily fluids, the patient's pain, and the smell of the operating room—are left out of the case study. The field report builds on the widespread, familiar genre of medical case studies, stripped of the phenomenological, cultural and intersubjective qualities of medicine. The medical case study features detailed exposition of the body "as a common locus of understanding and sensibility" (Lacquer 1989, 201). Though the Global Links field report resembles a medical case study, it is clearly written for nonspecialists and leaves out, for example, technical terms that would more precisely describe the patient's condition. Yet it endeavors to produce the effect for the audience of feeling as if they share in the doctor's technical knowledge and orientation to the medical problem.

II. HEROIC PRECARITY IN BIOSPIRITUAL IMAGINARIES   The field report establishes Malagasy physicians like Dr. Adrianarijaona as heroic figures in their provision of life-saving care. Yet several double binds can also be seen to characterize this heroism, thus contributing to its cultural instability. In the field report, life-saving intervention happens through the timely arrival of US-donated sutures. Thus, SALFA doctors' ability to carry out necessary medical procedures partly hinges in the Global Links accountability document on US collaboration from afar. Moreover, part of what makes Malagasy doctors heroic in this context—the practice of a technologically spare medicine closer to the humanitarian ideal—is also something the aid program seeks to change by building a resource chain for Malagasy clinics. This contributes to the precarity of the doctors' heroism, as a phenomenon partly elaborated through the aid program: with more US technological support, a primary justification for this kind of heroism—resourcefulness under medically challenging conditions—could conceivably disappear.

   Malagasy doctors' masculinity can also be understood as a component of their perceived heroism and self-sacrifice in these accountability documents, yet this characteristic is also influenced by broader cultural discourses in the aid program. In her analysis of European and US medical missionary memoirs that were published in the 1950s and 1960s, Megan Vaughan (1991, 156) traces how ex-missionary doctors—who are almost entirely men in her study—constructed themselves through the dramatic storyline that "the doctor is empowered to 'save' patients." In this narrative framing, often associated with surgery and the role of the battlefield medic, the doctor's masculinity attains value through, and

subtly genders, the power of medicine and technology to give and recover life itself. According to Vaughan (158), missionary narratives of
work in African communities frequently portrayed the white doctor doing "battle" with the African landscape, rife with dangers of the natural
environment like snakes and crocodiles and the perceived social pathologies of disease and immorality.

With contemporary Malagasy physicians, similar notions of heroic
masculinity in an inhospitable or challenging environment are signaled
to US readers through the Global Links description of the spare operating room, as well as the case study's triumph of technology and surgical expertise. Although the actors have importantly shifted from a white
US doctor to a Malagasy physician, it is striking that the outline and
content of the narrative, particularly the heroic masculinity of surgical
care, cleaves quite closely to the medical missionary genre described by
Vaughan (1991). SALFA physicians' masculinity can be interpreted as
part of what enables them, through a US cultural lens, to be perceived as
heroic medical figures, and part of what in turn consolidates that heroism as a gendered phenomenon, building on a US cultural history of venerating white male doctor "hero figures" (Vaughan 1991, 155).

It is also possible to see in doctors' moral heroism more covert, less
apparent processes of racialization. Cultural discourses and images that
seem on the surface to not be "about" race, from those of an operating room without electricity to the normalization of high-risk obstet-
rics, can nonetheless encode and prefigure racial difference. As Jemima
Pierre (2013, 5) cogently argues, "The very production of 'Africa'—its
colonial history, its geographical, political and cultural mapping, as
well as ongoing discursive configurations of the continent's incorrigible
difference—occurs through ideas of race." Among the multifaceted cultural work performed by US moral discourse on Malagasy doctors, we
can also interpret it as a Euro-American moral overcorrection linked
to the racial inequality associated with the colonial legacy (described in
chapter 1).

By culturally elevating the moral status of SALFA doctors, US aid
partners indirectly fashion themselves as white antiracist actors, in contrast with the widely recognized structural racism of colonial missions.
Paradoxically, this move quietly racializes anew SALFA doctors, who
authenticate this antiracist discourse through their embodied racial and
cultural identities. Such a moral overcorrection can place SALFA doctors in a kind of model minority position, a cultural role that erases the

white gaze that produces it. This covert racialization sheds light on faith-based aid programs as global sites in the production and reconfiguration of race as a transnational phenomenon, which draws on some of the structural power associated with US colonial and imperial domination (Pierre 2013). The role of race does not necessarily diminish in such post-colonial interactions but may take on less perceptible, reworked forms.

SALFA Physicians as Proxy Missionaries

Within the aid program, SALFA doctors were imagined as not only medical heroes but also as those who help secure the Christianness of medicine and as individuals who act on behalf of larger collectives of Malagasy and Americans. I use the term *proxy missionaries* in this section to highlight how, for US aid workers, SALFA doctors seemed to continue certain aspects of the cultural role of mid-twentieth-century US missionaries. Through this culturally and historically constructed position, US aid workers fostered a composite view of Malagasy doctors as those who represent US NGO interests in the clinic and authenticate Malagasy Christian medicine by virtue of their cultural, professional, and religious identities.

The forty-eight SALFA clinics across Madagascar treat patients regardless of their religious affiliation but employ only Christian doctors and nurses. My Malagasy and American informants consistently characterized Christian physicians as key figures in the SALFA system who ideally provided a moral example of Christian behavior and delivered spiritual counsel to their patients at opportune moments. When I once asked the former SALFA director Mr. Rajoanary what he thought needed to be done to secure SALFA's future, he answered without hesitation that SALFA needed a strong class of young Christian doctors; many current physicians were close to retirement or "endangered species," he joked, using a conservation discourse particularly well worn in Madagascar. Mr. Rajoanary added that SALFA should market its uniqueness in providing holistic Christian care that tends to spiritual and bodily needs and distinguish itself from secular, government-run clinics. In a 2006 email correspondence written to US supporters and circulated at an IHM fundraiser, the SALFA financial officer Clement described SALFA's work as a "combination of commercial and social work, in which is added its main job: spreading the Gospel."

Though medical care was viewed by both Malagasy and US aid participants as spiritual work, the US aid workers in my research seemed especially concerned about ensuring that their funds and supplies contributed to an *authentic* Christian practice of medicine in Madagascar rather than a secular medicine with Christian window-dressing. Their anxieties are not necessarily new, for such concerns were the focus of substantial discussion in earlier European and US medical missions. Vaughan (1991, 74) reports that missionary discourses in Africa in the early to mid-twentieth century often debated how to ensure that patients recognized the Christian God at the center of mission medicine. Medicine could appear powerful in practice, having the capability to heal with an injection or regimen of antibiotics; missionaries therefore worried that patients would take the material medicine on its own as a powerful force and, in their eyes, misrecognize the otherwise immaterial source of healing power. In a 1979 ethnohistory of the Manambaro Hospital in southeast Madagascar, the missionary pastor-author prominently states on the first page that the hospital "seeks not to be just another hospital, not just a repair shop for broken bodies, but a *Christ*-ian hospital: a place where healing is seen as part of the ministration to the whole person in the name of Jesus, the Christ" (Vigen 1979, 43, italics in original). Moreover, in the same document, the author approvingly quotes Norwegian American missionary doctor J. O. Dyrnes (described in chapter 1) who said that if given the choice between evangelism and medicine he would "without hesitation" choose evangelism (1979, 48). Today, US aid workers demonstrate concern for remarkably similar issues yet they now focus on Malagasy doctors as standard bearers of the spiritual authenticity of Christian medicine.

I. AID BROKERS' PROXY ROLE AND SPIRITUAL PRECARITY Specific US narratives and events, including Malagasy physicians' US visits, culturally shaped SALFA doctors' proxy missionary role. During his October 2005 visit to Minneapolis, Dr. Rafolo, introduced at the beginning of the chapter, told the Malagasy Partnership volunteers that evangelism was the "most important piece of all" in the SALFA operation, a phrase that Gene quoted with emphasis in several later conversations. Since Gene and the other US volunteers understood their aid work as a kind of spiritual labor, which reinforced their Christian identity and relationship with God, they often sought verification that they were doing

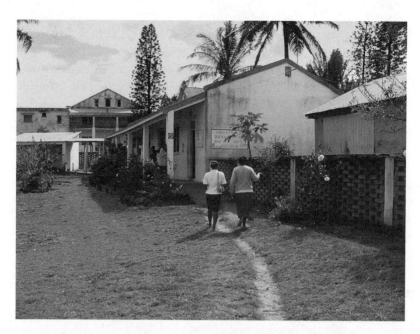

FIGURE 5.1. Worn path leading to SALFA's Tolagnaro–Ft. Dauphin dispensary.

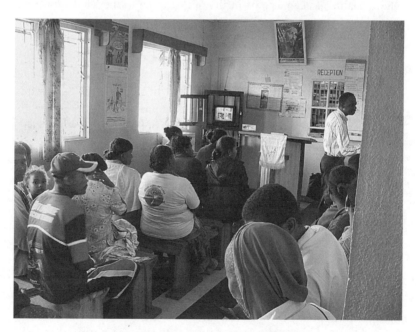

FIGURE 5.2. An evangelical video plays on a small television while patients wait to be seen, Tolagnaro–Ft. Dauphin.

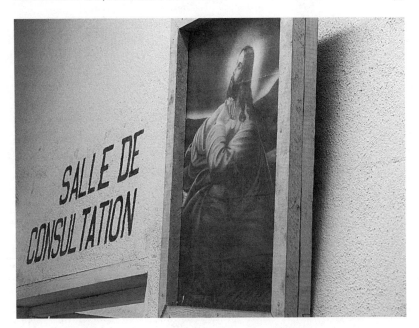

FIGURE 5.3. Entrance to one of the dispensary's two treatment rooms, Tolagnaro–
Ft. Dauphin.

God's work. In this framework, a range of small acts, such as Dr. Rafolo's words or Clement's written prioritization of evangelism mentioned
earlier, were reassuring to US volunteers and interpreted as signs of
SALFA's spiritual authenticity. In this context, it could be observed that
Malagasy physicians needed to appropriately communicate their Christian commitment to their US partners, as Dr. Rafolo did. If they failed
to verbally or in writing prioritize the Gospel, which I admittedly never
witnessed, it could be taken by US aid workers as a sign of an inadequate
prioritization of spirituality in the medicine they practiced.

Sometimes, SALFA physician–aid brokers successfully navigated
this complex moral terrain to advance their own political and religious
goals. After Dr. Rafolo's US visit and his recommendations, Gene an-
nounced in January 2006 that he had solicited US funding to pay for
the salaries of three Malagasy evangelists for three years (US$60 per
month per evangelist). The evangelists lived around Ejeda in southwest
Madagascar, an area reported to have experienced several villagewide
conversions to Christianity in the past decade. Evangelists hold specific
positions in the FLM; they are lay preachers who frequently teach read-

ing and writing to rural villagers, usually improving literacy with the aim of introducing specific biblical lessons. Sometimes they also assist nurses in small, understaffed rural clinics. For Gene and Dr. Rafolo, the Ejeda evangelists' work would strengthen the spiritual witness possible through the physicians and nurses at Ejeda Lutheran Hospital. That is, in their eyes, the evangelists' work in the local community would help to ensure that the doctors' physical care was interpreted by patients as a sign of the more encompassing spiritual and cultural work of Christian faith. As a long-time physician at the Ejeda Hospital, Dr. Rafolo played a central role in designing and implementing this program, using his US visit to spark conversation about securing the necessary funding.

In addition, US discourses affirmed the cultural and spiritual authenticity of current SALFA physician–aid brokers by strikingly aligning them with a historically rooted ontological conflict between Christian medicine and Malagasy ritual healing, as described in chapter 1. On a few occasions, US narratives about Malagasy physicians made explicit this ontological conflict. One evening, in the group prayer that closed the Malagasy Partnership work session, Gene noted that it was about 6 a.m. in Madagascar "now" and "people are already up." As though experiencing a vision, Gene said a person could be "traveling in an oxcart" and on his or her way to a SALFA clinic at "this very minute" as a "last resort." The person had "already paid an *ombiasa*" all they had and sought medical treatment after traveling overnight from a far distance. Through the movement of the approaching oxcart, Gene built for his US listeners a feeling of anticipation as the SALFA clinic staff—aligned with the US volunteers—awaited the person as he or she entered the Christian world of the clinic. Through its narrative view from above, Gene's prayer story prompted awareness of the divine hand uniting these two space-times and sets of Christian and non-Christian actors.

Less explicitly, Gene's words also illustrate how Malagasy medicine (*fanafody-gasy*) and biomedicine (*fanafody vazaha*) have been "entangled objects" (Thomas 1991 cited in Hunt 1999, 7) in US missionary discourse, mutually constituted and reliant on each other to produce the value of the other though ostensibly opposed. As we saw in Gene's prayer, US discourses portray *ombiasa* as those who take money from the Malagasy individuals who consult them; this implies that a dishonest commercial transaction lies at the core of the *ombiasa*'s work, in contrast with the more upright quid-pro-quo of biomedical care (i.e., payment for services). In fact, ethnographers report that, among contemporary

Tanala and Betsileo respectively, people consult *ombiasa* because they can afford to do so, in contrast with state-run and private biomedical clinics (Harper 2002; Legrip-Randriambelo and Regnier 2014).[12] If their relative's condition improves, the ailing person's family often gives the *ombiasa* remuneration in the form of rice, rum, meat from a slaughtered animal, and sometimes money; while *ombiasa* partake in these exchanges, they sometimes frame them as offerings to the ancestors who aid in healing's effectiveness (Legrip-Randriambelo and Regnier 2014, 32).[13] Through these ethnographic portraits of *ombiasa*, as well as my earlier discussion in the chapter, it becomes apparent that the *ombiasa* of missionary discourse is a selective US construction and often serves to draw out the value of Christian biomedicine.

In sum, Gene's prayer culturally and morally aligned US aid workers with SALFA physicians-qua-proxy missionaries and distinguished them from the *ombiasa*. In the weekly group prayer, at least one Malagasy Partnership volunteer routinely prayed for Malagasy Lutheran physicians, asking God to bless them and to allow them to awake on the following day renewed in energy. Physician–aid brokers were imagined in these narratives as collective proxies or collaborators who shared interests with US laypeople, as US foreign missionaries were conceptualized in the early to mid-twentieth century. Moreover, praying for foreign missionaries, as Malagasy Partnership volunteers do now for SALFA doctors, was something that US congregants long did as companions to missionaries "at home."[14] Through reading stories "from the field" in church periodicals and viewing missionaries' church-basement slide shows while on leave, US laypeople long occupied the role of moral spectators of twentieth-century US missionaries' foreign work, a cultural role now placed in the service of medical aid. In contrast with earlier US mission work, the aid relationship fosters a sharper emphasis on Christian medical care and features Malagasy aid brokers. As we can see among US aid workers, however, it extends select cultural narratives and subject positions, such as the spectacle of the mission field and the US-produced category of *ombiasa*, from the earlier work of US missionaries.

II. MIDDLE FIGURES REVISITED   In her influential book *A Colonial Lexicon* (1999), historian Nancy Hunt coined the term "middle figure" to characterize the cultural translator role of African Christian medical specialists in the Belgian Congo. Revisiting this concept will help shed light on the differences and similarities between this colonial work and the contemporary role of SALFA physician–aid brokers in the Minnesota-Madagascar aid program. As in Hunt's work, Merina and Betsileo physicians often translate biomedical care to Malagasy populations across the island. As we saw in Dr. Andry's clinical stories, some of these patients have infrequent interactions with biomedical clinics and more regular visits with *ombiasa* (ritual healers) and other Malagasy medical specialists. Moreover, many contemporary Merina and Betsileo Protestant physicians actually practiced medicine side by side with US missionaries in Madagascar in the late 1970s and 1980s and succeed by one generation Malagasy nurses and doctors who, like the "middle figures" of Hunt's book, worked with colonial missionaries. Today, they represent the first Malagasy generation to fully run Malagasy Lutheran medical institutions with no US or Norwegian foreign missionaries on staff. As Clement pointed out in chapter 1, however, SALFA is still casting off colonial and US mission structures of authority and emerging as an independent or Malagasy-run network of medical institutions. Thus, the complex legacy of missionary interactions, described so richly in Hunt's work, is not of the far distant past but, as I have argued in this book, part of the lived experiences of SALFA aid brokers.

Although it is important to note the aid program's colonial missionary origins, which prompt comparisons with Hunt's work, the current relief endeavor also differs from Hunt's colonial-era research in several significant ways. The contemporary aid broker role does not solely involve establishing the authority or veracity of biomedical views of healing, the body, and treatment, as Hunt (1999) documented in the Belgian Congo. Rather, since such biomedical views are already well established (though certainly not universally espoused), Merina and Betsileo doctors are frequently characterized as conveyors of the Christianness of Lutheran biomedicine. Among US aid participants, Merina and Betsileo aid brokers appear to combine the role of the US foreign missionary with that of the cultural translator that Hunt attributes to "middle figures." Yet, rather than translating between foreign biomedical and indigenous medical understandings as Hunt described, Merina and Betsileo physicians today often translate Malagasy medical settings to foreign aid organizations. Simultaneously, rather than being prototypic "local" actors as Hunt primarily characterized Congolese middle figures, Malagasy doctors emerge in the current aid program as cosmopolitans aligned with a broader, transnational field of Christian health care.

In sum, the Minnesota-Madagascar aid program selectively borrows and extends some of the cultural resources of the evangelical missions that preceded it while ostensibly problematizing—but not necessarily extricating itself from—other elements of the colonial context, particularly asymmetries of institutional authority and autonomy. Indeed, as we have seen, the colonial legacy serves as more than a "context," and viewing it as such could mistakenly lead us to miss finer traffic in representations and practices between the so-called colonial and postcolonial periods. As I have shown, imageries and practices of the colonial, both as reworked historical forms and as negative images, are thoroughly enmeshed in the small-scale intimacies of contemporary aid interactions.

Global Health Conferences as Performative Spaces

Global health conferences and other US visits constitute a third cultural space—in addition to medical case studies and narratives of SALFA doctors as proxy missionaries—where Merina and Betsileo physicians were fashioned, and cast themselves, as aid partners. Global health conferences professionalize Christian medical aid, amplifying the expertise and standards of Christian medical work. At the same time, they trade in symbols and discourses of both secular and faith-based global health, bringing them together and recombining them into a new form. As in secular global health meetings, where foreign physicians are called upon to present (and represent) overseas work, Merina and Betsileo Malagasy physicians supply credibility to US Christian medical work during their Minneapolis visits. Such events fit the broader notion among US aid workers involved with Malagasy Partnership that their Malagasy partners should be brought to the United States for "cultural exchange" but—in contrast and response to the colonial mission legacy—US participants should remain in a supportive, noninterfering role in the United States, with only their medical materials circulating from the US Midwest to Madagascar. Through my analysis of one IHM global health conference, I examine in this section how the conference operates as a performative space, establishing partnership as an ethical and moral project while smoothing out the potential tensions and contradictions that surround the aid program.

The IHM conference pitches the long-standing practices of mission medicine into a new framing—that of global health—with particular social capital for US participants. By characterizing their work as "global health," US agency leaders legitimate Christian efforts through the moral authority and cachet now cohering around global health as a field, in contrast with international public health, mission medicine, and tropical medicine. They also place their work professionally on par with secular initiatives, implying they adhere to similar standards of expertise, social justice, and professional rigor. In her book *Scrambling for Africa*, medical anthropologist Johanna Crane (2013) points out that the increasing number of global health programs initiated by US universities frequently pivot their work around claims to partnership, as does the Minnesota-Madagascar aid program. Global health emerged from international public health in the 1990s, a field that, in turn, has roots in the colonial practice of tropical medicine. Global health, as Crane (2013) maintains, is in some ways a North American relabeling of these predecessor fields. Global health practitioners often claim a more egalitarian approach than their predecessors yet still primarily pursue northern-initiated or northern-funded medical programs that typically happen outside of North America and Western Europe. Important questions thus remain about what partnership means in global health programs; these questions include the degree to which nonnorthern physicians and scientists define the priorities of global health programs and benefit from the immense resources put toward global health initiatives (Crane 2013).

At the 2005 global health conference that I attended, the SALFA physician Dr. Rafolo and his wife Honore were selected as the featured guests and were flown to Minneapolis by IHM. The couple, normally stationed in Ejeda in southwest Madagascar but at the time doing a surgical skills program in Cameroon, gave the keynote address for the conference, which was titled "Expanding Our Borders: Growing in Mission." Dr. Rafolo and Honore's address, "Sharing the Good News through Health Outreach—Experiences from Madagascar," was attended by approximately fifty, predominantly Euro-American, laypeople and former missionaries. Dr. Rafolo had donned a dark-toned business suit for the occasion, and Honore wore a dress with a highland Malagasy *lamba* wrapped tightly around her shoulders. Their address was held in the sanctuary of the Grace Lutheran Church in St. Paul, where a greeting, welcome, and devotions framed the conference as a spiritual event. In contrast to secular global health meetings, which establish program priorities through biostatistical portraits and reported program "outcomes," I was surprised by how much Dr. Rafolo's address defined the "urgency" of IHM programs through the need to bring the Gospel to rural populations of southwest Madagascar.

As part of their presentation, Dr. Rafolo and Honore sang in English a hymn they had composed for the event, titled "Waiting for Us," and circulated a handout with the English lyrics so the audience members could add their voices to the performance. The hymn, like the address, which Dr. Rafolo spoke in English with Honore accompanying him on stage, delineated how the Gospel message could be communicated through health care outreach, or through organizing from SALFA medical centers like the Ejeda Hospital mobile teams of community health workers and evangelists. Indeed, the hymn lyrics characterized "distant people" as being "eager to hear the Holy Word of God" and linguistically aligned the Euro-American audience with Dr. Rafolo and Honore ("us") in the shared pursuit of "reveal[ing]" it. Notably, at no point in the address or hymn did Dr. Rafolo or Honore explicitly refer to their work as "global health," a term that seemed more to characterize the US initiatives. After the keynote address, the conference program featured an afternoon of breakout sessions in adjoining rooms; illustrating IHM's mixture of secular and faith-based aid approaches, these sessions covered a range of spiritual and medical issues and included programs on IHM volunteer opportunities, health care management and accountability, news about the old contract (the "Old Covenant" or Old Testament), and successes and challenges in the global fight against AIDS. Two of the four breakout-session speakers were former US missionaries to Madagascar.

Global health conferences in North America like IHM's annual event create a space of exchange between Malagasy physicians and US agency leaders about clinical needs and funding priorities. Yet I could not help but notice that these events in the Minnesota-Madagascar aid program played an equally important performative and ritual role. Building on the classic work of sociolinguist Erving Goffman (1976, 1981), linguistic anthropologists have shown that people often perform multiple shifting roles in conversations and that conversations themselves are guided by intricate and dynamic, yet often socially unrecognized, "participation frameworks." Such interactive scaffoldings establish each participant's footing in relation to other participants, as well as foreshadowed, imagined, or past voices; collectively, though often not knowingly, individuals activate this dense nexus of relations and interpretive frameworks in "the participation structure of the moment" (Irvine 1996, 135). Participation roles are thus performed or culturally made and renegotiated through these contextually anchored but also somewhat fleeting cultural resources. When these insights are applied to humanitarian aid organizations, it is possible to see the underanalyzed role of these participation scaffoldings in a variety of humanitarian spaces, whether in global health conferences, program meetings, or site visits. Aid organizations use these linguistic and performative resources to create moral participation frameworks that function as ideological structures for their work and that have affective, moral, and political entailments for individuals.

The IHM global health conference selectively activates these embodied and linguistic structures to shape certain roles for Malagasy physicians and for US aid workers. The physical presence of SALFA physicians performs partnership and unity in the face of possible gaps of understanding and collaboration. As an embodied event, the global health conference draws attention to the geopolitical divides of the medical aid program and, by bringing American and Malagasy partners together in one space, attempts to at least fleetingly resolve the tensions presented by this cultural and geographic distance. For SALFA physicians, the conference also consolidates access to forms of social and political capital by confirming their role as important actors in the transnational field of Christian global health. Selected SALFA physicians like Dr. Rafolo are publicly recognized as aid partners. Because of their familiarity to US agency leaders, these physicians' participation can lead to economic capital, as well, facilitating greater access to funding sources for themselves and their clinics, as we saw with Dr. Rafolo and the Ejeda evangelists program.

Moreover, the conference publicly stages partnership as a moral and ethical endeavor. IHM representatives, US doctors, and other interested supporters, in addition to the Merina and Betsileo physician-guests, partake in the conference's transformative qualities. US participants hone their cultural identity as moral actors who partner with Malagasy physicians. In this setting, they morally witness to the organization's collective identity as an agency that seeks and values its partners' views. Yet it could be observed that SALFA physicians like Dr. Rafolo actively calibrate how they pitch their work for the context of the US audience. Malagasy aid brokers' heroic precarity derives partly from their need to reassure their US partners that they are "present with the Gospel," as Gene once described it. Attesting to the primacy of the Gospel in Malagasy medical programs, as Dr. Rafolo did, was a "message" that spoke to US concerns about the medical aid partnership. My intent in arguing this is not to question Dr. Rafolo's sincerity or genuineness in his testimony to the importance of the Gospel; Dr. Rafolo is a committed evangelical Christian. We must not overlook, however, how US aid workers' views and concerns may disproportionately shape the performance expectations for the aid broker role and infuse such performances with serious stakes for SALFA physicians, including their ability to secure funding for their work.

By comparison, US visits hosted by Malagasy Partnership fashioned slightly different qualities of SALFA physicians and administrators. During two-week-long visits, Clement and Dr. Remy each stayed at Gene's family's house in a northern Minneapolis suburb, and Gene, his wife, and their children hosted picnics, receptions, after-church coffees, and warehouse work sessions with them so they could get to know the US volunteers. It was clear to me that these visits were not viewed as pro forma cultural exchanges but rather such visits often fostered a sense of fondness and affection between the SALFA visitors and their US hosts. When I met with Clement in 2014 in Antananarivo, he independently brought up his 2004 Minneapolis visit during one of our conversations; perhaps influenced by my presence as an American researcher, he expressed his gratitude for Gene's hospitality and we laughed about Gene's fondness for volleyball, which Clement had found amusing. Likewise, Gene referred to Dr. Remy's and Clement's visits well after they had occurred, sometimes sharing an anecdote that came to mind with the other volunteers or marveling about Clement's love for soccer. Gene's and Clement's mutual emphasis on sportsmanship is, I would suggest, not coincidental. US aid workers espouse a spectatorlike admiration of these doctors and administrators, somewhat similar to the idolization of a heroic male athlete. Indeed, Gene once confessed that encountering SALFA physicians in person was "kind of like meeting heroes." US aid workers combine this sentiment with a deep appreciation of SALFA partners as role models in their Christian piety and in their gendered performance—like Gene and the other fathers of Malagasy Partnership—of a kind of family-based, heterosexual masculinity.

Thus, various activities and interactive spaces in the aid program drew forward and attributed different qualities and meanings to the category of Merina and Betsileo aid brokers. Simultaneously, these practices, which amplify SALFA physicians as (male) medical heroes, embodiments of Christian witness, and cultural translators, fostered slightly different roles and qualities for US participants, whether ethical actors or fans of admired heroes. It is important to note that each of these cultural identifications is a moral position in the aid program, socially performed by and sometimes conflated with individuals but not in fact intrinsic to them; these roles simplify the aid program's complex moral and political terrain by highlighting egalitarianism, intimacy, and shared moral aims while socially backgrounding less harmonious qualities. Such moral identifications demonstrate a fleeting quality in light of their connection to US visits and global health conferences, rare face-to-face meeting spaces in the aid program. Telling stories of those interactions is one way that American and Malagasy aid participants, in addition to SALFA doctors' correspondence and US narratives of doctors as proxy missionaries, attempt to make these moral relations more enduring.

Conclusions

In this chapter, I have described how the aid broker role of Merina and Betsileo Protestant physicians takes shape through a Malagasy history of ethno-regional differentiation and the nationalist protest tradition of Merina and Betsileo Protestant elites, which often relied on making strategic Anglo-Protestant alliances. Though contemporary Merina and Betsileo Lutheran physicians like Dr. Rafolo and Dr. Andry do not merely reproduce this historical role, it can be understood as a cultural resource among many that entitles them to access and build their position in the contemporary Minnesota-Madagascar aid program. In combination with their medical training, linguistic skills, and individual biographies, the historically organized role of national Merina and Betsileo Protestant leaders works to position them as appropriate aid brokers. In addition, I have suggested that, while this cultural identification is rooted in Malagasy cultural categories, it is simultaneously reworked and transformed through specific cultural activities in the aid program, such as global health conferences, narratives about doctors as spiritual workers, and accountability documents. In these transformative spaces and exchanges, American views and understandings play a disproportionate role, compelling and disfavoring certain performances of self-identification among SALFA doctors.

This complex political and moral terrain results in a situation in which a kind of precarious heroism encircles Merina and Betsileo physician–aid brokers. Their heroism favorably connects them to illustrious biblical acts of healing and, most important, to the work of the "Great Physician." Yet, in the aid program, SALFA physicians' heroism places them in a series of contradictory positions. Malagasy Lutheran doctors often come to be viewed by their US colleagues as authentic humanitarian actors and Malagasy Christians, becoming entangled in lingering images and narratives of mid-twentieth-century US foreign missions. They operate as both "objects and subjects" in a biospiritual imaginary of SALFA clinical practice, which builds on a century-long history of US discourses of missionary medical heroism and the pursuit of "risky," technologically spare African institutionalized medicine (Wendland 2012b). Yet as a result of this American reading of their cultural and professional identities and the fundamental instability of all authenticity claims, Malagasy doctors must often assure their US partners that they are genuine Christians and medical heroes, which makes precarious their cultural role in the aid program. Furthermore, SALFA doctors' heroism elevates them to a place where fairly small infractions of expected moral conduct, such as failing to supply an accountability report, can appear disappointing to their US colleagues. Physicians' highly visible role subjects them to greater US surveillance and required audit work, as I address in the next chapter. Audit work brings to the surface of the aid program divergent views of what partnership means in faith-based aid, and particularly to whom one is morally accountable.

CHAPTER SIX

Traversing Shadow Spaces of Accountability

We do not give *to* the Budget, but *through* the Budget.
—Evangelical Lutheran Church (US) pamphlet, circa 1960

Accountability in humanitarian aid is often taken to be synonymous with bureaucratic documents. Budgets, reports, and case studies seek to make "transparent" the use of donor resources and illustrate the specific "outcomes" of those resource flows. Ideally, they perform credibility and build trust with particular audiences in the process (Barnett and Duvall 2005; Ebrahim and Weisband 2007). But we can also view accountability, as anthropologists have long done, as a more basic and vital element of relationships. This form of accountability is something that in fact often emerges through a more widespread array of social practices than only those that are explicitly about accountability in bureaucratic terms. This broader notion of what it means to be accountable to others is, of course, the stuff of intimate social ties. It is in play when people make requests of and give gifts to each other and the divine, in keeping with prevailing values of mutuality, exchange, and reciprocity (Graeber 2011). In this chapter, I combine these two primary meanings of accountability to argue for finer attention to the interanimation of intimate and bureaucratic methods of moral accounting in humanitarian work.

In the Minnesota-Madagascar aid program, accountability work draws upon such culturally and historically rooted conventions and techniques of moral accounting and thus demonstrates how religious humanitarians selectively fuse the accountability procedures of the broader aid world with religious and cultural understandings of what it means to be morally accountable. Lutheran aid workers interestingly bring together both bureaucratic accountability's emphasis on transparency in the use of aid resources and a Bible-based model of moral accounting from Luke 24 that guides the aid partnership (discussed in chapter 1). US aid workers often interpret this biblical model of accountability to mean that they should minimize their interference in the church affairs of their overseas aid partners, sending relief aid and not humanitarian workers, and instead seek to establish an equitable partnership in contrast with the inequalities seen as characterizing colonial evangelism. Accountability requirements, however, certainly do travel and have been increasingly woven into each donation of medical relief, financial support, or equipment. Because they draw attention to the unequal and hierarchical qualities of aid, these accountability requirements sometimes problematically conflict with the tenets of Luke 24, which conceptualizes partnership in Christian aid alliances as a relational, mutually shared endeavor. My aim in this chapter is to illuminate how bureaucratic requirements are selectively socialized to or through preexisting cultural logics, opening up a wider cultural field than what is commonly analyzed in studies of humanitarian accountability. In what ways are religious and neoliberal reasoning on moral accountability combined or reconfigured, and with what effects? What implications does this have for transnational faith-based aid as both a form of humanitarianism and a site of religious engagement?

German sociologist Max Weber (1978, 225) famously called bureaucracy a form of "domination through knowledge." In his view, documents order institutions and reinforce techniques and hierarchies of information control. Yet taking the perspective of cultural actors negotiating bureaucratic forms reveals bureaucratic work to be filled with diverse trajectories and histories, to be more multiple, culturally contingent, and unpredictable than the ordered social systems Weber described. In her book *Humanitarian Insecurities*, for instance, anthropologist Erica James (2010) describes how, even as Haitian violence survivors performed *viktim* identity narratives to secure financial and emotional support from aid organizations, some characterized bureaucratic paperwork as a skilled practice—like witchcraft—for altering aid's unseen, seemingly distant funding channels. The meanings of bureaucratic work are thus not necessarily assured, nor are they of secondary importance. Rather, they are subject to diverse cultural interpretations that lay open to question the degree to which bureaucratic documents are "the same" material things in different cultural contexts. These insights challenge the common view, advanced by Weber himself (1978, 975), that bureaucracy epitomizes the depersonalized workings of modern life. Yet, even while taking this critical cultural perspective into account, bureaucratic documents clearly still hold significance as touchstones of modern efficiency and professionalism across many cultural spheres, including humanitarian aid.

Accountability work has been one of the main channels through which religious humanitarians—particularly post-9/11 Muslim agencies falsely accused of supporting terrorism—have sought to establish their credibility to federal and private funders, as well as professionalize their operations (De Cordier 2008; Benthall 2010). For Christian agencies like IHM and Malagasy Partnership (which emerged partly from early- and mid-twentieth-century lay projects of charitable giving), establishing themselves as professional has meant shedding a largely feminized history of nonprofessional charitable work within their own communities (Halvorson 2012b). Professionalization has also entailed adopting audit measures that facilitate an image of disinterested techno-efficiency while providing common standards of industry evaluation. Audit work appeals to both Minneapolis agencies precisely for its apparent "secularity," a quality that could perhaps better be glossed as disinterestedness or impartiality in matters of money and aid dissemination, in contrast with the organizations' obvious interestedness in matters of religion.[1] During my fieldwork, both IHM and Malagasy Partnership, in order to qualify for federal grants and for supply donations from larger aid organizations, were in the process of adopting a variety of bureaucratic procedures of the broader aid world, including more statistical record keeping on shipments, fiscal transparency measures, needs assessments, and accountability reports from aid recipients. Clustered with other historically associated secular values, the disinterestedness and techno-efficiency of such bureaucratic procedures—what Michael Herzfeld (1992, 5) has called the "secular theodicy" of bureaucratic discourse—emphasizes the professional equivalence of religious organizations with secular aid agencies.

I analyze accountability transactions in the chapter as cultural exchanges, which, though constrained by bureaucratic forms, involve a great deal more than bureaucratic artifacts alone, often evoking seen and unseen actors, spoken and unspoken ideals of moral comportment, and historically rooted moral subjectivities. Accountability in aid entails certain bureaucratic processes and crafts the subjectivity of those who participate in accountability work, as I will explore. Perhaps more fundamentally, though, it operates as a mutual request that the recipient and provider of aid make to each other to acknowledge the underlying terms of aid as an exchange.[2] Because it draws overt attention to these terms, accountability work is a revealing cultural space in which to investigate how power and authority are negotiated through small, even mundane, transactions in religiously motivated aid partnerships. For those involved in Lutheran medical relief, accountability elucidates an irresolvable tension between the ethical ideal of mutuality between global Christians based on equal footing and aid as an asymmetrical exchange.

In what follows, I focus mainly on accountability as experienced by US agency leaders and SALFA administrators, rather than on the views of US lay volunteers. Although volunteer workers morally accounted for aid through the labor and prayer activities I described in chapter 3, accountability took on additional meanings according to agency leaders' knowledge of and involvement with audit work. Both US agency leaders and SALFA administrators fulfilled accountability or audit work. The specific bureaucratic documents, conditions, cultural understandings, and effects of accountability work differed considerably, however, between US and Malagasy aid administrators. As I will first discuss, US agency leaders like Gene corresponded regularly with SALFA officials and participated in complex, multiparty needs assessments, often through email. From this bureaucratic correspondence, he then attempted, through the NGOs' donor contacts, to supply what equipment or technologies those working in foreign clinics had requested. Moreover, SALFA officials in Antananarivo like Clement were increasingly asked during my fieldwork to document the outcomes of US fiscal and in-kind supply donations with progress reports and medical case studies. These required procedures instilled new forms of accountable subjectivity among Malagasy clinicians and administrators and created tensions in the aid relationship because of the subtle inequalities they introduced. Moving in the chapter from the US Midwest to Madagascar, I therefore build a multisited portrait of accountability work as a "mobile" or traveling form of humanitarian governance (Pandolfi 2010, 239), understood and enacted in culturally distinct ways.

On the Matter of Appropriate Technology:
Combining Bureaucratic and Divine Persuasion

"You might be interested in the emails going back and forth," Gene told me while we stood outside the open Malagasy Partnership warehouse door in a northern Minneapolis suburb. As the sun sunk lower in the sky, the air gusts cooled our foreheads and arms. It was a hot summer day. The blasting heat of the 90-degree high made a balmy 75-degree evening feel practically chilly. I stood beside two regular volunteers in their twenties, Emily and Megan, at a long folding table pulled onto the asphalt of the driveway, next to a small stamp of bright green grass. Blood-pressure cuffs and pumps were strewn across the table's red lacquer surface. Gene had instructed us to carefully examine the thick black plastic tubing of each blood-pressure unit. If any deep cracks appeared on the surface, the tubing had to be pitched, but we were salvaging the units' small connectors, metal screws, and the cuffs themselves. We tested the units' pressure on our arms, inflating the cuff until it pinched our skin.

Gene explained to me, as well as to four listening volunteers, that he had been exchanging emails and reading the messages from a long needs assessment. The correspondence involved an IHM board member, a donor from a local hospital, Clement, Mark at IHM, and Gene; it debated whether an infusion pump that had been offered to SALFA was an appropriate donation. This equipment had already been donated to IHM and, as a local sister agency with ties to Malagasy Partnership, IHM was offering it to the agency to send to SALFA. Since Malagasy Partnership handled all aid shipments to SALFA, Gene was squarely involved in the email conversation about whether to send it. Gene summed up what to him was most troubling about the infusion pump as a possible donation. Each use of the pump for a patient required a cost of US$23, an amount of money Malagasy patients would not be able to pay. Moreover, the equipment, which administers intravenous fluids to patients, did a procedure that could conceivably be done by a nurse with less sophisticated technology. The pump would also require auxiliary items and specialized knowledge to safely maintain it, all things he worried SALFA would not be able to support. The equipment in his mind was symbolic of a US donor mindset in which people wanted to give things away but did not first ask the recipients about what would be most beneficial. Likewise, he worried that the SALFA liaison, Clement, might be unfamiliar with the technology yet not want to sour the aid relationship by rejecting a donation.

Just Asking Questions

I saw Gene again the following week and asked him about infusion pump donation. He said—haltingly and signaling some frustration—that the latest email messages in the needs assessment had concluded that perhaps it would be useful to have one pump in each of SALFA's nine large hospitals. Since we had last talked, Gene said he had separately contacted a US colleague at a large, TECH-member agency to get further statistics on the infusion pump model, a syringe cassette-driven pump. He had learned that the SALFA technician in Madagascar was not accustomed to the equipment and that it needs careful recalibration after each maintenance check to make sure the right amount of IV fluids are being dispensed to the patient. It also requires a special type of tubing, rather than regular IV tubing, which has to be replaced for each patient. Despite all these concerns, Gene said that he had had a "slight shift in thinking" during the previous week. He explained, "I got to thinking, 'Who am I to say whether this can be used or not?' It's probably a good idea to send one infusion pump and let SALFA people see whether it can be used and how. I'm not there. I don't know. *I just ask the questions.* I want them to make the decision, have a feeling of responsibility for it. Telling people what to do would be no help in the matter" [italics mine]. Gene added that SALFA physicians "deserve to have the best and newest equipment possible" and implied that US donors should not presume that second best is good enough for their overseas aid partners. Still, he expressed some unease in what he described as a trust in "equipment over human skill" among his Malagasy colleagues. Because of the uncertainty in the SALFA correspondence about how the equipment would be used, Gene thought the best solution was to send one infusion pump "for evaluation" in the next scheduled shipping container. He sometimes added one sample of a clinical item so that the SALFA liaison and technician could evaluate it for usefulness before sending a containerful. This assessment technique struck Gene as far more effective than the email dialogue.

Bureaucratic correspondence, such as the multiparty needs assessment in which Gene participated, carries an ideological aura of transparency that camouflages how its intersubjective qualities and power differentials often shape what can and cannot be stated. In his study of bureaucratic processes tied to the expropriation of land surrounding Islamabad, Pakistan, anthropologist Matthew Hull (2008, 505) observes that the material forms of official records are often presumed to be a "palpable sedimentation of the real." Although the email medium through which the infusion pump assessment was conducted may not carry the same authority as paper documentation, the genre conventions of needs assessments still imply that what is recorded in writing necessarily corresponds to the needs of Malagasy clinicians. Calling into question this assumed conflation of bureaucratic words and reality, Gene drew attention to the *ritual* and *performative* dimensions of such aid communications. In our conversations, he alluded insightfully to the way people perform particular roles in these communications, enacting graciousness and appreciation, for example, in the interest of maintaining the aid relationship and demonstrating respect for their correspondents. Yet these same qualities called the trustworthiness of the content into question. Hull (2008, 505) points to this phenomenon as well, labeling it a "bureaucratic irony" that written records that seek to concretize "the real" can actually, through their form, highlight the fundamental instability of the processes they seek to render legible or controllable.

Even though Gene indicated distrust in the bureaucratic form of the needs assessment, he still hoped to use language effectively in the email exchange and skillfully redirect the conversation to a kind of hidden truth, lurking beneath the surface. With written correspondence as a primary means for resolving issues, one of Gene's strategies for overcoming the weaknesses he recognized was to change the tone and style of his emails. Rather than stating his opinion directly, he often removed himself from the email exchange for a time or framed the written dialogue with leading questions rather than statements. Once I was aware of the infusion pump exchange, Gene forwarded me some of the emails while noting that, much to his chagrin, a series of misunderstandings about the infusion pump continued to skew the correspondence. As I saw, just two days earlier, he had attempted to allay some of these misunderstandings by restating some basic information about the infusion pump. Notably, he did not offer his opinion on what should be done with it or intervene in any other way; he signed off with a simple "Please let me know if you have any questions." By removing himself from the decision-making process and using language to signal a tone of distanced professionalism, Gene endeavored to recognize the power differentials otherwise concealed in the exchange and present himself to SALFA employees as a listening person, one willing to learn from their views and experiences. These strategies treated bureaucratic correspondence as an intersubjective rather than objectified form, one that mutually constructed American and Malagasy roles in relation to one another.

In fact, the infusion pump exchange draws our attention to bureaucratic language itself as a form of ethical action through which American individuals signal their accountability for past misconduct. Conversational roles in audit work thus model and enact the Malagasy-US relationship writ large, providing a cultural site in which styles and roles of linguistic participation constitute vital matters of power relations. In a volume on language and ethical action, Michael Lambek (2010, 26) interestingly describes judgment—building on Hannah Arendt's work to distinguish perspectival and situated judgment from thinking—as the "fulcrum of everyday ethics." Gene clearly judges certain styles of American conversational participation to be more ethical than others. Strikingly, though, his ethical model actually precludes him from taking an overtly recognized, at least to him, stance or position *of* adjudicating participation styles. As we can see in the previous exchange, Gene's expression "I just ask the questions" is a metadiscursive label or categorical term about talk, meant to define a more encompassing style of linguistic participation. For Gene, "asking questions" means being respectful, courteous, equitable, nonauthoritarian, and noninterfering. His emphasis on "asking questions," rather than making statements, can also be seen, however, as a culturally shaped language ideology that does not necessarily do away with the power differentials shaping assessment correspondence (Irvine and Gal 2000).

Linguistic power dynamics are shaped by such factors as the social position of the people asking the questions and their relationship with the other conversational participants, as much as how "asking" styles are organized sociohistorically and imbued with differential value. As Foucault (1979) observed, many tools of modern bureaucracy in fact rely on the coercive power of the expert listening person (e.g., priest, police officer, judge, psychologist, state bureaucrat), who is poised to ask and elicit confessions from other parties. Highlighting the interrelationship of language use and power asymmetries, Pierre Bourdieu (1991, 79) has noted that the "form and content of a discourse depend on the relation between a habitus . . . and . . . the severity of the sanctions [the linguistic market] inflicts on those who pay insufficient attention to 'correctness.'"

In this passage, Bourdieu points out that the habitus, or prevailing linguistic style, associated with a particular discourse, such as the needs assessment, is itself a product of a linguistic marketplace rife with symbolic power, as people attempt to perform particular socialized communicative roles. Participating in a discourse, then, can often mean internalizing what Bourdieu (1991) calls "censorship" associated with nonnormative expressions and thereby reproducing the discourse's conventions. All this is accomplished with no explicit use of force, but rather through the power of a socialized and felt desire to conform to discourse conventions, professionalism, and the perceived range of appropriate responses. The assessment correspondence was similarly influenced by such discourse conventions and, as Gene inferred, participants' desire to uphold them, for all the reasons above as much as an awareness of the possible effects of not doing so.

Just Asking God

Among my American informants, Gene was especially attuned to the paternalism and power differentials of the colonial past and saw part of his role as empowering Malagasy religious and cultural authority. His attempt to simply "ask questions" thus represented a consciously articulated effort to rectify these historical imbalances. Yet the very existence of the aid relationship placed him in a series of contradictory positions. In the case of the infusion pump donation, Gene indirectly reintroduced his concerns about assessment correspondence during the first evening, as we sat in a circle before the group prayer began. (Prayer sessions always closed off the group work session in the warehouse, framing the work as service to God.) Gene told us, "With the blood pressure equipment, some still contain mercury. In some countries, it's not legal to send items with mercury. Because of the dangers of mercury, I've asked SALFA whether they have mercury spill kits for leakages, but no one at SALFA is prepared for that." By "just asking questions," Gene attempted to walk a fine line between raising these concerns in an indirect manner while recognizing the way bureaucratic correspondence is saturated with the power differentials of the aid relationship.

What I noticed in this delicate negotiation was that, for Gene, turning to prayer as a means of communication was a way to hand over these concerns and the power to persuade to the divine. It was also a way to attempt to influence decisions made by Malagasy colleagues through appealing to God rather than through bureaucratic correspondence. For instance, in prayer, Gene asked God to "prepare the people working for SALFA to face their work with a sense of knowing You" and asked that God "would guide" specific SALFA officials in the decisions before them. On another occasion, in a Malagasy Partnership board meeting in August 2005, which I describe later in the chapter, Gene explicitly stated, during a discussion of possible future projects, that it was not his role to determine which projects could or could not be done—that was the Lord's work—and that perhaps any potential project, big or small, should be given a hearing. "You never know how God will work," he added. Addressing his words to God rather than to his colleagues directly was a different way of persuading than "just asking questions," and one seen among his US colleagues as more neutral in the aid relationship because of God's hierarchical position in relation to both Americans and Malagasy.

Turning to God enabled US NGO leaders like Gene to displace anxieties about the opacity and coerciveness of bureaucratic correspondence. For US aid workers, handing things over to God reinforced the humility and obedience of the speaker while appealing to a ready and socially acceptable channel of power: prayer. Prayer holds many social functions, one of which is to affect action elsewhere. To do so, however, supplicants often use directives framed in appropriate forms that minimize the human speaker's agency in relation to the divine (Keane 1997). In fact, by asking questions or making requests of his Malagasy counterparts in an interrogative style, Gene amplified his humility and inability to decide matters, as one does through the conditional or subjunctive tense of prayer. Gene endeavored through question forms to construct his position as that of a divine client rather than a patron, in his relationship with Malagasy correspondents.

Surveillance Technologies

In addition to providing a socially valued, familiar participation role for the expression of humility, prayer also offers aid workers like Gene a mode of conveyance beyond the immediate space and time. One of prayer's less-discussed functions is its ability to surveil space-times outside the present moment and to effect change in them through divine intercession. For believers, prayer thus expands common modes of embodied perception that carry specific bodily limits. It enables a form of knowledge-gathering, as well as individual agency, outside the constraints of the embodied self. Such prayers, then, can also be perceived as a form of long-distance *perceiving* and *persuading* made socially acceptable because they do not call forth the inequalities of the aid relationship as overtly as bureaucratic forms do. Furthermore, even though prayer works through opaque or unseen channels, God's position as a present partner in the aid warehouse—a position solidified through the various kinds of evidence described in earlier chapters—often made these mechanisms seem more proximate and reliable than certain bureaucratic communications.

Like the kind of prayer I have described, bureaucratic forms also carry a role as surveillance mechanisms. This became clear in Gene's and the IHM operation manager Mark's concerns over their inability to visualize what was happening in foreign clinics or at the SALFA headquarters in Antananarivo. Their difficulty verifying what happened to the aid once it arrived in their partners' foreign offices meant they had to sometimes "read between the lines" of bureaucratic correspondence. Occasionally, they would get on-the-ground reports from US medical practitioners who did short voluntary stints in Malagasy clinics and from visiting Malagasy clinicians. Their concerns about this inability to confirm the usefulness of the aid, however, centered on the image of clinics' stockrooms full of a jumble of rotting, dusty, and disordered medical materials. Gene would sometimes ask people who had visited Malagasy clinics whether they "got a glimpse in the storeroom" to see what was there. This hidden space was the lurking, concealed underside of the transparency hoped for—but, they were acutely aware, not attained—through bureaucratic correspondence. That is, even as such forms promised an open accounting of the actual situation on the ground, they often seemed to produce new potential for distrust and misrepresentation. Gene's desire to see the Malagasy storerooms points, in turn, to the perceiving and surveying role of bureaucratic artifacts through which humanitarians not only communicate knowledge but attempt to visualize the conditions of their partners in the absence of other means.

Bureaucratic audit's moral authority across government, business, and humanitarian sectors draws strength from conventions and metaphors of visuality that stem from the European Enlightenment. Budgets, case studies, and reports form part of a much broader set of "sceptic regimes of modernity" in which seeing and being seen substantiate empirical truth claims as well as enact forms of governance through surveillance (Jay 1988, cited in Apter 2002, 564). Even if visuality plays little direct role in such bureaucratic artifacts (in contrast with photography, for example), vision metaphorically conjures the ground of truth. Most tellingly, transparency has become the ideological backbone of audit cultures, a claim to *see* "the real" *through* audit work even as many question its reliability (Strathern 2000). Religious communities, of course, frequently invert such visual conventions. For them, the unseen, or that-which-cannot-be-visualized, as well as the revelation or uncovering of the previously unseen, stores the greatest truth (Meyer and Pels 2003; West and Sanders 2003). It is interesting that aid practitioners like Gene juxtapose visual conventions drawn from bureaucratic artifacts, such as budgets and case studies, with religious sources of truth and knowledge gathering, such as prayer. Their selective reconfiguration of both forms shows how audit documents not only produce knowledge but bring with them specific participation frameworks, frameworks that presuppose and enact certain kinds of subjectivities and social relations (Bornstein and Redfield 2010; Nguyen 2010; Ticktin 2011). Looking closely at specific assessment exchanges shows how aid practitioners strategically move between and combine the diverse "accountable subjectivities" available to them through such technologies, which include the communication channels of prayer and of bureaucratic documents.

In sum, Lutheran aid workers thus perceive a dynamic field of visualizing and surveilling technologies in accountability work. The Minnesota aid organizations' leadership often felt stymied by the partial, sometimes incompatible, visions of aid's usefulness and effectiveness that were produced through their regular correspondence. Getting a glimpse of the storeroom sometimes promised a presumably truer, more complete picture of what was happening in the clinics themselves. In the absence of such on-the-ground reports, the storeroom of rotting supplies took on a life of its own as a real blind spot of bureaucratic surveillance. Navigating such blind spots often required turning to divine forms of persuasion, such as the prayer described earlier, as well as forms of moral accounting that combine religious and neoliberal methods, which I discuss later. In the next section, I shift my focus to practices of accountability among SALFA administrators and doctors. US accountability requirements increasingly asked for Malagasy aid partners to document the uses and outcomes of the medical donations, and these requirements began to configure among them a specific notion of accountable subjectivity.

Subjectivities and Tensions of Medical Aid Accountability

If US aid workers construct an accountable subject as one who scrupulously distinguishes useful aid from junk aid and continuously discerns God's will—materializing this ethical position through procured goods while vanishing oneself from the aid encounter—a different kind of Malagasy accountable subject has taken shape through the aid relationship. As I described in the previous chapter, a small group of primarily male, ethnically Merina and Betsileo physicians and administrators have rendered themselves, and been crafted by their US colleagues, as culturally elaborated "Malagasy partners." Certain physicians are known by name and prayed for by US volunteers. They correspond regularly with the NGOs and visit the United States as special guests for Christian global health conferences in Minneapolis–St. Paul. In contrast with efforts by those in the US NGOs to invisibly "accompany" Malagasy brethren, a kind of selective hypervisibility characterizes these Merina and Betsileo physicians and administrators among US volunteers. The IHM motto encourages this vision by ambiguously suggesting that individual laborers' hands fold together with those of the Christian doctor—and, ultimately, Jesus—in administering care and "helping the hands that heal." Likewise, SALFA advocates a comparable position through the words emblazoned on the walls of all its clinics: "*Izahay mitsabo; Jesosy manasitrana*" (Malagasy, We treat [medically]; Jesus heals).

If physicians and administrators were positioned as already accountable for the most significant aspects of the Christian medical partnership, it seemed fitting to US agency leaders that some of these same individuals would absorb additional accountability paperwork as both agencies began to professionalize their operations. IHM had long derived some 80 percent of its operating budget from small individual donations (at the US$5 or $10 level).[3] With its expanding aid program and a predominantly elderly US support base, however, in the fiscal year 2004–5 it applied for and received from USAID $36,000 in ocean freight reimbursement for ten shipments, which brought with it additional record-keeping requirements.[4] A primary measure of NGO credibility for government and private donors is, of course, fiscal transparency, as well as low overhead costs (e.g., staff salaries, office upkeep) in relation to program expenses. IHM worked to establish this kind of trustworthiness by sending its eighteen thousand mailing-list recipients an annual report, which included paragraph-length narrative summaries of special programs by country, a financial statement, and an overview of the year's financial activities. In 2006, for example, IHM received $910,284 in financial grants for project support and estimated the value of its shipped medical supplies at $1,061,096; the annual statement emphasized budget transparency by offering supporters "a complete copy of audited financial statements" upon request and by noting that "over the years the [program expense to total expense] ratio has averaged 95%, demonstrating the efficiency with which [IHM] utilizes its resources to fulfill its mission."

Though Malagasy Partnership, as a volunteer-based agency, did not produce elaborate layouts of fiscal transparency, it, too, had begun inquiring into grant eligibility and embarking on partnerships with other, larger medical aid organizations. In fact, Malagasy Partnership often received funding from IHM. In 2006, for example, IHM paid $10,347 of the agency's shipping costs.[5] One retired Malagasy Partnership volunteer, Susan, who had worked in a university outreach office focused on reducing waste in Minnesota industries and whose daughter was a

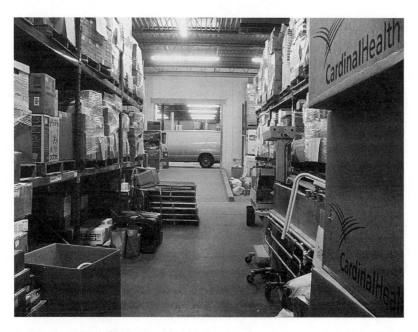

FIGURE 6.1. The IHM warehouse in 2006, with its expanded capacity for storing and shipping medical materials.

Peace Corps volunteer in Madagascar, began in 2005 to consider writing a grant application to the USAID Faith-Based Initiative. When I later asked Gene about the application, however, he said that he and Susan had determined Malagasy Partnership was ineligible, perhaps because it occasionally shipped proselytizing materials.[6] He added that as a small agency he probably could not sustain federal grant work because it was hard to "know what Washington wants." Malagasy Partnership nonetheless continued to partner with other medical aid agencies. After the Pittsburgh-based NGO Global Links donated seven thousand surgical sutures to SALFA via Malagasy Partnership in 2005, it required substantial documentation on the uses and effectiveness of the suture donation, triggering an unprecedented chain of accountability documentation among SALFA, Malagasy Partnership, and Global Links. In summer 2005 Global Links highlighted SALFA as the featured story in its national newsletter, prominently displaying SALFA physician-written medical case studies and photographs on the way the sutures were being used (as described in the previous chapter). Reflecting on the positive press SALFA gained through the newsletter, Gene called the Global Links donation a "success story." He told me he hoped it would alert SALFA personnel to the ability of prompt and thorough accountability work to yield substantial future donations.

The sheer volume, time constraints, mandatory character, and genre specificity of this accountability work, however, distinguished it from most prior and ongoing correspondence sent by SALFA personnel to US organization leaders. Such communications, often written in the style of an intimate letter between believers, had long verified the Christian basis of the work as a shared endeavor while less exactingly acknowledging the receipt of materials or funding. At the close of 2005, for example, Clement, the SALFA financial officer well known to US volunteers from a Minneapolis visit a few years earlier, wrote a letter to Malagasy Partnership board members and volunteers in which he relayed news from the recent Madagascar visit of a Seattle-based couple who also sit on the agency's board. Clement wrote that his family, the visiting Seattle-based board members, and a SALFA physician and his family from Antsirabe spent the day after Christmas together, during which they prayed "for the continuation of the work. We put the whole work at [Malagasy Partnership] and in Madagascar in the hands of our Lord and Savior Jesus Christ." Reporting on the previous year, Clement pointedly thanked each US volunteer by name and concluded, "Thank you for bringing love and life to the patients whom you do not always see but whom God gives to you to [take] care of." In January 2006 the Manambaro Hospital administrators, a husband and wife team, used a new Malagasy Partnership–donated digital camera and sent US supporters seventeen photographs of the hospital grounds in southeast Madagascar, including images of a recently refurbished linoleum floor in the in-patient recovery room, with a New Year's greeting written in English. "Dear Brothers and Sisters in Christ," the message read, "Thanks to God and thanks for all of you for your ongoing supportive help and prayers!" It was signed "God bless you all now and always, Manambaro Hospital's Staff."

Though Malagasy administrators and physicians had long sent communications such as these voluntarily, specific documents were now becoming *required* components of individual donations. It was this shift —in which Malagasy were slightly more restricted in how they could acknowledge or handle donations—that created some friction in the aid relationship. Although Malagasy and Americans had built social solidarity through a religious discourse that emphasized their shared footing in relation to God—in which neither party can ever "repay" the greatest gift of Jesus's self-sacrifice except to acknowledge it—audit work subtly destabilized these claims to complete mutuality. In effect, through audit work, US aid workers asked Malagasy aid workers for specific kinds of acknowledgment of aid being sent, giving donations overt qualities of market exchange. Where before there had been a sense of common human circumstance in which there could be no squaring of accounts in relation to Jesus's self-sacrifice, audit work made more explicit the hierarchical qualities of aid and periodically and openly placed Malagasy in a position of temporary indebtedness to their US brethren (Graeber 2011). It could be argued that American and Malagasy aid workers had long seen the aid relationship as unequal. On the whole, however, such feelings were socially submerged and did not seriously affect Malagasy practices until accountability work aligned receiving with a position in which equality could only temporarily be restored by fulfilling demands for paperwork.

Two Instances of Accountability Conflict

Two examples will illustrate how a specific kind of accountable subjectivity was being socialized among Malagasy clinicians and SALFA administrators perhaps as much through conflicts of accountability as through donation success stories. One SALFA physician, whom I call Remy, was well known for his adept management of a large hospital in Antsirabe and had earlier been a special guest of Malagasy Partnership in the United States. Yet he once came under a kind of negative scrutiny when he did not supply reports on time. Malagasy Partnership had secured an external grant for Remy to build a new surgical recovery room, making an arrangement to funnel the money to him in a series of installments. The funding was contingent, however, on the submission of regular progress reports. When Remy failed to send the first required report, Gene halted the money transfer. A few weeks later, Gene told me, Remy submitted the first progress report and continued to promptly send each monthly report, notifying Gene if it would be even a day late. Gene told me he had reluctantly "forced a record keeping" on the part of Remy yet felt "guilty" for doing so. As Omri Elisha (2008, 157) observes, one dominant exchange ideology among evangelical US Protestants emphasizes the social value of giving yet obscures the conditions of receiving, "to the point where givers . . . are often surprised or flustered to have to manage [the conditions of receiving] at all." Gene implied that Remy had breached certain cultural and moral expectations for receiving aid, but he also expressed moral ambivalence with his newfound ability to enact a form of power such as stopping payment. By needing to get Remy to acknowledge the request for paperwork, Gene had to make explicit that aid was a transaction predicated on a required return for the medical relief given and not solely based on a kind of communistic mutuality.

Another case occurred during my 2005–6 fieldwork. Rumors were regularly reaching the US NGOs, circulated through letter and email by SALFA clinicians in southern Madagascar via retired US missionaries, that certain supplies designated for hospitals in southern Madagascar, such as the Manambaro Lutheran Hospital, had not reached them. Alternately, Gene once explained to me that the reason Global Links initially sent sutures to Madagascar was that they "heard" that SALFA was charging the Manambaro Hospital the full market price for sutures, something the hospital clearly could not afford. Although it was hard for me to gauge the veracity of these claims and was not necessarily my aim to do so, what is clear is that some clinicians stationed outside the capital and central highlands, many of whom were themselves Merina, held the perception that Merina Lutherans and other SALFA workers in Antananarivo were disproportionately and unfairly accumulating aid resources. This perception echoes long-standing discourses of ethno-regional inequality in Madagascar that have pitted highland peoples such as Merina and Betsileo against *côtiers* (coastal peoples).[7] Rumors like these can be understood as a commentary on the unseen workings of power. They make visible long-standing forms of economic and political inequality that operate in Madagascar, inequalities that are woven into and yet tear at the very seams of the centralized SALFA operation. Bureaucratic procedures in this view attest to unseen channels and sources of power perhaps more than their ostensible claim to enact transparency and efficiency, paralleling Erica James's (2010) arguments about "bureaucraft" among aid workers in Haiti.

Concerns over SALFA's institutional accountability raised a conflict for US aid workers between the ethical ideal of invisibly accompanying brethren overseas and deploying audit as a means of bureaucratic surveillance. Such concerns prompted US board members to consider new mechanisms to hold SALFA administrators accountable for their dissemination of aid and thus advanced new forms of accountable subjectivity in the aid program, as I address later in the chapter. Rumors of corruption and expectations of how SALFA should run drew on an ideal of bureaucratic functioning as a "transparent" and seamless dispensing of aid, unimpeded by competing cultural claims to resources that are common in situations of "improvising medicine" (Livingston 2012). As an unseen or unauthorized redirection of resources, corruption allegations overlook the structural reasons why the scarcity of resources fuels multiple demands for them. Instead, such allegations often frame corruption as merely an individual moral or cultural issue, problematically leaving aside fundamental political-economic inequalities in access to resources.

Still, concerns over institutional corruption in Madagascar are not unfounded. State and nonstate entities in the capital are often viewed warily as sites of elite graft and favoritism, of which SALFA itself has suffered (as I pointed out in chapter 4). In a study of development NGOs and corruption in Nigeria, anthropologist Daniel Jordan Smith similarly observes that among many Nigerians, "local NGOs are simultaneously viewed as beacons of hope and change and bastions of corruption perpetuating the inequality of the status quo" (2010, 248). In Madagascar, ample evidence substantiates Malagasy suspicion about the unequal dissemination of aid. One study of the Malagasy Republic's distribution of relief after the 2004 Cyclone Gafilo, for example, found that areas with a high percentage of support during the 2001 elections for then-president

Ravalomanana were more likely to receive aid from the government (Francken, Minten, and Swinnen 2011).[8] The authors also discovered that wealthier communities in Madagascar tended to receive more aid, not because they suffered more serious damage from the cyclone, but because they had more developed "response mechanisms" for aid, such as storage facilities and basic infrastructure like passable roads (Francken et al. 2011, 496).

Early- to Mid-Twentieth-Century American Discourses on Malagasy Institutions

The American concerns over the SALFA distribution system that I have described, which ultimately resulted in additional US accountability requirements for medical donations, may also have gained traction through prevalent Eurocentric tropes of African institutional corruption or ineffectiveness. Among mid-twentieth-century US missionaries, Malagasy institutions were frequently depicted in written reports as immature or ineffectual versions of European and US models, a characterization that may continue to color US aid workers' images of SALFA. One 1957 issue of *Lutheran Herald*, a church-produced weekly for US congregants, marked seventy years of mission work in Madagascar with a series of articles on the FLM, officially founded seven years earlier. The magazine's table of contents characterized the FLM in a reductive, racializing developmental paradigm: "The Malagasy Church, child of our work, is now a thinking adult."[9] Another pamphlet of the American Lutheran Church's Division of World Missions, likely written in the early to mid-1960s, noted that "the local churches have reached various stages of self-support ranging from 75 to 100 percent, and, as it matures, the Malagasy Church undertakes its own home mission program of sending out evangelists into new territory."[10] The missionary author of a 1979 history of Manambaro Hospital, referring obliquely to a recent budgetary crisis the hospital had just suffered, editorialized that "church politics or tribal differences must *never* be allowed to hamper the highest standards of professionalism which are absolutely necessary if the best, lifesaving diakonia [service] is to be provided to the people of Madagascar" (Vigen 1979, 73, italics in original).[11]

Earlier missionary writings show that this paternalistic discourse of institutional development was originally interwoven with a parallel racialized discourse on Euro-American missionary efforts to instill individual fiscal responsibility among Malagasy congregants. As in other early-twentieth-century US and European missionary encounters in African societies, foreign notions of self-betterment were pervasive components of US Lutheran mission work in Madagascar. Missionaries sought to reform an array of Malagasy cultural practices that they viewed as an obstacle to the spread of the Gospel and the establishment of Christian community. By identifying numerous everyday arenas of Christian conduct, they implicitly, and at times explicitly, argued that being Christian meant performing Euro-American ideals of, for example, agricultural labor, companionate marriage, bodily dress, fiscal accounting, and civic participation. Social performances of moral comportment in these realms were evaluated and viewed as evidence of the parallel development of an interior, otherwise unseen Christian moral self (Halvorson 2008; see also Comaroff 1993; Keane 2007).

Scholars contend that the socialization of a self-disposed, autonomous Christian subjectivity, accountable for its actions, has been foundational to colonial Protestant missionary encounters and their multifaceted legacies (Keane 2007; Nguyen 2010). By establishing the notion that numerous everyday practices were externalized signs of unseen interior moral states, European and US foreign missionaries propagated this interiorized moral selfhood, which has roots in European Pietism, across the world throughout the late nineteenth and early to mid-twentieth centuries. These ideals of moral comportment, intertwined with how earlier US Lutheran missionaries interacted with Malagasy congregants *and* institutions, bear striking similarities to current American discourses on SALFA.

An additional factor in contemporary concerns over SALFA is that missionary families involved in the two Minneapolis aid organizations tend to see themselves as historically aligned with Tanosy, Tandroy, and Mahafaly people in predominantly rural southern Malagasy communities such as Manambaro, where most US missionaries and their families were stationed. Many former missionaries in Minneapolis–St. Paul perceive Merina in the capital city as having unfairly disproportionate access to Malagasy resources. In one of our recorded interviews, Gene spoke directly of this sense of connection US missionary supporters maintained to clinics in southern Madagascar, rather than those in the capital city region or other areas of the island: "There's been a lot of questioning of what we do. For the group that goes from the '70s and back, Madagascar is southern Madagascar. Wasn't anything above

Tana. Questioning about why we would send supplies to Mahajanga in the northwest and not send it all to Manambaro where the blood, sweat, and tears of many missionaries have gone into. That's been a hard thing. Where we come from . . . is we've always gone by the decisions of the Malagasy rather than our programs." Though former US missionaries regularly voiced their enthusiasm to me concerning the national growth of the FLM, some were ambivalent about the fact that it was Merina Malagasy in predominantly urban areas who led this effort. Gabriel, a Minneapolis-based Merina Malagasy evangelist and medical doctor from Betafo (introduced in chapter 2), once told me that he and long-term US missionaries "do not perceive the same Madagascar." He went on to explain that many see him as part of a "privileged class," a point he did not dispute. But he also implied that he disagreed with US missionary preconceptions of Malagasy cities and their focus on rural populations, citing rural-to-urban migration and the experiences of the Malagasy urban poor as equally important concerns for the church. Views of SALFA among former missionaries in Minneapolis involved with IHM and Malagasy Partnership thus build on long-standing, ambivalent American missionary images of Merina Malagasy and of elite, urban Malagasy Christian activities.

In sum, current accountability discourse actually taps into, and draws upon, a multistranded, influential set of moral understandings that shaped Malagasy-US interactions in the mid-twentieth century. In particular, these include culturally specific American ideas about Malagasy institutional and individual moral responsibility, as well as urban spaces in Madagascar and initiatives run by Merina Malagasy. These understandings may continue to shape American anxieties and narratives about SALFA's institutional ineffectiveness. Accountability in the historical encounter between Americans and Malagasy can thus be conceptualized, to adapt Daniel's (1987) image of semiosis or meaning making, as a bundle of cables with latent and manifest meanings, some of which have been pulled forward at select sociohistorical moments while others recede to the background. This meaning-making process does not necessarily do away with the less activated meanings, but rather pulls them along as a form of historical detritus that remains selectively influential and available for uptake by various cultural actors. For instance, direct reference to the notion of individual fiscal responsibility, and its accompanying racialized imagery, is explicit in missionary writings from the 1930s. By the late 1960s, however, it is no longer present, perhaps submerged or excised as a result of the independence and civil rights movements sweeping the African continent and the United States. SALFA corruption allegations, which resurfaced in several forms during my research in Minneapolis–St. Paul, can be interpreted as discourses that contain and rework some of these ethno-regional missionary allegiances and earlier notions of accountable subjectivity, as well as ambivalent notions of elite Merina Malagasy in particular.

Revisiting SALFA's Institutional Accountability

SALFA's institutional accountability resurfaced as a concern in a Malagasy Partnership business meeting I attended in August 2005. At the time, Malagasy Partnership's board was mainly composed of former short-term medical missionaries, members of Gene's ELCA church, and Christian medical professionals who collectively had fewer ties to the Minneapolis–St. Paul missionary community. This situation meant that the board combined local missionary discourses and more far-reaching evangelical Christian notions of moral conduct in the way they conceived of and related to SALFA. At the business meeting, I witnessed Gene and the other board members grapple at length with how to hold SALFA employees in Antananarivo responsible for their distribution of the US medical aid donations. The meeting conversation revealed that, for the US board members, what was at stake was not only a kind of bureaucratic accountability, but also a specific notion of Christian moral propriety.

Sitting across from me at Gene's kitchen table, one board member, Rick, suggested that each SALFA clinic receiving supplies from a Malagasy Partnership container or suitcase should know what is being sent to them and receive an email to that effect. Then, if the supplies do not arrive, those clinicians can follow up with the SALFA headquarters, serving as a "check" on the distribution system. At Gene's request, another board member who was on the telephone, Steve (a manager at the corporate headquarters of a large pharmaceutical company), "weighed in" on the subject. People are "beneficiaries of goodwill from" Malagasy Partnership, he said, and Malagasy Partnership "has a practical role in making them accountable. Also, there's a moral, Christian responsibility to hold brothers and sisters accountable for their actions." What was interesting was how Steve wove several kinds of responsibility together in his response, perhaps bringing to light what others were considering as well. Accountability was more than a business or fiscal responsibility. It was also a moral responsibility of SALFA employees as Christians. The conversation, however, framed this responsibility as a general Christian duty, presumably involving all Christians, American and Malagasy, rather than a process imbalanced by the aid relationship. Placed in these terms, US board members appeared in fact to be doing what they should do as Christians, rather than establishing a hierarchical exchange that unsettled the desired mutuality of the aid partnership. This universalizing Christian moral discourse naturalizes accountability as a matter of individual moral propriety and thus dovetails with neoliberal accountability logic, as Omri Elisha (2008) has found among megachurch members in Knoxville, Tennessee.

Accountability is a striking example of what political theorist Timothy Mitchell (1990, 567) calls "enframing," referring to the naturalization of new forms of domination as "fixed" and "enduring," rather than as overtly reproduced or negotiated. To US NGO leaders, accountability work often carried the quality of an assumed social good, required as it was by some of the NGOs' own patrons and endorsed by the broader aid world. As something that almost seems beyond reproach or question, accountability reproduces its own authority. As Mitchell notes, "These new modes of power, by their permanence, their apparent origin outside local life . . . appear . . . as a framework that enframes actual occurrences" (1990, 569). Providing examples of state security forces, far-reaching commercial syndicates, and market pricing mechanisms, Mitchell attributes their everyday power to their "metaphysical effect" or "transcendental" quality, as compared with forms of authority that must be actively reestablished, such as relations between landowners and tenant farmers (569). Accountability as an ideal enframes some of the particular interactions between Malagasy and Americans, appearing to both in some cases as a framework, the justification of which "stands outside of actuality" (569). Considering what Mitchell calls the "metaphysical effect" of these frameworks, as well as their moral authority, it seems quite understandable that they would be culturally connected to other, far-reaching and unseen sources of moral authority, such as obedience to God.

Yet, even if accountability has the effect of appearing to "stand outside of actuality," what I have made a case for here is that these accountability requirements draw from older notions of the morally accountable self, a pervasive component of early-twentieth-century US

Lutheran mission work in Madagascar. As Mitchell argues, the appearance of standing outside actuality is an *effect and mode of power* that makes the accountability requirements introduced by humanitarian organizations seem ahistorical and acultural, even as they accrue meaningfulness through their position within specific social and historical landscapes of moral reasoning. In the medical aid program, neoliberal audit culture and the late-nineteenth- and early-twentieth-century US-Malagasy missionary encounter converge in a shared genealogy of the morally accountable self. A sociohistorical approach is therefore necessary to counter the notion that accountability or audit is a new cultural framework, only specific to late-twentieth-century secular neoliberalism. It is a social and historical formation shared in certain respects with colonial Protestant missionaries and their modern-day descendants.

US church funds spent in Madagascar were accounted for until recently by US missionaries on the ground there. Some bureaucratic procedures—needs assessments, progress reports, and financial activity logs—are thus new to the Minneapolis organizations' interactions with Malagasy Lutherans, who are now their aid partners. As with other cultural practices, however, making these bureaucratic procedures salient dimensions of fiscal trustworthiness has meant recognizing, transforming, and embedding them through prevailing cultural practices and understandings of accountability. At the same time, bureaucratic requirements redefine culturally pervasive norms of moral accounting, sharpening and enlivening certain rationales while making other styles of communicating trustworthiness seem less urgent, persuasive, and compelling.

Malagasy Discourses of the "Pure Gift" as Accountability Critique

Just as Americans interpret accountability requirements through pervasive historically and culturally shaped conventions of moral selfhood, so, too, do SALFA administrators. One afternoon, while we sat in Clement's basement office in the Andohalo neighborhood of Antananarivo, he explained, with a slightly conspiratorial smile, that he often compares his donor accounting work with the Malagasy practice of *fihavanana* (kinship). Drawing an analogy, Clement suggested that one must be morally obligated to donors and respectful of the aid structure in ways similar to *fihavanana*. Yet when I asked him whether he viewed aid relations as similar to kinship relations, he quickly replied that he did not. To him, *fihavanana* espouses the same principle of being morally accountable to others but—and this is the key—without necessarily being asked.

At its core, *fihavanana* is a Malagasy system of advantageous social ties that are spontaneously offered during a time of need: people are both givers and receivers, rather than one or the other. Clement gave as an example that, if someone has suddenly died in a small village, the closest kin will be consumed by sadness and by all the work that has to be done. Community members would ideally sweep in, without being asked, to bring rice, clothes, and money. Clement specified that asking for help is not *fihavanana*, but rather offering has to be done spontaneously and through an implicit sense of moral obligation. In our conversations, Clement emphasized the "communistic principles" (Graeber 2011) of mutual aid by suggesting that *fihavanana* (kinship) does not operate on the basis of keeping track of gifts given nor involve being accountable to an individual kinsperson. His comparison separated the moral obligations of kinship from something more closely resembling market exchange (Cole 2009, 118). Clement suggested that *fihavanana* or kinship facilitates the building of mutual ties, whereas, in audit practices, a transaction occurs that forecloses social solidarity based on theoretically equal footing.

The ethnographic literature on Merina communities in Madagascar has closely examined the concept of *fihavanana* or *havana*, sometimes understood as consanguineal or blood ties. At the center of analysis is the paradox that, within Merina communities, *fihavanana* has alternately symbolized equality and hierarchy and, in fact, served to "illustrate corporate equality" in Merina political discourse, including twentieth-century nationalist movements (Bloch 1986b, 218; also 227). Merina communities have historically been organized around hierarchical associations between castes, such as *andriana* (lords), *hova* (commoners), and *andevo* (slaves), as well as between parents and children, older and younger siblings, and consanguineal and affinal (in-law) relations. Yet in specific rituals, such as the famous *famadihana* ("turning of the dead"), Malagasy take great pains to emphasize unity and equality within a community and between the living and the dead.

Scholars like Maurice Bloch (1986b, 218) point out that this sentiment of equality and sharedness is carefully produced and managed and stands in stark contrast to the reality of a society that is, in fact, highly hierarchical and asymmetrical (also Graeber 2007b). *Havana*, Bloch argues, is particularly effective at dealing with differential rank by emphasizing corporateness through, for instance, the avoidance of reciting genealogies that would highlight hierarchical relations. As a framework through which other social relationships are conceptualized, Clement's point about *fihavanana* can also be interpreted as a subtle criticism of how accountability requirements evoke or handle the hierarchical relations of the aid relationship. Both Americans and Malagasy may recognize these asymmetrical dimensions, but, in light of broader Merina understandings of *fihavanana*, what matters is perhaps the degree to which they are made more or less explicit (see also Graeber 2007b, 50–51).

On many occasions Clement certainly emphasized the common spiritual basis of SALFA's work with US aid participants, found in a shared love of Jesus. Unlike his US counterparts, however, he did not appear to characterize his required accountability work primarily as part of an individual Christian's accountability to God. When we talked about the US NGOs' concerns about the SALFA distribution system, Clement expressed uncertainty about why certain US NGO leaders had thought SALFA workers were hiding something, or redirecting supplies in a dishonest or inappropriate way. Clement hinted that the problem, from his point of view, lay not in the actual redistribution of the materials nor, importantly, in his coworkers' sinfulness, but rather in cultural miscommunications about accountability work. Using the example of *fihavanana* to draw a sharp cultural contrast, Clement told me that the direct "American" style of accounting for materials—saying "thank you"—was at odds with a more indirect, observational "Malagasy" sensibility of reciprocation-in-kind for things given rather than reciprocating by directly acknowledging them (see also Keenan 1974 on this point). Within this distinction arguably lies what Graeber (2011) identifies as the key difference between mutuality based on moral obligation and a more hierarchical exchange that requires gratitude. Giving thanks can imply that the gift giver has a choice to give or not and that, above all, the request for the recipient to acknowledge the gift makes the exchange's hierarchical dimensions, however slight, explicit.

For other SALFA employees, accountability requirements in which the US NGOs requested acknowledgment of certain donations or placed restrictions on how they were used, signified a particular kind of transaction that conflicted with US discourses in which the aid was framed a charitable gift. Mr. Rajoanary, the former SALFA director, told me that his US colleagues have sometimes expressed the concern that SALFA may be profiting from medical-supply donations, something I also heard occasionally in US NGO meetings. This relates to moral anxieties over the SALFA distribution system. When specially procured donations did not arrive at a SALFA hospital or clinic that was to receive them, one possibility was that SALFA workers had resold or "profited from" them. Rather than address that particular concern, however, Mr. Rajoanary took issue with the idea that US donations are "free" gifts that exist outside medical commerce. They say the donations are free, he said one morning as we sat in his office in Antananarivo. He laughed and paused with a dramatic flair. "Nothing is free," Mr. Rajoanary declared pointedly in English, before explaining further. SALFA absorbs many in-country expenses for distributing the donated supplies, including transportation costs from Antananarivo to SALFA clinics, the storage of unused items, customs fees, and the labor costs of handling the supplies from the shipping container in the Tamatave port to Antananarivo.

Mr. Rajoanary also pointed to the problem of having to account for specific US-donated medical materials—perhaps referring to the seven-thousand-suture donation that Malagasy Partnership orchestrated in 2005–6—which otherwise end up in the general clinical stock. When the clinic writes up a bill for a surgery, he said, how do they manage or value the Malagasy Partnership–donated suture versus one they received through another means? The two sutures look the same on the surgery bill, which includes items like equipment, supplies, and the surgeon's time. Mr. Rajoanary's comments dispute the notion that profiting from the donations should be a concern on the part of US donors, as SALFA is always situated in a for-fee medical environment in which donated supplies have economic value. Free supplies, he implied, do not really exist. They are a fiction created by the aid system, in which materials always bear exchange value or exist in a capitalist context in which the labor to use and transport them is commodified. Mr. Rajoanary is also suggesting here that the US-donated medical discards are not necessarily unique *on their own*—subtly countering the American construction of the individual discards as gifts that communicate with Malagasy brethren—but accrue value in the broader SALFA clinical system, itself part of global medical commerce.

It is worth pointing out that Mr. Rajoanary's views were not necessarily typical of other SALFA employees and, as a successful businessman who went on to run a large Malagasy medical nonprofit called Salama ("well" in Malagasy), his take on the aid partnership in our conversations often carried a strong market-based perspective. As noted earlier, many SALFA personnel indicated that, to some degree, they did generally view US donations as based on a shared partnership of faith, even if they debated the worth of particular individual supplies and placed greater emphasis on the partnership itself. Mr. Rajoanary, however, suggests that the donated materials have all along been a commercial transaction in disguise as a charitable gift. Part of his basis for this claim is that, by requiring acknowledgment of the aid in the form of accountability documents, US NGOs evoke an exchange that resembles a market transaction. That is, this arrangement places Malagasy in a relation of temporary debt that can only be squared by submitting the paperwork, much as one might pay for a commodity in a store (see Graeber 2011). In making this point, Mr. Rajoanary, like Clement, evokes a categorical division between gifts and the market, something that scholars have contended is an ideological opposition created by capitalism itself (Parry 1986). Besides the clear market worth of the aid, which Mr. Rajoanary describes, audit work, a form of required reciprocation, proves the aid from his perspective to not be a "free gift" with no strings attached.

Anthropologists have suggested that, if giving is understood as a form of exchange, the notion of a "free gift" central to charitable giving has paradoxical dimensions. Marcel Mauss (1990, 10) famously held that every gift is theoretically a relation that carries forward an obligation to reciprocate, sometimes compelling the recipient through what Maori of New Zealand called *hau*, the "spirit of the thing given." In her foreword to Mauss's *The Gift*, anthropologist Mary Douglas (1990, vii) writes of charitable gifts that "the whole idea of a free gift is based on a misunderstanding. . . . What is wrong with the so-called free gift is the donor's intention to be exempt from return gifts coming from the recipient." Contra Douglas, it can be argued that religiously motivated charitable gifts often presume a third party, a divine being, from which return gifts flow. Nonetheless, a fundamental tension in charitable giving is a giver's attempt to forestall the exchange cycle and mutuality associated with giving when the gift is characterized as "free."

Mr. Rajoanary upholds the moral model of the "free gift" rather than dispute its existence but asserts that US medical aid does not constitute that type of gift. Drawing from his twenty-five years of experience as a SALFA administrator, Mr. Rajoanary suggests that if the aid were recognized as a market exchange, without the trappings of gift discourse,

SALFA might be able to put the aid to whatever use the clinic has, whether this means revaluing the aid as part of a for-fee medical procedure or even reselling the medical donations if they are not clinically useful. Mr. Rajoanary's strong views, which were a source of debate at SALFA (as I discuss in chapter 4), can be interpreted as a claim to Malagasy autonomy and decision making in what Erica James (2010, 184) has described as an increasingly "results-oriented" audit culture. When Mr. Rajoanary characterizes donation as an increasingly audit-driven commercial exchange, he draws out the idea that these audit terms impinge on SALFA's clinical and administrative autonomy.

Conclusions

Although scholars of humanitarianism have cast attention mostly on the subjectivities and disjunctures of bureaucratic accountability work among aid recipients, in this chapter I have focused on both aid recipients and aid providers to illuminate how bureaucratic practices of humanitarianism are transforming global religious communities from within. Geographically dispersed religious adherents understand and contest these accounting measures through diverse cultural and moral logics. My approach to accountability parallels the recent work of scholars such as Andrea Muehlebach (2013), who has endeavored to show how neoliberal welfare-state reform has been pursued in Italy "through idioms of the Catholic imaginative universe" (452). Catholic charitable work, Muehlebach shows, is "both critical of and complicit in projects of neoliberalization" (454). As in the welfare-state reform efforts Muehlebach describes, the Lutheran aid program propounds a relational model of mutual care drawn from the theology of "accompaniment" in Luke 24:13–35. This model is meant to speak to global market inequalities in biomedicine and rectify power asymmetries associated with the colonial Lutheran missionary encounter. Yet the aid program also carries less explicit, though still deeply rooted, Pietistic understandings of the individualistic, morally accountable self, which impede the principles of mutuality contained in the "accompaniment" model.

In the medical aid program linking Christians in the United States and Madagascar, audit work thus brings forward contradictions between the discourse of partnership, based on Christian mutuality and solidarity before God, and a hierarchical exchange in which one party is at least temporarily indebted to the other. These unequal dimensions of the aid relationship have been present all along, but audit work makes them explicit by literally requesting Malagasy to acknowledge the terms of the exchange. For both Americans and Malagasy, this creates moral unease because it contravenes claims to communistic principles of mutual aid based on spiritual kinship and equal footing before the Lord. As I have described here, one way US aid workers attempt to restore this balance is by invoking God as the ultimate accountant to which both American and Malagasy aid workers are responsible. But audit work continually destabilizes these claims; this necessitates work on the part of both Malagasy and American aid workers to affirm solidarity through a religious discourse that identifies a shared love for Jesus as the common basis of the work. Since the aid relationship is built on a fundamental inequality between American and Malagasy aid participants, though, this work is never complete and forms an ongoing source of tension in the aid program.

I have examined accountability in this chapter as an ongoing series of transactions in aid programs, of requests for acknowledgment of exchanged goods and for the performance of accountable moral selves. Through these interactions, the terms of aid as an exchange are variously made explicit, disputed, reworked, and submerged. Looking more closely at these activities reveals that accountability is far from an insignificant issue in aid partnerships such as the one on which I focus. Rather, accountability constitutes an area in which the moral basis of partnership—and the potential for solidarity in global religious communities—is perpetually being negotiated. Accountability is thus not merely the fulfilling of bureaucratic requirements, but a more urgent and precarious moral terrain in which aid participants continually work to put the mutuality of the endeavor back on top, striving to have that win out over the economic inequality upon which it is based. Each of these interactions arguably prompts reflection on the moral hazards of sliding into—or making fully explicit—that inequality.

As I have discussed in previous chapters, US aid workers are also indebted to Malagasy in a more ambiguously defined moral endeavor that works, through the aid program, to tip the scales from the abstracted, inequitable past to a more even contemporary position. Yet as David Graeber (2011, 120) points out, moral debt is of course much harder to rectify than other forms of debt because of the inability to calculate what it takes to square the balance sheet or identify when a debt has been forgiven. I use the term *calculate* loosely here, not to signal that everything is quantifiable or imply that aid workers are rational choice actors in disguise, continually tabulating the best possible return for themselves. Instead, pointing to the incomplete and partial way that capitalist sensibilities and logics shape moral accounting, I have endeavored to highlight (as Graeber 2011 does) how debt concepts are socially and historically embedded with phenomena that are both culturally manifest and inscrutable, innumerable and countable, precise and inchoate. As I explore next in the book's conclusion, these complex issues of accountability—so intertwined with the relation of past and present—have continued to play a prominent role in the aid program, ultimately transforming it considerably since the end of my fieldwork.

Aid's End Times

R eligiously-based aid programs operate as multistranded conversionary sites that rework geographically dispersed religious communities' relationships with each other and engender novel understandings
of religious participation. As I have argued, such alliances inflect and
shape more sprawling, deeply rooted, and culturally variable notions of
the past, moral selfhood, risk, imaginaries of connectedness, and power
relations within and across global religious communities. The long duration of my fieldwork, from 2003 to 2014, provided an especially good
vantage point for observing religious aid alliances as vehicles of global
religious community, rather than merely functions of it. Surprisingly, I
have gained a special appreciation for the ephemeral quality of these alliances. SALFA's prolonged financial crisis (described in chapters 4 and
6) ultimately resulted in the closure of one of the two US NGOs that
I have profiled, Malagasy Partnership. The closure happened gradually
toward the end of the political coup and its five-year aftermath in Madagascar (2009–13). IHM has since absorbed most of Malagasy Partnership's programs. Here, I describe some of the events that have transpired
since the end of my fieldwork. These events spark two, even bigger, questions: What is aid's end, and what futures can be imagined through its
termination? In these closing lines, I consider how aid is a practice of
world making for religious actors.

SALFA's increasing troubles through the 2000s, which came to a
head in 2009–11, stem not only from the Malagasy political instability I
described in chapter 4, but also from a marked increase in global shipping costs and changing relations between church and state in Madagascar. Around 2000, as the cost of shipping was on the rise globally, the

Malagasy government started to assess taxes on the shipping containers of medical donations. These fees gradually increased, making it more difficult for SALFA to claim shipments in port. Around 2007–8, such fees had become so unwieldy that they amounted to approximately 20 million ariary (US$7,466) per container. Since SALFA received three to five containers per year from Malagasy Partnership, its annual customs fees came to nearly US$30,000. The customs control agency would accept only cash or immediate payment for these fees, no credit. SALFA simply could not afford to pay the fees and had to appeal for help from its outside partners, such as IHM and Malagasy Partnership.

Around this time, Clement believes, there came to be a misunderstanding on the part of some US partners that SALFA was profiting from the containers, ably accruing service fees from everything sent or even selling off the excess supplies on the market in Madagascar. Building on the concerns over SALFA distribution that I described in chapter 6, people wondered why SALFA was unable to pay for the containers. Yet Clement reiterated several times that these customs fees were a total loss for SALFA—money thrown into a hole, so to speak. The money accrued from needed medical supplies just could not make up for that large an expenditure. Even as he pointed out these difficulties, Clement said that he was grateful for the help that Malagasy Partnership has provided SALFA and, were it not for Malagasy Partnership paying some of the fees, the organization would have been in even worse financial shape. As of 2014, SALFA has changed its tack. As I speculated might happen (in chapter 4), SALFA currently buys most of its medical supplies from Salama and other discounters, who purchase in bulk from manufacturers in China and India. It is also adding a larger cost to each SALFA medical center for each medical item it receives from the International Dispensary Association.

US shipping containers have been few and far between since 2013, though IHM has continued its financial support for specific community health and medical education programs such as the Nursing School and Antanosy Villages Integrated Actions (described in chapter 4) and the purchase of medical supplies. When I visited him in October 2014, Clement described one US sea container that was packed for Manambaro Hospital. Political upheaval in the FLM synod structure in southern Madagascar, in addition to the problem of steep tariffs, had kept it stuck at IHM in Minneapolis for a year. Malagasy tariffs remain a big stumbling block for US donations: the government seeks to accrue as much money as possible from shipments into Madagascar to refill coffers that were emptied during the long-standing political crisis (2009–13). As a registered not-for-profit, SALFA should qualify for some tax exemption for medical relief. It has tried to apply for this exemption with the government but has not been successful. The reason, Clement explained, is that many churches in Madagascar now *are* for-profit businesses. When he and others plead their case with the government for tax exemption, government leaders suspect that SALFA—like so many other churches—are actually using foreign ties for profit. According to Clement, some 90 percent of government officials are Christian, so they have direct experience with many of these newer, for-profit churches that operate as businesses. He hopes that SALFA and a foreign partner, like IHM, will together plead the case for tax exemption with the Malagasy government. SALFA was unsuccessful doing so on its own.

It is interesting that the professionalization of aid in the two Minneapolis organizations, and with it the adoption of neoliberal audit procedures (described in chapter 6), resulted in more sustained, and in some cases irresolvable, moral concerns in the aid partnership. Malagasy Partnership folded as these audit procedures were becoming routine components of the aid program. What lingers in my conversations with SALFA officials—and through email and in-person exchanges with Gene—is that Gene struggled with the emerging terrain of accountability, both in enforcing audit practices and in his concerns over SALFA's distribution system. For Gene, who was always deeply attuned to the importance of an equitable partnership, the imbalances sparked by accountability work may have ultimately proven too much for the kind of agency he wished to run. IHM, on the other hand, has worked closely with SALFA officials since 2011 to help SALFA establish its own system of "good governance." IHM leaders guided SALFA in creating a new board in 2011 with members drawn not only from the FLM but also local businesspeople and officials from the Ministry of Health, all in an effort to seed a kind of neoliberal oversight within SALFA's work. Though I am inclined to see this mostly as a sign of the expansive reach of neoliberal audit culture, Clement views it differently. He tells me it is a good thing in his eyes, in that now he has been assured by his US colleagues that accountability is not an individual responsibility per se but ultimately a collective, shared endeavor.

Imagining Aid's End

SALFA's financial problems during the coup period played a direct role in Malagasy Partnership's closure. The "long-term lack of a viable government and the difficulties in getting containers into the country" were the primary reasons, Gene told me over email. Nonetheless, decisions like the closure are often complex and cumulative, and I wonder whether Gene's discomfort with scaling-up aid, which was never his aim, factored into the decision. Religiously-based aid partnerships like the Minnesota-Madagascar program raise a series of vexing questions about their duration or end: Do the moral obligations of religious community mean that aid partnerships last into perpetuity? Who or what decides when they end? Does aid based on religious commitment in fact prolong forms of problematic dependency, rather than the sustainable development and self-reliance prized in the aid world?

These questions have been discussed extensively by scholars of humanitarianism. For example, in her book *Having People, Having Heart*, anthropologist China Scherz (2014) argues that, among Sebandan residents in Uganda, sustainable development techniques required villagers to invest considerable labor and time in the initiatives of the organization Hope Child. Villagers, however, viewed the arrangement as a patron-client relationship that would in time give them returns. This situation led to villagers waiting and then feeling disappointed when the organization tailored its initiatives to self-perpetuating, "sustainable" aid but failed to focus on the community's priorities. Dependency is not inherently bad, Scherz suggests, and a narrow ideological focus on sustainability can actually do more harm than building a responsive, mutually beneficial relationship.

Questions about aid's duration and ultimate purpose were shared concerns of Minnesotan agency leaders during my fieldwork. Reflecting on the aid program in 2006, already twenty-five years since it had begun, Gene observed that Malagasy Partnership "isn't set up to perpetuate very well. And you know that has never bothered me because I have really felt that our presence and our need should have a definite termination point. There is this dependency or reliance on us to come through . . . in a way." Gene added that Malagasy Partnership was "there to help [SALFA] get going" and it would be a "positive thing when we don't exist anymore." Gene openly dreamt of a time when Malagasy

Partnership would not be needed, a time when in his eyes SALFA would be self-sustaining. He was never an ideologue of sustainable development, however. In the same conversation, Gene oscillated, admitting that, though he was still working as an information technology supervisor, a "dream of retirement would be doing this full-time." Gene's vision of the future can be interpreted through the lens of the present moment and the ethics of aid that he avidly promoted. He envisioned a desirable time when SALFA would not need donated medical materials, a position that emphasized Malagasy autonomy and expertise as he had done on other occasions. Furthermore, his effort to highlight the transience of Malagasy Partnership can be understood as a position of humility, a way of acknowledging one's smallness amid unpredictable forces and the need to ultimately relinquish control to God's plan. Gene embraced these futures, whatever they might be, and he described them with affection, even longing (Piot 2010). Talking about aid's end was, like other Christian eschatologies or end-time philosophies, a conversation that shaped specific virtues and dispositions of Christian subjectivity in the present moment.

But virtues are multiple and the question of whose version of aid's future and, by extension, which virtues were more correct was not a straightforward matter. Pastor Curt, the IHM executive director, emphasized that, in his view, aid fulfilled the moral obligation of accompaniment from Luke 24 or of long-term solidarity between Christians in separate national churches. Though Curt affirmed IHM's commitment to "sustainability," the time frame for this overarching moral obligation appeared to be an enduring present with no foreseeable end. He once said that Lutheran foreign institutions may always require funding from outside the countries in which they reside as a result of inequalities in global capitalism, adding, "How do we work for a just distribution of the world's resources?" From this long-term or even timeless moral obligation he distinguished the time quality of the donations themselves, which he said should ideally foster those institutions' self-reliance. Thus, even in the matter of aid's duration was a subtle conflict between the strictures of the aid world—its thinly disguised market language of individualism and autonomy found in sustainability discourse—and the more relational, biblical model of interdependence from Luke 24 that, in Curt's terms, could last indefinitely. Between the two US NGOs that I have profiled, we see two distinct paths for navigating the neoliberal logic contained in professional aid work: Malagasy Partnership ended because of sizable political and economic obstacles in pursuing its mission while IHM has embraced neoliberal policies and helped SALFA increase its self-accountability.

Relief aid is thoroughly shaped by entrenched inequalities in global capitalism, but the various visions of aid's future described by the two organization leaders touched only obliquely on such matters. Nonetheless, medical relief is ambivalently embedded in the market fluctuations and ramifying inequalities of neoliberal capitalism. Resource inequalities in global medicine have not abated during the nearly thirty-year-duration of the aid partnership. Medical relief of this sort has no easily identifiable end, in contrast with the short-term crisis temporality common in many aid interventions (Bornstein and Redfield 2010; Redfield 2013). Although basic medical equipment and facilities can certainly become "self-sustaining," the need to acquire expendable medical supplies like bandages, sutures, and medicines will not go away. Producing medical supplies in Madagascar could relieve Malagasy clinics from the economic hurdles of purchasing items on the international market, but, in the absence of the means and materials to do so, SALFA could be emboldened to, in the very least, sell donated items that it does not find clinically or financially useful and use the revenue for other purposes. The Minnesota-Madagascar aid program appears to be shifting away from the medical discard trade regardless. In 2006 Curt said he foresaw a future in which IHM contributed financially to public-private ventures that shared the cost burden of medical care.[1] Ten years later, this future is becoming a reality in Madagascar and elsewhere, further solidifying IHM's role as a foreign financial donor (rather than a contributor of medical materials).

Aid as a Practice of World Making

Even amid the enduring structural inequalities in global medicine that I have described, aid program participants were remarkably undeterred, joyful, deeply committed, and energetic. I suggest this vitality comes from the sense among both my Malagasy and American informants that they were doing important work in the world, work that was in fact world making. As I described in chapters 2, 3, and 4, aid work often drew attention metadiscursively to the wider seen and unseen spheres in which individuals acted. Many of these glimpses of a wider world-in-progress drew from, and shaped, value conversions, often of the medical discards themselves. Scholars have indicated that what we call religion may in fact hinge on religious authorities' ability to translate value or, in some way, manage value differences across diverse arenas of exchange, thereby catapulting such value forms into seemingly encompassing projects of world making (Graeber 2013, 233; Coleman 2004; Harding 2000). Because of the diverse forms of value in the medical discard trade, medical aid work seemed replete with such conversionary moments, or efforts to manage value differences. Medical relief workers utilized these gaps or incommensurabilities in value as creative spaces for generating relations, subjectivities, and economic resources, seizing upon the productive uncertainty that stems from these leaps across value asymmetries. Whereas medical waste practices equally reveal the limits of remaking relations between Christian communities, as I have argued, the value-focused activities of medical relief energized the work with an awareness of its ties with an interconnected though unseen whole, an orchestrated world-in-the-making.

Aid work often appeared timely in other ways, too. Several people framed aid labor as a form of "preparation" for the end times, a contribution that could help establish one's lot for the rapture. This framing brought a sense of urgency to Christian aid work. One evening at Malagasy Partnership, a retired Madagascar missionary, Karl, and his wife, Astrid, stationed for years in Ampanihy, stopped by for a visit with the volunteers. At Gene's invitation, Karl, then ninety years old, led the evening's group prayer. Coming on the heels of a niece's sudden passing and his wife's release from the hospital, Karl prayed that each volunteer would see how their faithfulness had "prepared them to meet the Lord. The blessings are all the same" regardless of exactly where one serves God, he concluded. Such a focus on one's passing or on the impending rapture can also become a "template for reading global politics" (Piot 2010, 65). When I participated in Gabriel's Minnesotan house church in St. Paul in 2004–6, the eight regular members eagerly dissected signs that the rapture was near. Hurricane Katrina and the 2004 tsunami figured prominently; many agreed they were "immense cosmic disturbances" foretold as part of the Second Coming in Matthew 24:29. Taking a more playful approach, Theo, the Malagasy Partnership volunteer, ran competitively with his teenage son and two friends on a four-person relay team they called "Not Left Behind."

Anthropologist Charles Piot (2010) suggests that, among Togolese charismatics, end-time forecasts and narratives reflect an exhaustion with previous narratives of colonial and Cold War politics and a desire to start anew and end time itself, to radically "forget" what was. Though I have often characterized Christian medical relief as a process of reworking pasts, it is equally one of setting forward-looking paths. I see these two cultural processes as intertwined rather than separate ones, even though one dimension can be selectively emphasized in a given context. Yet perhaps because of sectarian and cultural differences among my informants, I perceived less than Piot (2010) of a desire to fully forget and jump into the abyss of the end of history itself. Sentiments were pulled strongly in both directions, as Tanzanian theologian Richard Lubawa described in chapter 1, recognizing moral problems of the past while carving the "right direction for the future." Evangelicals were of course readying themselves for the rapture, as described earlier, but with the exception of Gabriel's house church in St. Paul, they spent less time immersed in end-time scenarios.

Religiously-based aid may itself shape these temporal orientations among aid participants. Such aid alliances are, however flawed, a refusal to ignore the world's inequalities and jump into the abyss. They are premised on the idea that doing the hard work of tackling social problems may lead to a better world worthy of the divine. For some, Christian aid is a slow repairing of the world that acknowledges humans' sinfulness and anticipates the world to come but that also makes Christian identity a project of this-worldliness. Nevertheless, at a time when neoliberal policies favor horizontal, transnational alliances, one can understandably feel some déjà vu: Christian communities that established ties with one another under colonial-era evangelism appear especially well suited, even primed, to take up the reins of these neoliberal and ultimately unequal projects. In these moments, time itself appears not as an arrow, a circle, or a rupture. Instead, it seems somewhat like a muscle memory, reigniting a bodily connection.

Acknowledgments

All writing projects bear many influences, and this book is no different. First and foremost, I owe a special debt of gratitude to the Lutherans in Minneapolis–St. Paul, Antananarivo, and elsewhere who opened their lives to me. Several former Madagascar missionaries, agency leaders and Malagasy Lutherans, particularly "Gene," "Clement," "Dr. Fosse," "Rose," "Pastor Gabriel," "Mark," and "Lois," took me under their wing and understood the value of studying the transforming connections between Lutherans in the United States and Madagascar, even though it at first seemed unusual for an anthropologist. I am in awe of the expertise, thoughtfulness, energy, dedication, and spirit of generosity they bring to their work. I was fortunate that they were willing to share some of their experiences with me. Numerous other US laypeople, former US missionaries, Malagasy Lutherans, and SALFA administrators spent hours talking with me; taught me about medical technologies, Malagasy history, and aid work; invited me to join their families for meals, trips, and worship services; and shared their hardships and joys. Though I am not naming each individual here, I have not forgotten these great kindnesses. *Misaotra betsaka*!

Early on, I was lucky to have a warm, supportive, and invigorating intellectual community to guide me through this research. Molly Mullin has always been an inspiring mentor, opening up the world of anthropology and setting a high bar through her intellectual play and curiosity. The research was supported by the Center for the Ethnography of Everyday Life (CEEL) at the University of Michigan, which was funded by the Alfred P. Sloan Foundation. Under the directorship of Tom Fricke, CEEL was an important intellectual home. Together with events coordinated by Tom, I found a wonderful community of anthropology students there: Sallie Han, Cecilia Tomori, Josh Reno, Jessica Smith Rolston, and Rebecca Carter. We read and discussed books and talked through ideas about our research, and they each set an impressive standard with their scholarship and collegiality. This project was also influenced by other faculty at the University of Michigan who gave helpful comments on my writing in progress, introduced me to key texts, or took the time for conversation, including Fernando Coronil, Stuart Kirsch, Judy Irvine, Bruce Mannheim, Katherine Verdery, Andrew Shryock, and Webb Keane.

As this project developed, it has been enriched by substantive comments on conference papers and other written contributions. I thank Elizabeth Dunn, Julie Livingston, Michael Lambek, Pierre Minn, Debbora Battaglia, Janet Carsten, Catherine Alexander, Joëlle Bahloul, David Graeber, Sherine Hamdy, Richard Parmentier, Elizabeth Koepping, Ben Peacock, Jennifer Cole, Doug Holmes, Ian Whitmarsh, and Fred Klaits for their comments on earlier pieces of writing that become components of this book. In addition, the work has benefited from conversations with faculty during presentations at SUNY Binghamton, Mount Holyoke, Bates College, the "Asking and Giving in Religious and Humanitarian Discourses" conference at SUNY Buffalo, Loyola University, the Brown University "Global Relations: Kinship and Transnationalism" conference, the "Marginal Conversions" Workshop at University of London–Goldsmiths College, and with my outstanding colleagues in Anthropology and Global Studies at Colby College. I am appreciative of intellectual exchanges with Mark Auslander, China Scherz, Hillary Kaell, Pier Larson, Chika Watanabe, Lesley Sharp, and David Boarder Giles along the way. I formed a writing group while at Mt. Holyoke with the unparalleled Chris Dole and Caroline Melly, and their comments on earlier writing, as well as friendship, left a strong imprint on this work. At Colby, I am grateful to Natasha Zelensky and Brett White for their supportive engagement with my work. Paul Sager, Laura Bevir, Colby College research assistants Jennifer Gemmell, Alisha Lee, Joshua Maillet, and Katie Ryan, and Colby research librarian Marilyn Pukkila each provided support on the long road to writing the book.

Gillian Feeley-Harnik is an incomparable mentor and scholar, as many people are fortunate to know. She shaped this project from its very early stages with long conversations and encouraging, incisive comments on writing. Like a great mentor, she also planted the seeds for me to take the research in new directions. Her critical empathy and intellectual inquisitiveness remain an inspiring example. Tom Fricke gave me crucial encouragement and advice when this project was in its early stages and led me to important sources on religious history in the Midwest US. Erik Mueggler's mentorship was a significant backbone of my graduate education, and this book bears his intellectual influence. In addition, I am grateful to Paul Johnson for his unwavering interest in my work and his support on the journey to assembling this book.

I thank Zed Books, Brill, and Palgrave Macmillan for permission to print in this book revised sections of earlier published work. An earlier version of chapter 3 appeared in "'No Junk for Jesus': Redemptive Economies and Value Conversions in Lutheran Aid," in *Economies of Recycling: The Global Transformation of Materials, Values, and Social Relations*, edited by Catherine Alexander and Joshua Reno (Zed Books, 2012). An earlier version of the section of chapter 2 on Pastor Gabriel previously appeared in "Translating the *Fifohazana*: The Politics of Healing and the Colonial Mission Legacy in African Christian Missionization," *Journal of Religion in Africa* 40 (Brill, 2010). Also, selected, revised sections of chapter 6 were included in "When God Is a Moral Accountant: Requests and Dilemmas of Accountability in U.S. Medical Relief in Madagascar," in *The Request and the Gift in Religious and Humanitarian Endeavors*, edited by Frederick Klaits (Palgrave Macmillan, 2017). I am also thankful to archivist Paul Daniels and his staff at the Evangelical Lutheran Church in America Region 3 Archives in St. Paul, Minnesota, for help with my archival research and wonderful, wide-ranging conversations about missionary history, Lutheranism, and much more.

A tapestry that hung for years in my grandmother's apartment in Sweden says "Glatt sällskap gör livet lättare" (Good company makes life lighter). I am especially thankful for the companionship of Debbora Battaglia, Yolanda Covington-Ward, Joshua Reno, Sallie Han, Cecilia Tomori, Kerry Boeye, Emanuela Grama, Chandra Bhimull, Nadia El-Shaarawi, Winifred Tate, Meghan Piersma, and David Cuddohy. Many friends and family provided meals and listening ears along the way, particularly my brother Bengt and mother Berit and the extended Halvorson and McCoy clans. Though I have not named everyone here, I trust they know that I am grateful for their support. For long-term engagement with my writing, I am especially indebted to Josh Reno, Cecilia Tomori, and Ema Grama. They have been an influence on this book at every step. In addition, I am grateful to Priya Nelson, David Brent, Dylan Montanari, Ellen Kladky, and their editorial team at the University of Chicago Press for the time and insight they invested in the manuscript. I also thank two anonymous reviewers for the University of Chicago Press for their careful readings and encouraging remarks. All remaining errors are my own.

Finally, words cannot express my profound gratitude for the support in writing this book of Jonathan McCoy. I feel fortunate to have his wit and wisdom in my life.

Notes

Introduction

1. Throughout this book, I refer to "Americans" involved in the aid endeavor, an admittedly problematic term. Wherever possible, I use US in its adjective form, rather than *American*, to destabilize US imperialist claims over two continents and the Euro-American displacement of Native Americans historically encoded in the term *American*. While bearing in mind these problematic qualities, I have opted to use the term in its noun form for several reasons. One is that this term is in keeping with the self-identifier used by many of my US informants, who situationally identify as "American" or "Norwegian American" for example. Another is that the term *American* draws attention to Christian foreign mission work as an historically nationalist religious imperial project, and thus fosters useful comparisons and contrasts with contemporary discourses of national church sovereignty in the aid program. Finally, the primary alternatives to the term *Americans* introduce a host of issues that have made them more disfavorable to me. One example is the term "US nationals," which problematically draws attention to a citizenship claim and implies that non-US nationals are not participants in the aid endeavor on US soil. This is not the case, as I show that Malagasy émigrés are substantial participants in US-based aid activities. In my discussion of these US based activities, I distinguish the various participants in the aid endeavor by referring for instance to Malagasy émigré-evangelists and American aid participants.

2. This figure counts only the officially "called" missionaries of the American Lutheran Church (after 1988, the ELCA) in 1960, which typically included single female missionaries and male missionaries. The wives and families of married male missionaries often were not listed as official employees or were considered part of a married "unit." I have included male missionaries' wives in the calculation of total ELCA missionaries to Madagascar in chapter 1.

3. Although it is an independent Lutheran agency, IHM cooperates with the ELCA and its Companion Synod Program. Under this program, which began in 1988, the church establishes partnerships between Lutheran synods that participate in the Lutheran World Federation (Lubawa 2007). Congregants make exchange visits and complete service projects for their "companions," which sometimes includes packaging medical supplies at IHM for hospitals that exist within the companion synod.

4. In quantitative terms, in 2005 volunteers worked more than 8,000 hours for IHM, the equivalent of four full-time employees (fieldnotes, 7 February 2006).

5. I also periodically use the terms *mainline Protestant* and *mainline Lutheran* to make the point that I refer to the American Lutheran Church, the Evangelical Lutheran Church in America, or its predecessors, rather than other Lutheran denominations in the United States. By using these terms, I do not wish to imply that certain Lutheran churches are mainstream while others are not; rather, the terms signal that the ALC/ELCA arose at a specific historical moment in the early and mid-twentieth century when US Protestant denominations, including Methodists, Episcopalians, Presbyterians, and Lutherans, were organizing large, national, and bureaucratic establishments.

Chapter 1

1. This figure includes both the officially "called" and paid missionaries of the American Lutheran Church (after 1988, the ELCA), which typically included single female missionaries and male missionaries, and the often uncounted wives of married male missionaries. Madagascar Missionary Collection, ELCA Region 3 Archives, St. Paul, Minnesota.

2. The previous Merina sovereign, Queen Ranavalona I, had banned missionaries, traders, and diplomats from Madagascar between 1835 and 1861, in an effort to diminish the increasing incursion of Westerners on the island (Covell 1995, 149; Raison-Jourde 1995, 292). Written accounts of her reign by British Protestants, which emphasized the persecution of Christians, were read widely in Europe and in Norway as the mission movement there gained prominence and thus served as an impetus for it (Feeley-Harnik 2001, 42; Nyhagen Predelli 2003, 17).

3. Such statistics should be interpreted cautiously; the act of counting Christians is encumbered by regional and local complexities of Christian practice and variations in Christian affiliation. These include whether those who mainly follow the "ways of the ancestors" (*fomban-drazana*) but have ties with Christian communities are counted as "Christians." This syncretic practice is commonplace and accepted across many Lutheran and Catholic congregations but not among charismatic *fifohazana* (awakening) revivalists and other Pentecostalist churches.

4. Norwegian American Lutheran missionaries were initially sponsored by two separate Lutheran churches in the US Midwest (the Lutheran Free Church and the Evangelical Lutheran Church).

5. See, e.g., Bjelde 1938, 41, 85; Burgess 1932, 189-90; Ose 1979, 26.

6. In making these arguments, missionaries may have been fulfilling genre conventions in missionary writing for lay US audiences; in my review of hundreds of missionary-written articles, published stories often feature a dramatic storyline of foreign mission work replete with clear, morally suspect opponents and "obstacles" to overcome.

7. Dyrnes Papers, Madagascar Missionary Collection, ELCA Region 3 Archives, St. Paul, Minnesota.

8. It is a historical irony that US Lutherans once instructed *ombiasa* to cast off their medicines, devaluing them, and now send US medical discards to Madagascar to be infused with new value by Malagasy practitioners through the aid program. I thank David Graeber for sharing this observation in 2010 during a workshop at Goldsmiths College, University of London.

9. Mission archival records are full of stories of US missionaries instructing gendered moral standards of timeliness, stewardship of personal property, and wage labor. I discuss fiscal accountability in chapter 6. But lessons that fostered a subjecthood compatible with a capitalist economy extended into other areas as well. For example, the Manafiafy Girls School, founded in southern Madagascar in 1895, enrolled hundreds and taught cooking, handwork, healthfulness, and homemaking. School lessons instructed the formation of a Christian female bodily subjectivity that, in the idealized mission understanding of gender relations, facilitated labor participation among men through the establishment of "Christian homes" (Burgess 1932, 220).

10. One retired missionary pastor, who sent a newsletter to the Madagascar missionaries and their families, told me that in 2005–6 he had 150 recipients on his mailing list. Mailing list recipients are only a small fraction of the total of people connected through kin, personal involvement, or churches to US Lutheran mission work in Madagascar.

11. Missionaries and their children are internally divided along several professional and ideological axes, which periodically cause conflict: short-term and lifelong missionaries, or "lifers"; liberal and conservative Lutherans; and a number of social and theological issues, including the sanctification of same-sex unions, the inerrancy or critical historical interpretation of the Bible, and the beginning of life debates.

12. This couple was stationed at Manambaro from 1983 to 1988.

13. Although IHM has since expanded its programs to include Lutheran churches in many other world regions, I focus on the perspectives of these Madagascar-connected Americans because they have been influential figures in both NGOs.

14. Pastor Curt had paraphrased the well-known passage of Matthew 7:15–23, which characterizes false prophets as "wolves in sheep's clothing." All biblical quotations in this text, unless otherwise noted, derive from *The New Oxford Annotated Bible with the Apocryphal/Deuterocanonical Books* (Metzger and Murphy 1991).

15. Thus, by 1984, it was not unusual to see a different approach to *fanafody-gasy* and Malagasy medical specialists in missionary publications. Rose, the registered nurse and wife of Dr. Fosse, who was active in primary health care visits to rural villages in the southwest, wrote in one September 1984 letter, "We foreigners also have much to learn from villagers about their customs." She went on to extensively describe how mothers in Andranomena (Morondava region) did not commonly cut the umbilical cord (*mamatotra*) and that this method may provide the newborn with extra oxygen and higher immunity from the mother's bloodstream (American Lutheran Missionary Fellowship Newsletter, ELCA Archives, Chicago, 48-54-70-190).

16. The Manambaro Hospital, opened in southeast Madagascar in 1954, had three Malagasy nursing aides on its original staff—Rasamy, Rabenjamina, and Rawilson—but, in my reading of the archival records, Americans held nearly double the number of these medical positions. Ejeda Hospital, opened in 1960, also had three Malagasy nurses—Sylvain, Melanie, and Narson—on its original medical staff, though, as with Manambaro, it appears that Americans initially occupied the majority of positions in the hospital's medical hierarchy.

17. For example, in a transcribed 1985 address that Rafam'Andrianjafy Mahavatra gave at a Bezaha synod conference of the FLM, he said one contemporary debate among church members was whether to send American missionaries home and request their salary plus institutional subsidies to run Malagasy churches or keep missionaries because they come with substantial US church funds that would otherwise be lost ("Aleo ihany aloha tazonina ireo Misionery ireo sitrany ahay hahazoana vola sy fitaovana"; correspondence from "Dr. Fosse," SALFA, to Rev. Jack Reents, DWMIC-ALC, July 17, 1985, ELCA Archives, Chicago, 48-54-40-100).

18. By 1971, the majority of the Manambaro Hospital operating budget, a striking 83 percent, came from assessed patient fees. This figure did not include salaries for Americans on the hospital staff, nor foreign donations for equipment, building repairs, or the hospital's poor fund (Vigen 1979, 65).

19. November 4, 1947, from R. Delavignette, director of political affairs of France overseas, by order of the Ministry of Overseas Territories, addressed to, Mr. M. J. Brun, France Forever, P.O. Box 291, Station G, New York 19, NY. It appears Brun had, in Delavignette's words, "transmitted to [him] a demand from Mr. Rolf A. Syrdal, Secretary General of the Lutheran Evangelical Mission asking to be authorized to open a hospital in Madagascar." Delavignette conveys

the Ministry's permission to build the hospital on the condition that the American missionary doctors not practice medicine outside the hospital to which they are assigned. He also notes that the approval was reached through an agreement between the Ministry and the High Commissioner of the Republic of Madagascar. Madagascar Missionary Collection, ELCA Region 3 Archives, St. Paul, Minnesota.

20. During World War II, rural Malagasy populations had been squeezed for nearly double the previous tax rate, which had increased hardship and sowed the seeds of unrest (Harper 2002).

21. For example, in his 1937 yearly report, Evangelical Lutheran Church mission superintendent O. P. Stavaas wrote, in a particularly obsequious tone, "I wish to express appreciation for the splendid attitude the government shows in all our dealings with it. This is not only a spirit of tolerance but of friendly co-operation" (Board of Foreign Missions 1937, 91). Such statements can be read as performances of hoped-for treatment from the French administration, coming as they did from official representatives. Nonetheless, this tradition of affirming remarks continued well into the mid-1950s.

22. Since 1988 the ELCA has paired together the sixty-five US church synods with overseas "partners" in the Lutheran World Federation, an umbrella organization representing 140 churches in seventy-eight countries. These church relationships, called the Companion Synod Program, involve humanitarian service, prayer, regular communication, and exchange visits between the partner churches.

23. I am grateful for the written comments on this point of an anonymous reader for the University of Chicago Press.

24. Janet served as a missionary from 1977 to 1988.

25. As I demonstrate in subsequent chapters, this ethical practice extends to many other cultural activities, including the selection of "useful" versus "junk" medical aid.

26. FLM leaders were specifically concerned about losing the payroll benefits of US missionaries who were already paid by the US church, as I described in a previous section.

27. Horning (2008, 427, citing Callaghy 1988, 14) even writes that, between 1979 and 1986, Madagascar "held the record number of IMF assistance programmes." These reforms paved the path for many other aid programs, as well, such as a World Bank and US government or Anglo-Saxon–endorsed conservation agenda (Horning 2008).

28. Several of my Malagasy informants, including Clement, half-jokingly referred to Dr. Fosse as "Malagasy." They explained that they viewed him as more Malagasy than American because he was born and grew up in Madagascar, had lived in Madagascar for the vast majority of his life (more than fifty years), spoke

Malagasy fluently with no detectable accent and, from their perspective, often appeared to behave in accordance with "Malagasy" rather than "American" sensibilities.

29. I am indebted for this phrasing to an anonymous reader for the University of Chicago Press.

Chapter 2

1. Political discourses also sometimes use hand imagery to ensconce activities of imperialism and war in a more benign-sounding nationalistic language. In his address to Congress on June 18, 1945, General Dwight Eisenhower identified relief projects during World War II as exemplifying the "friendly hand of this nation, reaching across the sea to sustain its fighting men" (quoted in Becker n.d.).

2. To my knowledge, only one of the signs directly referred to patients, and it stated, "We provide hospital patients . . . with a bed."

3. The practice of bandage making has a long, gendered history as an activity performed "at home" in American Lutheran Women's Missionary Federations and many Protestant aid societies, which in turn originated in Red Cross bandage campaigns during the US Civil War (Halvorson 2008, 2012b; Hutchinson 1996).

4. These designations risk becoming empty signifiers in the United States, where the middle class is an aspirational category. Drawing primarily on occupation rather than volunteers' own self-designations, however, I aim to gesture here not to volunteers' performance of class per se but rather to their financial status; some of the forms of bodily insecurity I describe stem from privatized health care and its costs.

5. Their own work with discards contributes to US medical profit-making, as I describe in chapter 3; making medical discards into medical relief is a process that paradoxically strengthens the very medical regime that sometimes exacerbated the insecurity of volunteers and their families.

6. Many people in the Imerina region converted to Protestant Christianity after 1869 when it became the state religion of the Merina kingdom (see, e.g., Ellis 1985, 18; Graeber 2007b, 102).

7. In using the term "house church," I am referring to a small group that meets within a residential house, rather than a sanctuary, often but not always in conjunction with a specific church congregation. House churches often become the kernel for an independent congregation that splits from its original institutional home.

8. Gabriel's wife could not be ordained in the Malagasy Lutheran Church (FLM), for it does not permit the ordination of women.

9. The ELCA Research and Evaluation data on baptized membership by

race/ethnicity for 2007 showed that 96.77 percent of participating congregants self-reported being white (http://www.elca.org/News-and-Events/6293?_ga=2 .15623989.206854504.1503686565-761237300.1503686565).

10. This is Gabriel's English translation of SALFA's Malagasy motto: "Izahay mitsabo; Jesosy manasitrana" (We treat; Jesus heals). It may be a reworking of a well-known, sixteenth-century expression attributed to French physician Ambroise Paré: "Je le pansai, Dieu le guérit" (I bandaged him and God healed him).

11. Syringes of course also carry a range of negative associations with the bodily discomfort and pain of medical procedures. Such risks may heighten the significance of the bodily encounter Gabriel implies in which medicines or spirit agents make contact with the individual body and promote some kind of unseen transformation.

12. The incumbent Didier Ratsiraka had refused to recognize the election results, which resulted in a six-month political crisis. Many *mpiandry* protested in the streets of the capital in support of Ravalomanana and thus "played a leading role in the transition of power" (Keller 2005, 56). I refer to Ravalomanana's presidency and the 2009 coup that removed him from office in chapter 4.

Chapter 3

1. Such portraits are complicated by a lack of clarity about what measures are being employed to compare disparate waste forms, ranging from air emissions to municipal solid waste. Though the precise claims must be viewed critically, my goal is to convey the vast waste produced by the US medical industry; this waste stream often is overlooked because it is institutionally and not individually produced garbage and, as I show, because a substantial portion gets reclaimed as medical relief.

2. Rosenblatt, Ariyan, et al. (1996, 631) report that the nonprofit Yale–New Haven program, entitled REMEDY, accrued operating room supplies valued at $500,000 between the inception of the recovery program in June 1991 and the date of publication. At the April 2006 Technical Exchange for Christian Healthcare (TECH) meeting, several people expressed concerns that a multinational corporation may organize a used medical-supply market and siphon off the charitable donations they receive into a lucrative for-profit trade. One could observe, then, that there is a separate incentive for nonprofits in calculating the monetary value of the medical donations only for the purposes of their financial records, as required by law, but in not doing so for any other reason. Some of the TECH members pointed out that it also is fiscally beneficial for hospitals to make charitable donations rather than sell their supplies in a used market. They are able to value these supplies at their fair market price when they claim them as charitable donations, whereas they may not be able to acquire the fair market price if

they were to sell them used. In this calculation, the tax credit is worth more than the direct sale.

3. Volunteers also sometimes brought attention to the ecological value of recycling discards. Some IHM leaders, however, like Mark, avoided referring to the agencies' work as recycling because, to him, this characterized the discards as already used rather than often unused castoffs and, in my interpretation, diminished their moral and clinical value in the aid partnership (see Halvorson 2012a).

4. I am grateful to one of two anonymous University of Chicago Press readers for the latter reading.

5. AMSCO, originally known as the American Sterilizer Company, was at the forefront of the Pasteurian revolution, having been founded in 1894. The company was involved in creating the sterile operating room and has continued to manufacture sterilization and surgical equipment, though the Erie manufacturing plant has since been closed.

6. I have been unable to completely verify the attribution to Mother Teresa. She is often attributed comparable statements that highlight how Christian giving should treat every person as if he or she is a reflection of Jesus.

Chapter 4

1. I am grateful to an anonymous University of Chicago Press reader for this point.

2. The only divergence from this observation that I found is that SALFA employees, as well as the small number of remaining ELCA missionaries in Madagascar, often work together to unpack the contents of the shipping container, sometimes saying a prayer at the beginning of the work session. This practice began in the early to mid-1980s, when the US NGOs sent their first shipping containers.

3. The World Health Organization Action Programme on Essential Drugs revised these guidelines in 1992, 1996, and 1999 (World Health Organization 1999, 4).

4. By the time I began research at Malagasy Partnership in 2005, the organization was not sending any expired medicines to Madagascar. Several times I witnessed Gene instructing other volunteers to throw away expired medicine bottles that had been donated with other items.

5. Among the many translations of this passage, another English version is "Teach me, O Lord, the way of your statutes, / and I will observe it to the end" (Metzger and Murphy 1991, 779).

6. By revolving fund structure, I am referring to the system described earlier in the chapter in which SALFA headquarters replenishes its finances continually through the service fees paid for medical items by individual SALFA clinics. In

turn, because they receive discounted medical donations, individual clinics ideally replenish their funds through the fees patients pay for medical services.

7. To my knowledge, IHM has taken no official stance on either the ordination of gay and lesbian clergy or the sanctification of same-sex unions. Josette may assume that IHM does not support the ELCA's position because it has not taken a formal position on those matters. It could also be that her impression here draws from specific, personal conversations with some IHM officials who may have presented their own individual views but left ambiguous the degree to which those views are espoused by others affiliated with IHM. My research at IHM suggests a broad range of opinions and views exists among staff and volunteers on everything from "correct" Lutheranism to the relationship of Christianity and social justice to the sanctification of same-sex unions.

Chapter 5

1. The overall HIV rate is low in Madagascar, with a 0.2 percent prevalence rate in 2013 among adults age 15 to 49. In Cameroon, where Dr. Rafolo was doing a short-term surgical-skills program and was struck with a needle used in treating an HIV-positive person, the HIV positive prevalence rate was 4.2 percent in 2013 among adults age 15 to 49 (World Health Organization/UNAIDS, HIV Prevalence, Country Data Sheets, http://aidsinfo.unaids.org/).

2. I became acquainted with only one female physician who collaborated occasionally with the US NGOs; when I met her in Madagascar in 2005, she was stationed with her husband in the southeast hospital at Manambaro, built by US missionaries in former times. Though she never visited the United States to my knowledge, she sometimes wrote emails to US supporters with digital photographs of US-funded improvements to the hospital.

3. Some of these ethnonyms foster dynamic insider–outsider distinctions within communities and have come to be associated by people themselves with specific, defining features of an ethnic category: taboos (*fady*) on food, marital and burial customs, and local animal or plant life; dialects of the Malagasy language; territories; dynastic or royal lineages; and practices of agriculture or animal husbandry (Sharp 1993, 56).

4. Portraits of this sort of course mask the diverse socioeconomic experiences of those considered Merina or Betsileo; communities in the central and southern highlands have been described as highly stratified, with castelike groupings of landholders or lords, a status encoded in one's surname (*andriana*), commoners (*hova*), and descendants of former slaves (*mainty-andevo*).

5. As in other parts of the world, research shows that wealth differences in Madagascar manifest in health disparities. In their analysis of ten years (2000–9) of national health data, Sharp and Kruse (2011) point to marked regional

differences in child, infant, and maternal mortality in Madagascar. They note, "Compared with the highlands, children are exposed to a higher mortality risk by 43 percent in the coastal areas and by 85 percent in the desert south" (2011, 9). One 2003–4 survey strikingly claims that child mortality is about 70 percent higher in rural areas of Madagascar than in the capital (cited in Sharp and Kruse 2011, 9). What emerges in this statistical portrait is the disproportionate communicable disease burden of rural areas and predominantly rural "coastal" regions such as southern Madagascar, in which the population faces a higher prevalence of chronic malnutrition, anemia, malaria, and diarrheal diseases, particularly among children, than in most areas of the central highlands.

6. Bloch (1986a, 30) points out that VVS had no Catholic members, something disputed in Brown (1995). Bloch (1986a, 30) and others scholars argue that Catholics were associated with French colonial rule and French clergy held more positions for longer in the Catholic Church than foreign clergy in Protestant churches, some of which created greater opportunities for Malagasy leadership. Though VVS may have had some Catholic members, such as Venance Manifatra (Brown 1995, 245), those involved were predominantly Merina Protestants.

7. This suspicion was also stoked by the French, as part of their strategy for rule involved destabilizing Merina political power (Feeley-Harnik 1991, 128) and fostering a "crude" ethno-regional division of highland and coastal peoples (Randrianja and Ellis 2010, 159).

8. This also forms a noteworthy contrast to Legrip-Randriambelo and Regnier's (2014) recent observation of *fifohazana* lay preachers' (*mpiandry*) denigration of the work of *ombiasa* in Betsileo country. They write, "In contrast to the *ombiasa*'s attitude towards Christian healing practices, the *mpiandry* never miss an occasion to virulently condemn the *ombiasa*'s work and influence in their [preaching] and healing sessions" (33). The authors also describe a Lutheran doctor and *mpiandry* practicing in Fianarantsoa who, like Dr. Andry, approves of prayer healing and exorcism techniques but, unlike Dr. Andry, actively disavows the healing practices of the *ombiasa* (2014, 34).

9. This asymmetry is reflected in the national organization (*Association nationale des tradipraticiens malgaches*) established in Madagascar in 1997 to register *ombiasa* as "traditional practitioners" and assign them a membership card (Legrip-Randriambelo and Regnier 2014, 34–35); as is the case among *sangomas* or ritual healers in South Africa, this state apparatus carries a regulatory purpose, registering and monitoring *ombiasa* through local biomedical clinics, and does not appear to have been successful thus far (2014, 35).

10. Wendland (2012b, 114) reports a similar situation in Queen Elizabeth Central Hospital in Blantyre, Malawi.

11. Read on its own, this individual case, which details an unusually "difficult labor," tends to obscure the pluralistic medical environment in Madagascar

in which an estimated 65 percent of Malagasy women do not give birth in medical centers but rather consult midwives and female birth attendants (Sharp and Kruse 2011, 12). Caesarean sections are rare overall in Madagascar because of the lack of surgical infrastructure in the country. In 2008 a World Health Organization study estimated Madagascar's caesarean section rate to be a low 1.0 percent, well below the report's 10 percent benchmark for appropriate use (rather than overuse) of caesarean sections (Gibbons et al. 2010, 16). Madagascar has a high maternal mortality rate (498 per 100,000 live births), some of which is attributed to a lack of access to prenatal care and institutionalized medical care during delivery, in addition to other influential factors like malnutrition ("Health-Madagascar" 2012).

12. As I discussed in chapter 4, SALFA clinics charge one comprehensive fee for pharmaceuticals, services rendered, and tests, which tends to range from 1,000 to 3,000 *ariary* per visit (approximately US$0.37 to 1.12). I was told that, though ostensibly free, government-run clinics often charge separate fees for pharmaceuticals and for necessary tests; in addition, some require under-the-table bribes to clinicians. Some of my SALFA informants thus argued that SALFA clinics actually charge less overall than government-run clinics.

13. The authors also give an example of an *ombiasa* who, at least in their translation to English, does frame the hoped-for amount of 25,000 Malagasy francs (approximately US$1.56) as a "payment" for the therapeutic consultation (Legrip-Randriambelo and Regnier 2014, 35).

14. The US Lutheran missions to Madagascar encouraged US laypeople to pray for missionaries through a vast publishing enterprise that included pamphlets, missionary-authored articles in church periodicals, letters to congregants, and books and films on Madagascar. These diverse media were crucial to nurture and sustain US financial support for the Madagascar missions. One Norwegian Lutheran Church in America (NLCA) church pamphlet from 1943, for instance, featured photographs of each missionary and Bible passages for each day of the month that would guide that day's prayer; another titled "Daily Prayer for Foreign Missions" included quick statistics on the number of foreign missionaries, church members, and "native workers" for each of the church's three major mission fields (Madagascar, South Africa, and China). Madagascar Missionary Collection, ELCA Region 3 Archives, St. Paul, Minnesota.

Chapter 6

1. The secular value of these bureaucratic measures is not static or given but, when contrasted with the religious, it is part of a dynamic, continually made and remade set of values, sensibilities, and stances.

2. I owe a special debt to Fred Klaits for influential comments that contributed to this formulation.

3. The IHM executive director provided this figure in our August 2005 recorded interview.

4. Mark worked on the next USAID grant application for fiscal year 2006–7. He explained to me that it required him to, for example, project the IHM shipping schedule for two years, duties and customs' fees for each port to which IHM ships, and to disclose whether IHM qualified for duty-free status in any of those countries.

5. This figure was provided on page B of IHM's 2006 "Annual Report Summary" mentioned earlier.

6. Proselytizing materials, meant explicitly for religious purposes, are prohibited by the U.S. Faith-Based Initiative. This small provision is the US government's effort to maintain the separation of church and state in the Faith-Based Initiative, which gives federal funds to religiously-based US domestic and international social service organizations. Malagasy Partnership on occasion sent items for religious buildings, such as stained-glass windows for a Lutheran church in Madagascar, and explicitly religious materials, like French-language health booklets with Christian evangelical messages. Although aid providers are allowed to individually interpret the Faith-Based Initiative stipulations in borderline cases, thus in many ways determining eligibility themselves, Gene and Susan may have viewed these items as violations of the prohibition against explicitly religious material.

7. See my longer discussion of this distinction in chapter 5.

8. The relief aid consisted of water, medication, blankets, and makeshift shelters, as well as cash-for-work programs to rebuild damaged infrastructure, such as schools and health centers. The relief came from international agencies like CARE, Catholic Relief Services, SAHAFA, the United Nations, and the World Bank's Development Intervention Fund. The government's National Disaster Management Agency of the Ministry of the Interior managed the aid distribution (Francken et al. 2011).

9. "In This Issue," *Lutheran Herald*, October 8, 1957, p. 947, Madagascar Missionary Collection, ELCA Region 3 Archives, St. Paul, Minnesota.

10. "Madagascar," undated, folded booklet with one color accent, American Lutheran Church, Madagascar Missionary Collection, ELCA Region 3 Archives, St. Paul, Minnesota.

11. When considering how contemporary discourses may critically approach SALFA, we must not overlook the irony that Midwest US medical institutions, which may serve as exemplars of the unmarked modernity against which Malagasy bureaucracy is evaluated, produce so much waste as to easily sustain a thirty-year-old aid program.

Conclusions

1. Public-private partnerships like this one raise a number of questions. Among them are the extent to which the medical care pursued in those partnerships will remain Christian in focus, how such medicine will balance public and private or religious interests, and whether IHM supporters in the United States will want to fund ventures that do not prioritize Lutheran or Christian care.

Bibliography

Archives and Manuscript Collections

ELCA3—Evangelical Lutheran Church in America, Region 3 Archives, St. Paul, Minnesota
LSL—Luther Theological Seminary Library Collection, St. Paul, Minnesota
PC—Private collections loaned to the author

Works Cited

Adams, Vincanne. 2013. *Markets of Sorrow, Labors of Faith: New Orleans in the Wake of Katrina*. Durham, NC: Duke University Press.

Agamben, Giorgio. 1998. *Homo Sacer: Sovereign Power and Bare Life*. Stanford, CA: Stanford University Press.

Akinade, Akintunde. 2007. "Non-Western Christianity in the Western World: African Immigrant Churches in the Diaspora." In *African Immigrant Religions in America*, edited by Jacob K. Olupona and Regina Gemignani, 89–101. New York: New York University Press.

Alexander, Catherine, and Joshua Reno, eds. 2012. *Economies of Recycling: Global Transformations in Materials, Values, and Social Relations*. London: Zed.

Allen, Marshall. 2017. "What Hospitals Waste." *ProPublica*, March 9. https://www.propublica.org/article/what-hospitals-waste.

Andersen, Margaret Cook. 2010. "Creating French Settlements Overseas: Pronatalism and Colonial Medicine in Madagascar." *French Historical Studies* 33 (3): 417–44.

Appadurai, Arjun. 1986. "Introduction: Commodities and the Politics of Value."

In *The Social Life of Things: Commodities in Cultural Perspective*, edited by Arjun Appadurai, 3–63. Cambridge: Cambridge University Press.

Apter, Andrew. 2002. "On Imperial Spectacle: The Dialectics of Seeing in Colonial Nigeria." *Comparative Studies in Society and History* 44 (3): 564–96.

Barnett, Michael. 2011. *Empire of Humanity: A History of Humanitarianism.* Ithaca, NY: Cornell University Press.

Barnett, Michael, and Raymond Duvall, eds. 2005. *Power in Global Governance.* Cambridge, UK: Cambridge University Press.

Barnett, Michael, and Janice Gross Stein, eds. 2012. *Sacred Aid: Faith and Humanitarianism.* Oxford, UK: Oxford University Press.

Barnett, Michael, and Thomas G. Weiss. 2008. "Humanitarianism: A Brief History of the Present." In *Humanitarianism in Question: Politics, Power, Ethics*, by Michael Barnett and Thomas G. Weiss, 1–48. Ithaca, NY: Cornell University Press.

Battaglia, Debbora, ed. 1995. *Rhetorics of Self-Making.* Berkeley: University of California Press.

Bays, Daniel H., and Grant Wacker. 2003. "Introduction: The Many Faces of the Missionary Enterprise at Home." In *The Foreign Missionary Enterprise at Home: Explorations in North American Cultural History*, edited by Daniel H. Bays and Grant Wacker, 1–12. Tuscaloosa: University of Alabama Press.

Beck, Ulrich. 1992. *Risk Society: Towards a New Modernity.* London: Sage.

Becker, Paula. n.d. "Knitting for Victory—World War II." *HistoryLink.org Online Encyclopedia of Washington State History.* http://www.historylink.org/File/5722.

Beidelman, T. O. 1974. "Social Theory and the Study of Christian Missions in Africa." *Africa* 44 (3): 235–49.

Benjamin, Walter. 1968. *Illuminations: Essays and Reflections*, edited by Hannah Arendt. New York: Schocken.

Benthall, Jonathan. 2010. "Islamic Humanitarianism in Adversarial Context." In *Forces of Compassion: Humanitarianism between Ethics and Politics*, edited by Erica Bornstein and Peter Redfield, 99–122. Santa Fe, NM: School for Advanced Research Press.

Benthall, Jonathan, and Jérôme Bellion-Jourdan. 2003. *The Charitable Crescent: Politics of Aid in the Muslim World.* London: I. B. Tauris.

Besteman, Catherine, and Hugh Gusterson. 2010. Introduction to *The Insecure American: How We Got Here and What We Should Do about It*, edited by Catherine Besteman and Hugh Gusterson, 1–23. Berkeley: University of California Press.

Bialecki, Jon, and Eric Hoenes del Pinal. 2011. "Introduction: Beyond Logos: Extensions of the Language Ideology Paradigm in the Study of Global Christianity (-ies)." *Anthropological Quarterly* 84 (3): 575–93.

Biehl, João. 2010. "'Medication Is Me Now': Human Values and Political Life in the Wake of Global AIDS Treatment." In *In the Name of Humanity: The Government of Threat and Care*, edited by Ilana Feldman and Miriam Ticktin, 151–89. Durham, NC: Duke University Press.

Bjelde, P. A. 1938. "These Fifty Years." In *From Darkness to Light, 1938 Yearbook*, 27–57. Minneapolis: Norwegian Lutheran Church in America, Board of Foreign Missions. ELCA3.

Bloch, Maurice. 1986a. *From Blessing to Violence: History and Ideology in the Circumcision Ritual of the Merina of Madagascar.* Cambridge, UK: Cambridge University Press.

———. 1986b. "Hierarchy and Equality in Merina Kinship." In *Madagascar: Society and History*, edited by Conrad Phillip Kottak, Jean-Aimé Rakotoarisoa, Aidan Southall, and Pierre Vérin, 215–28. Durham, NC: Carolina Academic Press.

Board of Foreign Missions, Norwegian Lutheran Church of America. 1937. "Christ for the World." *Yearbook 1937.* Minneapolis: Norwegian Lutheran Church of America, Board of Foreign Missions. ELCA3.

Boarder Giles, David. 2014. "The Anatomy of a Dumpster: Abject Capital and the Looking Glass of Value." *Social Text* 32 (1): 93–113.

Bohannan, Paul. 1955. "Some Principles of Exchange and Investment among the Tiv." *American Anthropologist* 57 (1): 60–70.

Bongmba, Elias. 2007. "Portable Faith: The Global Mission of African Initiated Churches." In *African Immigrant Religions in America*, edited by Jacob K. Olupona and Regina Gemignani, 102–32. New York: New York University Press.

Bornstein, Erica. 2005. *The Spirit of Development: Protestant NGOs, Morality, and Economics in Zimbabwe.* Stanford, CA: Stanford University Press.

———. 2012. *Disquieting Gifts: Humanitarianism in New Delhi.* Stanford, CA: Stanford University Press.

Bornstein, Erica, and Peter Redfield. 2010. "An Introduction to the Anthropology of Humanitarianism." In *Forces of Compassion: Humanitarianism between Ethics and Politics*, edited by Erica Bornstein and Peter Redfield, 3–30. School for Advanced Research Advanced Seminar Series. Santa Fe, NM: School for Advanced Research Press.

Bourdieu, Pierre. 1977. *Outline of a Theory of Practice.* Cambridge, UK: Cambridge University Press.

———. 1983. "The Field of Cultural Production; or, The Economic World Reversed." *Poetics* 12 (4–5): 311–56.

———. 1991. *Language and Symbolic Power*, edited by John B. Thompson. Translated by Gino Raymond and Matthew Adamson. Cambridge, MA: Harvard University Press.

Brown, Mervyn. 1995. *A History of Madagascar.* London: Damien Tunnacliffe.

Burgess, Andrew. 1932. *Zanahary in South Madagascar*. Minneapolis: Augsburg. ELCA3/PC.

Butler, Jon, Grant Wacker, and Randall Balmer. 2000. *Religion in American Life: A Short History*. Oxford, UK: Oxford University Press.

Caldwell, Melissa. 2017. *Living Faithfully in an Unjust World: Compassionate Care in Russia*. Berkeley: University of California Press.

Callaghy, Thomas. 1988. "The State and the Development of Capitalism in Africa: Theoretical, Historical and Comparative Reflections." In *The Precarious Balance: State-Society Relations in Africa*, edited by Donald Rothchild and Naomi Chazan, 67–99. Boulder, CO: Westview Press.

Canadian Agency for Drugs and Technologies in Health. 2008. "Reprocessing of Single-Use Medical Devices: Current Practice, Safety, and Cost-Effectiveness." *Health Technology Update* 9: 4, https://www.cadth.ca/health-technology-update-issue-9-sept-2008.

Cannell, Fenella, ed. 2006. *The Anthropology of Christianity*. Durham, NC: Duke University Press.

Chidester, David. 2005. "The American Touch: Tactile Imagery in American Religion and Politics." In *The Book of Touch*, edited by Constance Classen, 49–65. Oxford, UK: Berg.

Cole, Jennifer. 1997. "Madagascar: Peoples and Cultures." In *Encyclopedia of Africa South of the Sahara*, vol. 3, edited by John Middleton, 82–86. New York: Charles Scribner's Sons.

———. 2001. *Forget Colonialism? Sacrifice and the Art of Memory in Madagascar*. Berkeley: University of California Press.

———. 2009. "Love, Money, and Economies of Intimacy in Tamatave, Madagascar." In *Love in Africa*, edited by Jennifer Cole and Lynn M. Thomas, 109–34. Chicago: University of Chicago Press.

———. 2010. *Sex and Salvation: Imagining the Future in Madagascar*. Chicago: University of Chicago Press.

Coleman, Simon. 2004. "The Charismatic Gift." *Journal of the Royal Anthropological Institute* 10 (2): 421–42.

Collier, Roger. 2011. "The Ethics of Reusing Single-Use Devices." *Canadian Medical Association Journal* 183 (11): 1245.

Comaroff, Jean. 1985. *Body of Power, Spirit of Resistance: The Culture and History of a South African People*. Chicago: University of Chicago Press.

———. 1993. "The Diseased Heart of Africa: Medicine, Colonialism, and the Black Body." In *Knowledge, Power, and Practice: The Anthropology of Medicine and Everyday Life*, edited by Shirley Lindenbaum and Margaret Lock, 305–29. Berkeley: University of California Press.

———. 2009. "The Politics of Conviction: Faith on the Neo-Liberal Frontier." *Social Analysis* 53 (1): 17–38.

Comaroff, John, and Jean Comaroff. 1992. "Homemade Hegemony: Modernity,

Domesticity, and Colonialism in South Africa." In *African Encounters with Domesticity*, edited by Karen Hansen, 37–74. New Brunswick, NJ: Rutgers University Press.

———. 2000. "Millennial Capitalism: First Thoughts on a Second Coming." *Public Culture* 12 (2): 291–343.

Connerton, Paul. 2008. "Seven Types of Forgetting." *Memory Studies* 1 (1): 59–71.

Covell, Maureen. 1987. *Madagascar: Politics, Economics, and Society*. London: F. Pinter.

———. 1995. *Historical Dictionary of Madagascar*. Lanham, MD: Scarecrow Press.

Crane, Johanna Tayloe. 2013. *Scrambling for Africa: AIDS, Expertise, and the Rise of American Global Health Science*. Ithaca, NY: Cornell University Press.

Csordas, Thomas. 2002. *Body/Meaning/Healing*. New York: Palgrave Macmillan.

Dahl, Nellie. 1934. *Stories from Madagascar*. Minneapolis: Augsburg. ELCA3.

Daniel, E. Valentine. 1987. *Fluid Signs: Being a Person the Tamil Way*. Berkeley: University of California Press.

De Cordier, Bruno. 2008. "Faith-Based Aid, Globalization, and the Humanitarian Frontline: An Analysis of Western-Based Muslim Aid Organizations." *Disasters* 33 (4): 608–28.

DelVecchio Good, Mary-Jo. 2001. "The Biotechnical Embrace." *Culture, Medicine, and Psychiatry* 25 (4): 395–410.

Douglas, Mary. 1990. "No Free Gifts." In *The Gift: The Form and Reason for Exchange in Archaic Societies*, by Marcel Mauss. Translated by W. D. Halls, vii–xviii. New York: W. W. Norton.

Ebrahim, Alnoor, and Edward Weisband, eds. 2007. *Global Accountabilities: Participation, Pluralism, and Public Ethics*. Cambridge, UK: Cambridge University Press.

Eggert, Karl. 1986. "Mahafaly as Misnomer." In *Madagascar: Society and History*, edited by Conrad Phillip Kottak, Jean-Aimé Rakotoarisoa, Aidan Southall, and Pierre Vérin, 321–35. Durham, NC: Carolina Academic Press.

Eiss, Paul and David Pederson. 2002. "Introduction: Values of Value." *Cultural Anthropology* 17 (3): 283–90.

Elisha, Omri. 2008. "Moral Ambitions of Grace: The Paradox of Compassion and Accountability in Evangelical Faith-Based Activism." *Cultural Anthropology* 23 (1): 154–89.

———. 2011. *Moral Ambition: Mobilization and Social Outreach in Evangelical Megachurches*. Berkeley: University of California Press.

Ellis, Stephen. 1985. *The Rising of the Red Shawls: A Revolt in Madagascar, 1895–1899*. Cambridge, UK: Cambridge University Press.

Engelke, Matthew. 2007. *A Problem of Presence: Beyond Scripture in an African Church*. Berkeley: University of California Press.

Erling, Maria. 2003. "The Lutheran Left: From Movement to Church Commitment." In *Lutherans Today: American Lutheran Identity in the 21st Century*, edited by Richard Cimino, 45–61. Grand Rapids, MI: Eerdmans.

Farmer, Paul. 2004. *Pathologies of Power: Health, Human Rights, and the New War on the Poor*. Berkeley: University of California Press.

Fassin, Didier. 2007. "Humanitarianism as a Politics of Life." *Public Culture* 19 (3): 499–520.

———. 2008. "The Humanitarian Politics of Testimony: Subjectification through Trauma in the Israeli-Palestinian Conflict." *Cultural Anthropology* 23 (3): 531–58.

———. 2010. "Noli Me Tangere: The Moral Untouchability of Humanitarianism." In *Forces of Compassion: Humanitarianism between Ethics and Politics*, edited by Erica Bornstein and Peter Redfield, 35–52. Santa Fe, NM: School for Advanced Research Press.

Feeley-Harnik, Gillian. 1986. "Ritual and Work in Madagascar." In *Madagascar: Society and History*, edited by Conrad Phillip Kottak, Jean-Aimé Rakotoarisoa, Aidan Southall, and Pierre Vérin, 157–74. Durham, NC: Carolina Academic Press.

———. 1991. *A Green Estate: Restoring Independence in Madagascar*. Washington, DC: Smithsonian Institution Press.

———. 1994. *The Lord's Table: The Meaning of Food in Early Judaism and Christianity*. Washington, DC: Smithsonian Institution Press.

———. 1997. "Madagascar: Religious Systems." In *Encyclopedia of Africa South of the Sahara*, bk. 3, edited by John Middleton, 72–73. New York: Charles Scribner's Sons.

———. 2001. "*Ravenala Madagascariensis* Sonnerat: The Historical Ecology of a 'Flagship Species' in Madagascar." *Ethnohistory* 48 (1–2): 31–86.

Feierman, Steven. 1985. "Struggles for Control: The Social Roots of Health and Healing in Modern Africa." *African Studies Review* 28 (2–3): 73–147.

Feldman, Ilana, and Miriam Ticktin. 2010. "Introduction: Government and Humanity." In *In the Name of Humanity: The Government of Threat and Care*, edited by Ilana Feldman and Miriam Ticktin, 1–26. Durham, NC: Duke University Press.

Ferguson, James. 2006. *Global Shadows: Africa in the Neoliberal World Order*. Durham, NC: Duke University Press.

Foucault, Michel. 1979. *Discipline and Punish*. New York: Vintage.

———. 2000. "The Subject and the Power." In *Michel Foucault: Power*, edited by James Faubion, 326–48. New York: New Press.

Francken, Nathalie, Bart Minten, and Johan F. M. Swinnen. 2011. "The Political

Economy of Relief Aid Allocations: Evidence from Madagascar." *World Development* 40 (3): 486–500.

Frow, John. 2003. "Invidious Distinction: Waste, Difference, and Classy Stuff." In *Culture and Waste: The Creation and Destruction of Value*, edited by Gay Hawkins and Stephen Muecke, 25–38. Lanham, MD: Rowman and Littlefield.

Ganti, Tejaswini. 2014. "Neoliberalism." *Annual Review of Anthropology* 43: 89–104.

Ghosh, Amitav. 1994. "The Global Reservation: Notes toward an Ethnography of International Peacekeeping." *Cultural Anthropology* 9 (3): 412–22.

Gibbons, Luz, José M. Belizán, Jeremy A. Lauer, Ana P. Betrán, Mario Merialdi, and Fernando Althabe. 2010. *The Global Numbers and Costs of Additionally Needed and Unnecessary Caesarean Sections Performed per Year: Overuse as a Barrier to Universal Coverage.* World Health Report Background Paper No. 30. Geneva, Switz.: World Health Organization.

Giddens, Anthony. 1990. *The Consequences of Modernity.* Stanford, CA: Stanford University Press.

———. 1991. *Modernity and Self-Identity: Self and Society in the Late Modern Age.* Stanford, CA: Stanford University Press.

Gifford, Paul. 1998. *African Christianity: Its Public Role.* Bloomington: Indiana University Press.

Gjerde, Jon. 1985. *From Peasants to Farmers: The Migration from Balestrand, Norway, to the Upper Middle West.* Cambridge, UK: Cambridge University Press.

Gjerde, Jon, and Carlton C. Qualey. 2002. *Norwegians in Minnesota.* St. Paul: Minnesota Historical Society Press.

Division for Global Mission, Evangelical Lutheran Church in America. 1999. *Global Mission in the 21st Century: A Vision of God's Faithfulness.* Chicago: Evangelical Lutheran Church in America, Division for Global Mission.

Goffman, Erving. 1976. "Replies and Responses." *Language in Society* 5 (3): 257–313.

———. 1981. *Forms of Talk.* Philadelphia: University of Pennsylvania Press.

Gow, Bonar A. 1997. "Admiral Didier Ratsiraka and the Malagasy Socialist Revolution." *Journal of Modern African Studies* 35 (3): 409–39.

Graeber, David. 2001. *Toward an Anthropological Theory of Value: The False Coin of Our Dreams.* New York: Palgrave Macmillan.

———. 2007a. "Army of Altruists: On the Alienated Right to Do Good." *Harper's Magazine*, January, 31–38.

———. 2007b. *Lost People: Magic and the Legacy of Slavery in Madagascar.* Bloomington: Indiana University Press.

———. 2011. *Debt: The First 5000 Years.* New York: Melville House.

———. 2012. "Afterword: The Apocalypse of Objects—Degradation, Redemption and Transcendence in the World of Consumer Goods." In *Economies of Recycling: The Global Transformation of Materials, Values and Social Relations*, edited by Catherine Alexander and Joshua Reno, 277–90. London: Zed.

———. 2013. "It Is Value That Brings Universes into Being." *Hau: Journal of Ethnographic Theory* 3 (2): 219–43.

Granquist, Mark. 2007. "Lutherans." In *The American Midwest: An Interpretive Encyclopedia*, edited by Richard Sisson, Christian Zacher, and Andrew Cayton, 753–55. Bloomington: Indiana University Press.

Guyer, Jane. 2004. *Marginal Gains: Monetary Transactions in Atlantic Africa*. Chicago: University of Chicago Press.

Halvorson, Britt. 2008. "Lutheran in Two Worlds: Remaking Mission from Madagascar to the United States." PhD diss., Department of Anthropology, University of Michigan.

———. 2010. "Translating the *Fifohazana* (Awakening): The Politics of Healing and the Colonial Mission Legacy in African Christian Missionization." *Journal of Religion in Africa* 40 (4): 413–41.

———. 2012a. "'No Junk for Jesus': Redemptive Economies and Value Conversions in Lutheran Medical Aid." In *Economies of Recycling: The Global Transformation of Materials, Values and Social Relations*, edited by Catherine Alexander and Josh Reno, 207–33. London: Zed.

———. 2012b. "Woven Worlds: Material Things, Bureaucratization, and Dilemmas of Caregiving in Lutheran Humanitarianism." *American Ethnologist* 39 (1): 122–37.

Hannerz, Ulf. 2004. "Cosmopolitanism." In *A Companion to the Anthropology of Politics*, edited by David Nugent and Joan Vincent, 69–85. Oxford, UK: Blackwell Publishing.

Hansen, Karen Tranberg. 1999. "Secondhand Clothing Encounters in Zambia: Global Discourses, Western Commodities and Local Histories." *Africa* 69 (3): 343–65.

———. 2000. *Salaula: The World of Secondhand Clothing and Zambia*. Chicago: University of Chicago Press.

Harding, Susan. 2000. *The Book of Jerry Falwell: Fundamentalist Language and Politics*. Princeton, NJ: Princeton University Press.

Harper, Janice. 2002. *Endangered Species: Health, Illness and Death among Madagascar's People of the Forest*. Durham, NC: Carolina Academic Press.

Haskell, T. L. 1985. "Capitalism and the Origins of the Humanitarian Sensibility." *American Historical Review* 90 (2): 339–61.

Hawkins, Gay, and Stephen Muecke, eds. 2003. *Culture and Waste: The Creation and Destruction of Value*. Lanham, MD: Rowman and Littlefield.

Hayden, Cori. 2004. "Prospecting's Publics." In *Property in Question: Value*

Transformations in the Global Economy, edited by Katherine Verdery and Caroline Humphrey, 115–28. Oxford, UK: Berg.

"Health-Madagascar." 2012. *African Research Bulletin* 49 (6): 19329A–C.

Hefferan, Tara. 2007. *Twinning Faith and Development: Catholic Parish Partnering in the U.S. and Haiti.* Boulder, CO: Kumarian Press.

Hefferan, Tara, Julie Adkins, and Laurie Occhipinti. 2009. "Faith-Based Organizations, Neoliberalism, and Development: An Introduction." In *Bridging the Gaps: Faith-Based Organizations, Neoliberalism, and Development in Latin America and the Caribbean*, edited by Tara Hefferan, Julie Adkins, and Laurie Occhipinti, 1–34. Lanham, MD: Lexington.

Henare, Amiria, Martin Holbraad, and Sari Wastell. 2007. "Introduction: Thinking through Things." In *Thinking through Things: Theorising Artifacts Ethnographically*, edited by Amiria Henare, Martin Holbraad, and Sari Wastell, 1–31. New York: Routledge.

Herzfeld, Michael. 1992. *The Social Production of Indifference: Exploring the Symbolic Roots of Western Bureaucracy.* Chicago: University of Chicago Press.

Hetherington, Kevin. 2004. "Secondhandedness: Consumption, Disposal, and Absent Presence." *Environment and Planning D* 22: 157–73.

Ho, Karen. 2009. *Liquidated: An Ethnography of Wall Street.* Durham, NC: Duke University Press.

Hodges, Sarah. 2008. *Chennai's Biotrash Chronicles: Chasing the Neo-Liberal Syringe.* GARNET Working Paper No. 44/08: Center for the Study of Globalisation and Regionalisation, University of Warwick, UK.

Horning, Nadia Rabesahala. 2008. "Strong Support for Weak Performance: Donor Competition in Madagascar." *African Affairs* 107 (428): 405–31.

Hovland, Ingie. 2007. "Who's Afraid of Religion? Tensions between 'Mission' and 'Development' in the Norwegian Mission Society." In *Development, Civil Society and Faith-Based Organizations: Bridging the Sacred and the Secular*, edited by G. Clarke, M. Jennings, and T. Shaw, 171–86. New York: Palgrave Macmillan.

Hull, Matthew S. 2008. "Ruled by Records: The Expropriation of Land and the Misappropriation of Lists in Islamabad." *American Ethnologist* 35 (4): 501–18.

Hunt, Nancy Rose. 1999. *A Colonial Lexicon of Birth Ritual, Medicalization, and Mobility in the Congo.* Durham, NC: Duke University Press.

Hutchinson, John F. 1996. *Champions of Charity: War and the Rise of the Red Cross.* Boulder, CO: Westview.

Irvine, Judith. 1989. "When Talk Isn't Cheap: Language and Political Economy." *American Ethnologist* 16 (2): 248–67.

———. 1996. "Shadow Conversations: The Indeterminacy of Participant Roles."

In *Natural Histories of Discourse*, edited by Michael Silverstein and Greg Urban, 131–59. Chicago: University of Chicago Press.

Irvine, Judith, and Susan Gal. 2000. "Language Ideology and Linguistic Differentiation." In *Regimes of Language: Ideologies, Polities, and Identities*, edited by Paul V. Kroskrity, 35–83. Santa Fe, NM: School for Advanced Research Press.

James, Erica. 2010. *Democratic Insecurities: Violence, Trauma, and Intervention in Haiti*. Berkeley: University of California Press.

Jay, Martin.1988. "Scopic Regimes of Modernity." In *Vision and Visuality*, edited by H. Foster, 3-23. Seattle: Bay Press.

Jenkins, Philip. 2002. *The Next Christendom: The Coming of Global Christianity*. New York: Oxford University Press.

Johnson, Paul Christopher. 2007. *Diaspora Conversions: Black Carib Religion and the Recovery of Africa*. Berkeley: University of California Press.

Jolly, Allison. 2004. *Lords and Lemurs: Mad Scientists, Kings with Spears, and the Survival of Diversity in Madagascar*. Boston: Houghton Mifflin.

Keane, Webb. 1996. "Materialism, Missionaries and Modern Subjects in Colonial Indonesia." In *Conversion to Modernities: The Globalization of Christianity*, edited by Peter van der Veer, 137–70. London: Routledge.

———. 1997. "Religious Language." *Annual Review of Anthropology* 26: 46–71.

———. 2003. "Semiotics and the Social Analysis of Material Things." *Language and Communication* 23 (3–4): 409–25.

———. 2007. *Christian Moderns: Freedom and Fetish in the Mission Encounter*. Berkeley: University of California Press.

Keenan, Elinor Ochs. 1974. "Norm-Makers, Norm-Breakers: Uses of Speech by Men and Women in a Malagasy Community." In *Explorations in the Ethnography of Speaking*, edited by Richard Bauman and Joel Sherzer, 125–43. Cambridge, UK: Cambridge University Press.

Keller, Eva. 2005. *The Road to Clarity: Seventh-Day Adventism in Madagascar*. New York: Palgrave Macmillan.

Klaits, Frederick. 2009. "Faith and the Intersubjectivity of Care in Botswana." *Africa Today* 56 (1): 3–20.

———. 2010. *Death in a Church of Life: Moral Passion in Botswana's Time of AIDS*. Berkeley: University of California Press.

Klaits, Frederick, ed. 2017. *The Request and the Gift in Religious and Humanitarian Endeavors*. New York: Palgrave Macmillan.

Klassen, Pamela. 2011. *Spirits of Protestantism: Medicine, Healing, and Liberal Christianity*. Berkeley: University of California Press.

Kopytoff, Igor. 1986. "The Cultural Biography of Things: Commoditization as Process." In *The Social Life of Things: Commodities in Cultural Perspective*, edited by Arjun Appadurai, 64–94. Cambridge, UK: Cambridge University Press.

Kwakye-Nuako, Kwasi. 2006. "Still Praisin' God in a New Land: African Immigrant Christianity in North America." In *The New African Diaspora in North America: Trends, Community Building, and Adaptation*, edited by Kwado Konadu-Agyemang, Baffour K. Takyi, and John Arthur, 121–40. Lanham, MD: Lexington.

Lacquer, Thomas. 1989. "Bodies, Details, and the Humanitarian Narrative." In *The New Cultural History*, edited by Lynn Hunt, 176–204. Berkeley: University of California Press.

Lambek, Michael. 2002. *The Weight of the Past: Living with History in Mahajanga, Madagascar*. New York: Palgrave Macmillan.

———. 2010. Introduction to *Ordinary Ethics: Anthropology, Language, and Action*, edited by Michael Lambek, 1–38. New York: Fordham University Press.

———. 2013. "The Value of (Performative) Acts." *Hau: Journal of Ethnographic Theory* 3 (2): 141–60.

Larson, Pier. 1996. "Desperately Seeking 'the Merina' (Central Madagascar): Reading Ethnonyms and Their Semantic Fields in African Identity Histories." *Journal of Southern African Studies* 22 (4): 541–60.

———. 1997. "'Capacities and Modes of Thinking': Intellectual Engagements and Subaltern Hegemony in the Early History of Malagasy Christianity." *American Historical Review* 102 (4): 969–1002.

———. 2000. *History and Memory in the Age of Enslavement: Becoming Merina in Highland Madagascar, 1770–1822*. London: Heinemann.

Legrip-Randriambelo, Olivia, and Dennis Regnier. 2014. "The Place of Healers-Diviners (Ombiasa) in Betsileo Medical Pluralism." *Health, Culture and Society* 7 (1): 28–37.

Lester, Rebecca. 2005. *Jesus in Our Wombs: Embodying Modernity in a Mexican Convent*. Berkeley: University of California Press.

Liechty, Mark. 2003. *Suitably Modern: Making Middle-Class Culture in a New Consumer Society*. Princeton, NJ: Princeton University Press.

Livingston, Julie. 2012. *Improvising Medicine: An African Oncology Ward in an Emerging Epidemic*. Durham, NC: Duke University Press.

López, A. Ricardo, and Barbara Weinstein, eds. 2012. *The Making of the Middle Class: Toward a Transnational History*. Durham, NC: Duke University Press.

Lubawa, Richard. 2007. *Shoulder to Shoulder, Bega kwa Bega: A Lutheran Partnership between Minnesota and Tanzania*. Minneapolis: Lutheran University Press.

Luhrmann, Tanya. 2004. "Metakinesis: How God Becomes Intimate in Contemporary U.S. Christianity." *American Anthropologist* 106 (3): 518–28.

Malkki, Liisa H. 1996. "Speechless Emissaries: Refugees, Humanitarian Aid, and Dehistoricization." *Cultural Anthropology* 11 (3): 377–404.

———. 2015. *The Need to Help: The Domestic Arts of International Humanitarianism*. Durham, NC: Duke University Press.

Mangan, Katherine. 2007. "Duke's Medical Surplus Finds New Life in Uganda." *Chronicle of Higher Education*, 21 September, A30.

Masuzawa, Tomoko. 2005. *The Invention of World Religions; or, How European Universalism Was Preserved in the Language of Pluralism*. Chicago: University of Chicago Press.

Mauss, Marcel. 1990. *The Gift: The Form and Reason for Exchange in Archaic Societies*. Translated by W. D. Halls. New York: W. W. Norton.

McDannell, Colleen. 1995. *Material Christianity: Religion and Popular Culture in America*. New Haven, CT: Yale University Press.

Metzger, Bruce M., and Roland E. Murphy, eds. 1991. *The New Oxford Annotated Bible with the Apocryphal/Deuterocanonical Books*. New Revised Standard Version. New York: Oxford University Press.

Meyer, Birgit. 1996. "Modernity and Enchantment: The Image of the Devil in Popular African Christianity." In *Conversion to Modernities: The Globalization of Christianity*, edited by Peter van der Veer, 199–230. New York: Routledge.

———. 2004. "Christianity in Africa: From African Independent to Pentecostal-Charismatic Churches." *Annual Review of Anthropology* 33: 447–74.

Meyer, Birgit, and Peter Pels, eds. 2003. *Magic and Modernity: Interfaces of Revelation and Concealment*. Stanford, CA: Stanford University Press.

Millar, Kathleen M. 2012. "Trash Ties: Urban Politics, Economic Crisis and Rio de Janeiro's Garbage Dump." In *Economies of Recycling: The Global Transformation in Materials, Values and Social Relations*, edited by Catherine Alexander and Joshua Reno, 164–84. New York: Palgrave Macmillan.

Miller, Daniel. 2005. "Materiality: An Introduction." In *Materiality*, edited by Daniel Miller, 1–50. Durham, NC: Duke University Press.

Miller, Donald E. 1997. *Reinventing American Protestantism: Christianity in the New Millennium*. Berkeley: University of California Press.

Mitchell, Timothy. 1990. "Everyday Metaphors of Power." *Theory and Society* 19 (5): 545–77.

Mol, Annemarie. 2002. *The Body Multiple: Ontology in Medical Practice*. Durham, NC: Duke University Press.

Morgan, David. 1998. *Visual Piety: A History and Theory of Popular Religious Images*. Oxford, UK: Oxford University Press.

Muehlebach, Andrea. 2012. *The Moral Neoliberal: Welfare and Citizenship in Italy*. Chicago: University of Chicago Press.

———. 2013. "The Catholicization of Neoliberalism: On Love and Welfare in Lombardy, Italy." *American Anthropologist* 115 (3): 452–65.

Munn, Nancy. 1992. *The Fame of Gawa: A Symbolic Study of Value Transformations in a Massim (Papua New Guinea) Society*. Durham: Duke University Press.

Myers, Fred. 2001. *The Empire of Things: Regimes of Value and Material Culture.* Santa Fe, NM: School of American Research Press.

Narayan, Kirin. 1997. "How Native Is a 'Native' Anthropologist?" In *Situated Lives: Gender and Culture in Everyday Life*, edited by L. Lamphere and P. Zavella, 23–41. New York: Routledge.

Nelson, E. Clifford. 1980. *The Lutherans in North America.* Rev. ed. Philadelphia: Fortress Press.

Nguyen, Vinh-Kim. 2010. *The Republic of Therapy: Triage and Sovereignty in West Africa's Time of AIDS.* Durham, NC: Duke University Press.

Nielssen, Hilde, and Karine Hestad Skeie. 2014. "Christian Revivalism and Political Imagination in Madagascar." *Journal of Religion in Africa* 44 (2): 189–223.

Nielssen, Hilde, Inger Marie Okkenhaug, and Karina Hestad Skeie. 2011. *Protestant Missions and Local Encounters in the Nineteenth and Twentieth Centuries: Unto the Ends of the Earth.* Leiden: Brill.

Nyhagen Predelli, Line. 2003. *Issues of Gender, Race and Class in the Norwegian Missionary Society in Nineteenth-Century Norway and Madagascar.* Lewiston, NY: Edwin Mellen.

Ochs, Elinor, and Lisa Capps. 2001. "Narrative as Theology." In *Living Narrative: Creating Lives in Everyday Storytelling*, 225–50. Cambridge, MA: Harvard University Press.

Okome, Mojúbàolú Olúfúnké. 2007. "African Immigrant Churches and the New Christian Right." In *African Immigrant Religions in America*, edited by Jacob K. Olupona and Regina Gemignani, 279–305. New York: New York University Press.

Olupona, Jacob K., and Regina Gemignani, eds. 2007. *African Immigrant Religions in America.* New York: New York University Press.

Ong, Aihwa. 1987. *Spirits of Resistance and Capitalist Discipline: Factory Women in Malaysia.* Albany: State University of New York Press.

———. 2006. *Neoliberalism as Exception: Mutations in Citizenship and Sovereignty.* Durham, NC: Duke University Press.

Ong, Aihwa and Stephen J. Collier. 2005. "Introduction: Global Assemblages, Anthropological Problems." In *Global Assemblages: Technology, Politics, and Ethics as Anthropological Problems*, edited by Aihwa Ong and Stephen J. Collier, 3–21. Oxford: Blackwell Publishing.

Orsi, Robert. 2005. *Between Heaven and Earth: The Religious Worlds People Make and the Scholars Who Study Them.* Princeton, NJ: Princeton University Press.

Ose, Roger. 1979. "A History of the South West Synod of the Malagasy Lutheran Church, 1889–1979." Unpublished manuscript. ELCA3.

Pandolfi, Mariella. 2010. "Humanitarianism and Its Discontents." In *Forces of*

Compassion: Humanitarianism between Ethics and Politics, edited by Erica Bornstein and Peter Redfield, 227–48. School for Advanced Research Advanced Seminar Series. Santa Fe, NM: School for Advanced Research Press.

Parmentier, Richard. 1997. "Semiotic Approaches to Meaning in Material Culture." Special Issue, "The Pragmatic Semiotics of Cultures." *Semiotica* 116 (1): 43–63.

Parry, Bronwyn, and Cathy Gere. 2006. "Contested Bodies: Property Models and the Commodification of Human Biological Artefacts." *Science as Culture* 15 (2): 139–58.

Parry, Jonathan. 1986. "The Gift, the Indian Gift and the 'Indian Gift.'" *Man, Journal of the Royal Anthropological Institute* 21: 453–73.

Peterson, Kristin. 2014. *Speculative Markets: Drug Circuits and Derivative Life in Nigeria.* Durham, NC: Duke University Press.

Petryna, Adriana. 2004. *Life Exposed: Biological Citizens after Chernobyl.* Princeton, NJ: Princeton University Press.

Pfeiffer, James. 2002. "African Independent Churches in Mozambique: Healing the Afflictions of Inequality." *Medical Anthropology Quarterly* 16 (2): 176–99.

———. 2003. "International NGOs and Primary Health Care in Mozambique: The Need for a New Model of Collaboration." *Social Science & Medicine* 56 (4): 725–38.

———. 2004. "Civil Society, NGOs, and the Holy Spirit in Mozambique." *Human Organization* 64 (3): 359–72.

Pierre, Jemima. 2013. *The Predicament of Blackness: Postcolonial Ghana and the Politics of Race.* Chicago: University of Chicago Press.

Piot, Charles. 2010. *Nostalgia for the Future: West Africa after the Cold War.* Chicago: University of Chicago Press.

Poewe, Karla, ed. 1994. *Charismatic Christianity as a Global Culture.* Columbia: University of South Carolina Press.

Porterfield, Amanda. 2005. *Healing in the History of Christianity.* Oxford, UK: Oxford University Press.

Povinelli, Elizabeth. 2006. *The Empire of Love: Toward a Theory of Intimacy, Genealogy, and Carnality.* Durham, NC: Duke University Press.

Raison-Jourde, Françoise. 1995. "The Madagascan Churches in the Political Arena and Their Contribution to the Change of Regime." In *The Christian Churches and the Democratisation of Africa*, edited by Paul Gifford, 292–301. Leiden, Neth.: Brill.

Rabary, Lovasoa. 2014. "IMF Restores Ties with Madagascar Five Years after Coup." *Reuters*, March 13.

Rakotojoelinandrasana, Daniel A. 2002. "Holistic Approach to Mental Illness at the *Toby* of Ambohibao, Madagascar." Doctorate of Ministry thesis. Luther Theological Seminary, St. Paul, Minnesota. LSL.

Randrianja, Solofo. 2001. *Société et luttes anticoloniales à Madagascar (1896 à 1946)*. Paris: Karthala.

Randrianja, Solofo, and Stephen Ellis. 2009. *Madagascar: A Short History*. Chicago: University of Chicago Press.

Rasolondraibe, Péri. 1998. "Healing Ministry in Madagascar." In *Baptism, Rites of Passage, and Culture*, edited by S. Anita Stauffer, 133–44. Geneva, Switz.: Lutheran World Federation.

Redfield, Peter. 2005. "Doctors, Borders, and Life in Crisis." *Cultural Anthropology* 20 (3): 328–61.

———. 2006. "A Less Modest Witness: Collective Advocacy and Motivated Truth in a Medical Humanitarian Movement." *American Ethnologist* 33 (1): 3–26.

———. 2010. "The Impossible Problem of Neutrality." In *Forces of Compassion: Humanitarianism between Ethics and Politics*, edited by Erica Bornstein and Peter Redfield, 53–70. Santa Fe, NM: School for Advanced Research Press.

———. 2013. *Life in Crisis: The Ethical Journey of Doctors without Borders*. Berkeley: University of California Press.

Reno, Joshua. 2009. "Your Trash Is Someone's Treasure: The Politics of Value at a Michigan Landfill." *Journal of Material Culture* 14: 29–46.

———. 2016. *Waste Away: Working and Living with a North American Landfill*. Berkeley: University of California Press.

Resnick, Elana. 2016. "Nothing Ever Perishes: Waste, Race and Transformation in an Expanding European Union." PhD diss., Department of Anthropology, University of Michigan.

Rice, Andrew. 2009. "Mission from Africa." *New York Times*, April 12, M8.

Rich, Cynthia Holder, ed. 2008. *The Fifohazana: Madagascar's Indigenous Christian Movement*. Amherst, MA: Cambria.

Riles, Annelise. 2000. *The Network Inside Out*. Ann Arbor: University of Michigan Press.

Robert, Dana. 1997. "From Missions to Mission to Beyond Mission: The Historiography of American Protestant Foreign Missions since World War II." In *New Directions in American Religious History*, edited by Harry S. Stout and D. G. Hart, 362–93. Oxford, UK: Oxford University Press.

Robbins, Joel. 2003a. "On the Paradoxes of Global Pentecostalism and the Perils of Continuity Thinking." *Religion* 33: 221–31.

———. 2003b. "What Is a Christian? Notes toward an Anthropology of Christianity." *Religion* 33: 191–99.

———. 2004. *Becoming Sinners: Christianity and Moral Torment in a Papua New Guinea Society*. Berkeley: University of California Press.

———. 2013. "Monism, Pluralism, and the Structure of Value Relations: A Dumontian Contribution to the Contemporary Study of Value." *Hau: Journal of Ethnographic Theory* 3 (1): 99–115.

Robbins, Joel, and Matthew Engelke. 2010. Introduction to "Global Christianities, Global Critique." Special issue, *South Atlantic Quarterly* 109 (4): 623–31.

Rose, Carol M. 1994. *Property and Persuasion: Essays on the History, Theory, and Rhetoric of Ownership.* Boulder, CO: Westview.

Rosenblatt, William H., Chris Ariyan, Viorel Gutter, Kelly Shine, and David Silverman. 1996. "Focused versus Operating Room–Wide Recovery of Unused Supplies for Overseas Reconstructive Surgery." *Plastic and Reconstructive Surgery* 97 (3): 630–34.

Rosenblatt, William H., Anthony Chavez, Dawn Tenney, and David G. Silverman. 1997. "Assessment of the Economic Impact of an Overage Reduction Program in the Operating Room." *Journal of Clinical Anesthesia* 9: 478–81.

Rosenblatt, William H., and David G. Silverman. 1992. "Recovery, Resterilization, and Donation of Unused Surgical Supplies." *Journal of the American Medical Association* 268 (11): 1441–43.

Rudnyckyj, Daromir. 2009. "Spiritual Economies: Islam and Neoliberalism in Contemporary Indonesia." *Cultural Anthropology* 24 (1): 104–41.

Sanneh, Lamin. 2003. *Whose Religion Is Christianity? The Gospel beyond the West.* Grand Rapids, MI: Eerdmans.

Scherz, China. 2014. *Having People, Having Heart: Charity, Sustainable Development, and Problems of Dependence in Central Uganda.* Chicago: University of Chicago Press.

Sharp, Lesley. 1993. *The Possessed and the Dispossessed: Spirits, Identity, and Power in a Madagascar Migrant Town.* Berkeley: University of California Press.

———. 1999. "Exorcists, Psychiatrists, and the Problems of Possession in Northwest Madagascar." In *Across the Boundaries of Belief: Contemporary Issues in the Anthropology of Religion,* edited by Morton Klass and Maxine Weisgrau, 163–95. Boulder, CO: Westview.

———. 2002. *The Sacrificed Generation: Youth, History, and the Colonized Mind in Madagascar.* Berkeley: University of California Press.

———. 2006. *Strange Harvest: Organ Transplants, Denatured Bodies, and the Transformed Self.* Berkeley: University of California Press.

Sharp, Maryanne, and Ioana Kruse. 2011. *Health, Nutrition and Population Outcomes in Madagascar, 2000–2009: A Country Status Report.* World Bank Working Papers. New York: World Bank.

Skeie, Karina Hestad. 1999. "Building God's Kingdom: The Importance of the House to Nineteenth-Century Norwegian Missionaries in Madagascar." In *Ancestors, Power and History in Madagascar,* edited by Karen Middleton, 71–102. Leiden: Brill.

Smith, Daniel Jordan. 2010. "Corruption, NGOs and Development in Nigeria." *Third World Quarterly* 31 (2): 243–58.

Smith, Erin A. 2007. "'What Would Jesus Do?' The Social Gospel and the Literary Marketplace." *Book History* 10 (1): 193–221.

Sodikoff, Genese. 2012. *Forest and Labor in Madagascar: From Colonial Concession to Global Biosphere.* Bloomington: Indiana University Press.

Stoler, Ann Laura. 2008. "Imperial Debris: Reflections on Ruins and Ruination." *Cultural Anthropology* 23 (2): 191–219.

Stoler, Ann, with David Bond. 2006. "Refractions off Empire: Untimely Comparisons in Harsh Times." *Radical History Review* 95: 93–107.

Strasser, Susan. 1999. *Waste and Want: A Social History of Trash.* New York: Metropolitan.

Strathern, Marilyn. 2000. "The Tyranny of Transparency." *British Educational Research Journal* 26 (3): 309–21.

Takyi, Baffour K., and Kwame Safo Boate. 2006. "Location and Settlement Patterns of African Immigrants in the U.S.: Demographics and Spatial Context." In *The New African Diaspora in North America: Trends, Community Building, and Adaptation*, edited by Kwado Konadu-Agyemang, Baffour K. Takyi, and John Arthur, 50–68. Lanham, MD: Lexington.

Terry, Fiona. 2002. *Condemned to Repeat? The Paradox of Humanitarian Action.* Ithaca, NY: Cornell University Press.

Theodossopoulos, Dimitrios, and Elisabeth Kirtsoglou, eds. 2013. *United in Discontent: Local Responses to Cosmopolitanism and Globalization.* New York: Berghahn.

Thomas, Nicholas. 1991. *Entangled Objects: Exchange, Material Culture, and Colonialism in the Pacific.* Cambridge, MA: Harvard University Press.

Ticktin, Miriam. 2011. *Casualties of Care: Immigration and the Politics of Humanitarianism in France.* Berkeley: University of California Press.

Tong, Xin, and Jici Wang. 2012. "The Shadow of the Global Network: E-Waste Flows to China." In *Economies of Recycling: The Global Transformation in Materials, Values and Social Relations*, edited by Catherine Alexander and Joshua Reno, 98–116. New York: Palgrave Macmillan.

Trouillot, Michel-Rolph. 1995. *Silencing the Past: Power and the Production of History.* Boston: Beacon Press.

Tsing, Anna Lowenhaupt. 2005. *Friction: An Ethnography of Global Connection.* Princeton, NJ: Princeton University Press.

Vaughan, Megan. 1991. *Curing Their Ills: Colonial Power and African Illness.* Stanford, CA: Stanford University Press.

Verdery, Katherine, and Caroline Humphrey. 2004. "Introduction: Raising Questions about Property." In *Property in Question: Value Transformations in the Global Economy*, edited by Katherine Verdery and Caroline Humphrey, 1–28. Oxford, UK: Berg.

Vigen, James. 1979. *Diakonia: A Short History of Manambaro Lutheran Hos-*

pital, Manambaro, Madagascar. Antananarivo: Trano Printy Loterana. ELCA3.

Vomhof, John Jr. 2010. "Report: Twin Cities Economy among Strongest Post-Recession." *Minneapolis–St. Paul Business Journal*, December 1. http://www.bizjournals.com/twincities/news/2010/12/01/report-minneapolis-economy-among.html.

Wacquant, Loïc. 2012. "Three Steps to a Historical Anthropology of Actually Existing Neoliberalism." *Social Anthropology* 20 (1): 66–79.

Walls, Andrew. 1996. *The Missionary Movement in Christian History: Studies in the Transmission of Faith.* Maryknoll, NY: Orbis.

Walsh, Andrew. 2003. "'Hot Money' and Daring Consumption in a Northern Malagasy Mining Town." *American Ethnologist*, 30 (2): 290–305.

———. 2012. *Made in Madagascar: Sapphires, Ecotourism, and the Global Bazaar.* Toronto: University of Toronto Press.

Weber, Max. 1978. *Economy and Society.* Berkeley: University of California Press.

Wendland, Claire. 2012a. "Animating Biomedicine's Moral Order: The Crisis of Practice in Malawian Medical Training." *Current Anthropology* 53 (6): 755–88.

———. 2012b. "Moral Maps and Medical Imaginaries: Clinical Tourism at Malawi's College of Medicine." *American Anthropologist* 114 (1): 108–22.

Werbner, Pnina, ed. 2009. *Anthropology and the New Cosmopolitanism: Rooted, Feminist and Vernacular Perspectives.* Oxford, UK: Berg.

West, Harry G., and Todd Sanders, eds. 2003. *Transparency and Conspiracy: Ethnographies of Suspicion in the New World Order.* Durham, NC: Duke University Press.

West, Michael O. 2002. *The Rise of an African Middle Class: Colonial Zimbabwe, 1898–1965.* Bloomington: Indiana University Press.

World Health Organization. 1999. *Guidelines for Essential Drugs.* Geneva, Switz.: World Health Organization.

Wuthnow, Robert. 1989. *The Struggle for America's Soul: Evangelicals, Liberals and Secularism.* Grand Rapids, MI: Eerdmans.

———. 2009. *Boundless Faith: The Global Outreach of American Churches.* Berkeley: University of California Press.

Zaloom, Caitlin. 2004. "The Productive Life of Risk." *Cultural Anthropology* 19 (3): 365–91.

Index